Praise for *Home Care Nursing*

"*Home Care Nursing: Surviving in an Ever-Changing Care Environment* should be required reading for all current or prospective home care providers. Tina Marrelli has written the definitive resource for anyone interested in the home care field. Her work is especially timely as home care navigates the transition to new care delivery and payment models requiring expanded care teams, new business models, and performance improvement. This book offers a critical guide to success in home care."

–Tracey Moorhead
President and CEO, Visiting Nurse Associations of America (VNAA)

"Tina Marrelli expertly captures the essence of providing home care in today's challenging and complex healthcare environment. Home care and hospice are unique niches of the healthcare continuum and their provision requires knowledge and understanding beyond basic clinical needs. This book encompasses the 'need to knows' and more for a home care clinician and conveys the information in an understandable and thoughtful manner. I envision this book in the bag of every home care nurse as their home care clinical companion."

–Jennifer Kennedy, MA, BSN, RN, CHC
Senior Director, Regulatory & Quality,
National Hospice and Palliative Care Organization

"Just as Tina Marrelli's *Handbook of Home Health Standards* has been a go to reference, *Home Care Nursing: Surviving in an Ever-Changing Care Environment* will become a classic resource. It is a helpful tool for those new to the field or as a refresher for the experienced home care nurse. It should also be a guide for non-clinicians that often serve as agency administrators or key operations staff in home care agencies."

–Barbara Piskor, MPH, BSN, RN, NEA-BC
President, CEO, BKP HealthCare Resources

D1103687

"A well timed gift to an industry experiencing widespread change! The information found in these chapters not only provides the new home care clinician with a basic foundation of home care concepts, it also identifies the current challenges in the industry and provides thoughtful strategies for successful care delivery and patient outcomes. A must read for everyone in home care!"

–Kim Corral, MaEd, BSN, RN, COS-C
Consultant, Chelta, Inc.

"Whether you are new to home care or have worked for years in that care environment, *Home Care Nursing* will provide the answers you have been looking for. The book reflects the diversity of nursing practice within home care, and the stand-alone chapters allow the reader to personalize the order in which the book is read. The author's many years of experience as a home care nurse and consultant make this the go-to resource every home care nurse needs."

–Maureen Anthony, PhD, RN
Professor, McAuley School of Nursing
University of Detroit Mercy
Editor-in-Chief, Home Healthcare Now

"This book offers a wonderful resource for home care nurses; nurses entering the specialty; and all levels of nursing students. The author is a long-time expert, which is demonstrated in the book. The book is critical. We need to adapt our nursing practice and provide quality services—patients need more services in their homes, reducing need for hospital days, readmission, and use of long-term care facilities when possible. The up-to-date content is easy to read and apply."

–Anita Finkelman, MSN, RN
Visiting Lecturer, Nursing Department
Recanati School for Community Health Professions
Faculty of the Health Sciences, Ben-Gurion University of the Negev

"Tina Marrelli brings her expertise in home care to address the complexity of providing patient-centered and value based care in the community setting—all within the current regulatory environment. This book pulls complex elements together to demonstrate a successful home based care model. This is a perfect resource for orientation, or reorientation, to home care."

–Cathleen "Cat" Armato, RN, CHPN, CHC, CHPC
Principal Consultant, Armato & Associates, LLC

"Once again, Tina Marrelli has made an informational book something that captures readers attention with personal stories and relevance. Home care is complex, but one can read this regardless of knowledge base and have sound, evidence-based, practical information. A must read for clinicians considering home care. Great training tool for any agency with questions at the end of each chapter and weaving of critical information in multiple chapters so one does not lose information."

–Dedee Culley, RN, COS-C
Legal Nurse Consultant

"Tina Marrelli's latest book is just on time as healthcare evolves away from acute care and into homes and communities. The reader is provided with a broad overview of the setting in which more than 90% of all long term care happens—the home. Progressive health professionals will want to dig into this book as we advance away from fee-for-service to value based purchasing, bundling, and ACOs. Don't miss the final chapter, "Where to From Here, or Welcome to the Most Exciting Healthcare Setting There Is!" Kudos to Marrelli and STTI for their foresight in addressing this important topic."

–Warren Hebert, DNP, RN, CAE
RWJF Executive Nurse Fellow (2006-2009)
Chief Executive Officer, Homecare Association of Louisiana

"Tina Marrelli's passion and commitment for providing the BEST possible care for patients continues to shine through in her new book *Home Care Nursing: Surviving in an Ever-Changing Care Environment*. Her depth of knowledge and understanding of regulatory issues, nursing practice standards, and clinical management challenges are unsurpassed in today's healthcare climate. She is definitely the 'go-to' person for all things home care and hospice!"

–Cathy L. Sasser, RPh
Clinical Pharmacist. Soleo Health
Former Editorial Board member, Home Healthcare Nurse

"Tina Marrelli's newest book makes an important contribution by providing thoughtful insights in the health care sector about the current state and future directions of home health care for professionals—both those just starting out and the more experienced leaders in the field."

–David. L. Jackson, MD, PhD
President, Jackson & Associates, Inc.
Adjunct Professor of Medicine, Division of Geriatric Medicine and Gerontology,
Johns Hopkins University School of Medicine

"This book is a practical, common-sense guide to remind us no matter how home care has changed in its many years of existence, there is always a need for the delivery of quality, accessible, and affordable care to our patients. The home is the most varied independent setting in healthcare, and the skills and knowledge of the clinician must be second to none. This book provides the information that is so needed to the newcomer and those more experienced to not only survive, but succeed!"

–Nancy E. Allen, BSN, RNC, CMC
Founder and President, Solutions for Care, Inc.
Author, Survivor!: 10 Practical Steps to Survey Survival, 4th Edition

"*Home Care Nursing: Surviving in an Ever-Changing Care Environment* is a relevant, on-point book that is well written. We highly recommend this book to anyone who is practicing in this field today. Tina Marrelli covers all the basics of home care nursing in a new, fresh way, and inclusion of Face to Face and homebound status issues make this a cutting edge resource for home care nurses, clinicians, managers, and administrators alike."

–Arlene O'Brien, MALS, RN
Alice Schroeder, MPA, RN
Executive Editors of the Journal of Community Health Nursing

"Tina Marrelli includes 'real-world' examples of the challenges and unique scenarios when providing care in the home, yet provides useful, practical information and a myriad of resources to address them. A must read for every new home care nurse, and a great resource for every veteran home care nurse."

–Mary McGoldrick, MS, RN, CRNI
Home Care and Hospice Consultant, Home Health Systems, Inc.

HOME CARE NURSING

Surviving in an Ever-Changing Care Environment

Tina M. Marrelli, MSN, MA, RN, FAAN

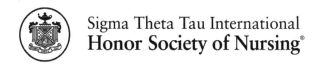

Sigma Theta Tau International
Honor Society of Nursing®

Nursing knowledge and best practices in home care are undergoing change. As new information, evidence, and research become available, there may be implications for practice, education, operations, or in other areas. It is for these reasons that it is very important that nurses, other clinicians, students, educators, and anyone involved in healthcare at home stay apprised of changes and improvements that impact practice and other facets of home care. In addition, the government sometimes updates tools, such as releasing new versions, or updates regulations with revised requirements or other directives for home care and/or other healthcare providers. It is for these reasons that all readers are advised to remain up-to-date and validate that the tools or other information they use contain the latest regulatory information.

The Honor Society of Nursing, Sigma Theta Tau International (STTI) is a nonprofit organization founded in 1922 whose mission is advancing world health and celebrating nursing excellence in scholarship, leadership, and service. Members include practicing nurses, instructors, researchers, policymakers, entrepreneurs, and others. STTI has more than 500 chapters located at more than 700 institutions of higher education throughout Armenia, Australia, Botswana, Brazil, Canada, Colombia, England, Ghana, Hong Kong, Japan, Kenya, Lebanon, Malawi, Mexico, the Netherlands, Pakistan, Portugal, Singapore, South Africa, South Korea, Swaziland, Sweden, Taiwan, Tanzania, Thailand, the United Kingdom, and the United States of America. More information about STTI can be found online at www.nursingsociety.org.

Sigma Theta Tau International
550 West North Street
Indianapolis, IN, USA 46202

To order additional books, buy in bulk, or order for corporate use, contact Nursing Knowledge International at 888.NKI.4YOU (888.654.4968/US and Canada) or +1.317.634.8171 (outside US and Canada).

To request a review copy for course adoption, email solutions@nursingknowledge.org or call 888.NKI.4YOU (888.654.4968/US and Canada) or +1.317.634.8171 (outside US and Canada).

To request author information, or for speaker or other media requests, contact Marketing, Honor Society of Nursing, Sigma Theta Tau International at 888.634.7575 (US and Canada) or +1.317.634.8171 (outside US and Canada).

ISBN:	9781940446714
EPUB ISBN:	9781940446721
PDF ISBN:	9781940446738
MOBI ISBN:	9781940446745

Library of Congress Cataloging-in-Publication data

Names: Marrelli, T. M., author. | Sigma Theta Tau International, issuing body.
Title: Home care nursing : surviving in an ever-changing care environment /
  Tina M. Marrelli.
Description: Indianapolis, IN : Sigma Theta Tau International, [2017] |
  Includes bibliographical references.
Identifiers: LCCN 2016021572| ISBN 9781940446714 (print : alk. paper) | ISBN
  9781940446721 (epub) | ISBN 9781940446738 (pdf) | ISBN 9781940446745 (mobi)
Subjects: | MESH: Home Health Nursing | United States
Classification: LCC RA645.35 | NLM WY 115 AA1 | DDC 362.140973--dc23 LC record avail-
able at https://lccn.loc.gov/2016021572

First Printing, 2016

Publisher: Dustin Sullivan
Acquisitions Editor: Emily Hatch
Editorial Coordinator: Paula Jeffers
Cover Designer: Tim Wurst
Interior Design/Page Layout: Rebecca Batchelor

Principal Book Editor: Carla Hall
Development and Project Editor: Kezia Endsley
Copy Editor: Kevin Kent
Proofreader: Erin Geile
Indexer: Joy Dean Lee

Acknowledgments

I thank my friends and family for their encouragement and support during work sessions that may have caused some hiccups in scheduling or otherwise changed plans—especially my hubby, Bill Glass!

The team at STTI are to be commended for organizational skills and their overall likability. They were a team that was coordinated, communicative, and made decisions in a timely manner. I am impressed!

Brit Stamey, BA, Managing Editor, has been a part of the Marrelli and Associates, Inc., team for over 10 years. Her editorial skills, access to hard-to-find data, and multifaceted organizational skills are to be commended. Brit—you are highly valued and we appreciate you!

I extend a special note to all the nurses, other clinicians, and administrative team members who asked really good questions about numerous aspects of home care and hospice care at home. I hope I answered those questions clearly and this content helps you become better at what you do—and helps patients and their caregivers!

Finally, healthcare in any setting, but perhaps especially in homes, given the personalized nature of the interactions, is truly all about performance improvement and having the "want to" to get better. For that enlightened mindset, a special thanks to Dr. David Jackson of Jackson & Associates, Inc.

About the Author

Tina M. Marrelli, MSN, MA, RN, FAAN, is the President of Marrelli and Associates, Inc., a publishing and consulting firm working in healthcare for more than 20 years. She is the author of numerous books, including the *Handbook of Home Health Standards: Quality, Documentation and Reimbursement*, which is in its fifth revised reprint edition. Other books include *The Hospice and Palliative Care Handbook* and the best-selling home health aide educational system *Home Health Aide Guidelines for Care: A Handbook for Care Giving at Home* and its accompanying *Nurse Instructor Manual*. She served on the workgroups that defined the first hospice nurse standards and also served as a reviewer in 2014 for the revised *Home Health Nursing: Scope and Standards of Practice* published by the American Nurses Association.

Marrelli attended Duke University, where she received her undergraduate degree in nursing. She also has master's degrees in health administration and in nursing. She has worked in home care, hospice, hospitals, nursing homes, and public health. She has practiced as a visiting nurse or managed in-home care and hospice for more than 20 years. She also worked at Medicare's central office (Centers for Medicare & Medicaid Services or CMS) for 4 years on Medicare Part A home care and hospice policies and operations, as well as serving as the Interim Branch Chief for Medicare Part B. She loves policy and the nuances that frame practice and delivery.

An international healthcare consultant, Marrelli specializes in home healthcare and models of care that are provided in the community to people being cared for at home. She and her team of specialized consultants have been in business since 2002 and provide services related to the design and implementation of challenges to providing home and community-based care. In that capacity, they have served more than 100 clients throughout the world, clients who represent varying segments of service to home care or hospice and/or related services and products.

Marrelli has been the editor of three peer-reviewed publications—most recently for *Home Healthcare Nurse* (now *Home Healthcare Now*), for which she served as the editor-in-chief for 8 years. She is also an emeritus editor for *Home Healthcare Now* and serves on the editorial boards of the *Journal of Community Health Nursing* and *The American Nurse*. She is also a member of the Duke University Nursing Alumni Council and in that capacity interfaces with nursing leaders, other alumnae, students, and others in efforts to improve health and healthcare.

Marrelli was the founding member of the International Home Care Nurses Organization (www.IHCNO.org), which was developed "to support a vibrant worldwide network of nurses to promote excellence in providing optimal care to patients living at home wherever they live in the world." The IHCNO was started with a small but "mighty" group of nursing leaders.

Marrelli is looking for educational institutions or healthcare centers of excellence that may wish to partner with the IHCNO for meeting venues and other opportunities. The Case Western Reserve University Frances Payne Bolton School of Nursing hosted and co-sponsored the IHCNO's inaugural conference in 2013. The 2014 IHCNO meeting was held in Singapore with the Tsao Foundation, and, similarly, the 2015 meeting was co-sponsored and held at the University of Illinois at Chicago's College of Nursing. The IHCNO has a unique vision—that these meetings be held at such sites to bridge practice and education and to introduce nursing and other students to home care and the many models of care at home across the globe.

Table of Contents

6 THE FUNDAMENTALS: THE INTERFACE OF LAW, REGULATION, AND QUALITY........123

7 THE HOME VISIT: THE IMPORTANT UNIT OF CARE 161

8 DOCUMENTATION OF CARE AND RELATED PROCESSES 207

9 WHERE TO FROM HERE? OR WELCOME TO THE MOST EXCITING HEALTHCARE SETTING THERE IS! .249

APPENDIXES

A HOME CARE AND HOSPICE/PALLIATIVE CARE ORGANIZATIONS/ ASSOCIATIONS 263

B RESOURCES FOR CLINICIANS AND PATIENT/CAREGIVER EDUCATION 277

C HOME HEALTH & HOSPICE MAC AREAS 301

D MEDICARE BENEFIT POLICY MANUAL . . .303

INDEX 401

Reviewers

Nancy E. Allen, BSN, RNC, CMC
CEO, Solutions for Care, Inc.
Jacksonville Beach, Florida

Cathleen "Cat" Armato, RN, CHPN, CHC, CHPC
Principal Consultant
Armato & Associates, LLC
Blairsville, Georgia

Kim Corral, RN, BSN, MaEd, COS-C
President, Chelta, Inc.
Mesa, Arizona

Mary H. Deeley, MHA, RN
Towson, Maryland

Joie Glenn, RN, MBA, CAE
Executive Director, New Mexico Association for Home and Hospice Care
Albuquerque, New Mexico

Lynda Hilliard, MBA, RN, CHC, CCEP
Compliance Consultant
Mt. Shasta, California

David L. Jackson, MD, PhD
President, Jackson & Associates, Inc.
Adjunct Professor of Medicine
Johns Hopkins University
School of Medicine
Baltimore, Maryland

Mary McGoldrick, MS, RN, CRNI
Home Care and Hospice Consultant, Home Health Systems, Inc.
Saint Simons Island, Georgia

Elizabeth "Ibby" Tanner, PhD, RN, FNGNA, FAAN
Associate Professor, Director of Interprofessional Education, Johns Hopkins School of Nursing and School of Medicine
Baltimore, Maryland

Patricia Zabell, RN, BS, MBA, CHCE, HCS-D, COS-C
Clinical Consultant
McBee Associates
Sarasota, Florida

Foreword

The 1980s were a time of great upheaval in home care, when agencies were being subjected to intense scrutiny that arose from the growing awareness of the need to protect the elderly, concerns about higher Medicare expenditures, and the rapid growth in the number of home health agencies in the United States. In response to these trends, Congress commissioned a study titled the "Black Box of Home Care Quality" in an effort to assess the state of affairs and develop recommendations to address the identified problems. The findings of this study resulted in reproach of home care providers and those responsible for their oversight. At the same time, many home health agencies found themselves in financial distress because Medicare contractors retroactively denied payment for large numbers of claims for services that had been appropriately delivered. This phenomena was known as the "denial crisis of the 1980s." It was during that time of confusion and consternation that I first met Tina Marrelli. We were colleagues, both working for home health agencies and serving together on the board of directors for the Maryland Association for Home Care.

One thing that was very clear to Tina and me in those days was that there was a severe shortage of guidance about the Medicare home health benefit including who qualified for home health services, what clinical services were covered by Medicare, and how services should be documented. Medicare instructions about home health were limited, vague, and loosely interpreted by contractors as well as providers. Since compliance was impossible without direction, the home health community's oft-repeated retort to payment denials was "tell us what we need to do, and we will do it." These pleas for clarity were eventually answered after the home care industry filed, and won, the landmark Medicare class action lawsuit, *Duggan v. Bowen*. As a result, the court directed Medicare to rewrite the home health benefit and to develop detailed policy descriptions for providers and contractors.

Although Tina and I went our separate ways in the early 1990s, we worked in parallel spheres where we both continued to pursue the goal of ensuring that proper policies were created and disseminated to home health agencies so that incorporation of the policies into agency practices was both reasonable and feasible. Armed with the belief that change at the source was also needed, Tina first worked as a senior policy analyst, and later acting branch chief, at what is known today as the Centers for Medicare & Medicaid Services (CMS). In those positions, she had a lead role in developing the policy guidelines for the home health benefit, ensuring that the Medicare contractors adopted them, and substantiating that proper payments were made. She played an active role in teaching the Medicare payment contractors about the coverage nuances in the updated Medicare manuals that were promulgated as a result of the lawsuit.

Since then, as consultant and author who still makes home visits, Tina has focused her attention on bolstering home health agencies' capacity to legitimately secure Medicare payment by serving as a guiding light for compliance. Meanwhile, I had moved on to become vice president of regulatory affairs at the National Association for Home Care & Hospice. There, and in my subsequent work as a consultant, I, too, have been able to support and help sustain the delivery of much needed services to patients by providing interpretation of regulations and policies to home health agencies through counseling, writing, and educational programs. Today, both Tina and I remain committed to assisting the home health community by providing the information needed to ensure compliance.

More than 30 years have passed since the "denial crisis of the 1980s," yet many of the issues of *then* are the issues of *now*. The elderly population continues to grow, as do concerns about Medicare expenditures, and a resurgence of growth in the number of new home health agencies. Denial of payment for services provided is again increasing. Control of fraud and abuse is the hot topic when Medicare expenditures are discussed.

When noncompliance is identified, there is no differentiation made by Medicare contractors and government oversight agencies between ignorance of the rules and outright fraud. Fulfillment of the many, ever-changing Medicare requirements is especially problematic in home health. Here, unlike in other healthcare settings, nurses and therapists are alone in the home, acting as sole decision-makers in determining patient needs and whether they qualify for Medicare payment. Therefore, it is critical that direct care workers are armed with the information needed to ensure compliance.

Home Care Nursing: Surviving in an Ever-Changing Care Environment will serve as a valuable tool to health care educators, home health managers, and orientation and in-service personnel to fulfill these needs. It delivers in-depth information in a manner than can be easily understood and applied by everyone who needs to be in the know. When it comes to knowledge of the Medicare home care benefit, ignorance is not bliss, nor is it an acceptable excuse for non-compliance. Tina Marrelli's new book dispels regulatory ignorance and provides the information necessary for solid decision making.

–Mary St. Pierre, RN, BSN, MGA
Former Vice President for Regulatory Affairs,
National Association for Home Care & Hospice
Home Health & Hospice Consultant

Introduction

This book provides an overview for those who are new to home care, as well as those who have been practicing or managing in this setting for some time and must now view home care in a different way. Readers may be nurses, administrators, physician assistants, clinical auditors, and hospital staff following patients back to home, as well as educators, policy makers, insurers, emergency medical technicians or paramedics, physicians, therapists, pharmacists, social workers, and others seeking to understand and/or move into the practice setting of the future—the patient's home.

After reading the contents of this book, I think you will also see that the practice setting is here now and will only grow in scope and importance. This is a fundamental shift in healthcare. Based on many calls I have received, home care for those making visits and the "scope" of those visits are all in flux. This is an exciting time to be in home care! We can all learn from each other.

The book was written so that each chapter can either be read as "stand-alone," even without reading the preceding chapter(s), or starting at the beginning of the book and continuing through to the end. If read the second way, from start to finish, each chapter builds on the information and content in the prior chapter. In that way, the first chapter sets the stage for the "biggest" picture of healthcare at home and then continues to get more detailed and directed toward more specific aspects of home care as the chapters progress. For example, if you need to know about home visits specifically, you can start with Chapter 7, "The Home Visit: The Important Unit of Care." Similarly, those with an interest in policy specifically, such as health-policy students or nursing educators, might be interested in Chapter 5, "The Environment of Care: The Home and Community Interface."

This book was also designed to be used as a part of the organization-specific orientation program. The organization has its specific policies and procedures and can integrate needed contents into the program to help with the standardization of care and processes among the team and across the organization.

There are no terms that are not clear or lingo that only home care or healthcare experts know. One overarching goal was to provide practical wisdom and information in common-sense language. This should also be passed on to our patients and their families, too. We should not need to explain what we mean whenever we explain something to them; it is hard enough to have effective communication and coordination considering the many facets and complexities of healthcare! The hope is that all who are caring for patients and families are understood, and for safety reasons, clarity becomes the watchword!

At the end of each chapter is a "Questions for Further Consideration and Discussion" section. These queries and activities are meant to encourage discussion and further thinking about given topics. There are also "For Further Reading" sections, which contain links or reports that provide more in-depth and thoughtful information about a specific facet of home care discussed in the text.

Fundamental information may be stated more than once and in multiple chapters. This was not done in error. I believe that some of the information is so important and/or required for many reasons that it bears repeating. In this way, information is "framed" in the context of that specific chapter in which the topic is addressed. Two topic areas that come to mind are physician orders and why the home and community environment is so different from other healthcare settings. These may be mentioned more than one time in the multiple areas where they apply.

The concept of this new book came after the 5th (latest) edition of the *Handbook of Health Standards and Documentation Guidelines for Reimbursement* (Marrelli, 2012) came in at 738 pages. That book, which is all about systems-based care planning and documentation and reimbursement, could not grow, but there was still so much more information needed for home care providers because the model of care is changing so much. This book then is "the rest of the story."

Sincerely,

Tina Marrelli
news@marrelli.com
www.marrelli.com

Reference

Marrelli, T. (2012). *Handbook of Home Health Standards: Quality: Documentation, and Reimbursement* (5th edition, revised reprint). St. Louis, MO: Mosby.

1

Healthcare: Overview of Change and Complexity

This chapter provides an overview of healthcare-related changes from a big-picture perspective. These are needed to best understand where home care fits into the bigger picture of healthcare as a whole. With this in mind, the overwhelming trend in healthcare can be summarized in one word: change.

This chapter seeks to identify some of these changes and their impact on home care. For purposes of this chapter and book, I am defining *home care* holistically *as any kind of health-related services provided at home.* A classic and comprehensive definition of home care is one by Claire F. Ryder Warhola from the U.S. Public Health Service, Department of Health and Human Services. It states that *home care* is:

> *"…that component of a continuum of comprehensive healthcare whereby health services are provided to individuals and families in their places of residence for the purpose of promoting, maintaining, or restoring health, or maximizing the effects of independence, while minimizing the effects of disability and illness, including terminal illness. Services appropriate to the needs of the individual patient and family are planned, coordinated and made available by providers organized for the delivery of home care." (1980)*

But where exactly does home care fit into and intersect with the bigger picture of healthcare and its delivery? And where exactly are the intersections in healthcare today that support this continuum and alignment with the "promoting of health" mentioned in this definition?

These and other questions may best be answered by reviewing where we are, how we got here, and how home care might be a solution or a large part of the answer to the major disruption of illness and some of the trends seen in healthcare. The following sections highlight some of those trends.

Drivers of Change in Healthcare: Factors and Forces

Many forces and factors are driving the needed changes to the healthcare system. As you read this chapter, try to pretend that you are a neophyte in healthcare—that you do not know much about healthcare and have "new eyes" to take in, thoughtfully review, and reimagine it as it could be. This fresh approach can help you have a better understanding of this chapter and bring new perspective to your work!

Cost, Quality, and the Affordable Care Act

Discussions about the pros and cons of the Affordable Care Act (ACA) will continue, but the focus must be about patients, quality, access, and cost. The passage of the ACA means generally mechanisms are now in place to help individuals access some kind of health insurance. Since the ACA was passed, 16.4 million formerly uninsured people in the United States now have health insurance (U.S. Department of Health and Human Services, 2015).

Parts of rural America still have challenges related to accessing healthcare, especially access to specifically needed levels of care or specialty services. This is important from a sheer volume perspective. According to the *2014 National Healthcare Quality and Disparities Report Chartbook on Rural Health Care* from the Agency for Healthcare Research and Quality (AHRQ, 2014a), "although rural residents make up less than one-fifth of the U.S. population, 65% of all U.S. counties are classified as nonmetropolitan" (p. 4).

This may be particularly problematic for home care organizations since this report also found that potentially avoidable hospitalizations are higher in rural areas than in other residential locations (AHRQ, 2014a). Though costly and sometimes unwieldy, the initiation of a process where more uninsured and underinsured Americans get some kind of health insurance and care helps in the promotion of health and health maintenance for millions of more Americans. Like all laws, such as those that created Medicare and Medicaid, there will be continued change and fine-tuning.

Sadly, many other countries had their healthcare reform many years before the United States did. In fact, the United States has the highest healthcare costs, but some of the poorest healthcare outcomes, in important areas such as infant morbidity and mortality and others (The Commonwealth Fund, 2014; PBS NewsHour, 2012). Simply put, we are paying more, but are not seeing "value" for that payment. It is for these reasons that the United States is moving toward a "value-based" reimbursement model.

The Population Is Aging

This is the first time in history that we have multiple generations of older adults, as well as tremendous growth in the number of the "oldest old" and *centenarians*, or people over 100 years of age. This has been called the "grey tsunami." What this means practically and from a care perspective is that we all need to know more about older adult care and need geriatric clinical nurse specialists on our teams! Americans are also living longer, and living sicker, often with chronic diseases.

To get an idea of the scope of the numbers, starting on January 1, 2011, and continuing for the next 19 years, 10,000 Americans are turning 65 every day (Pew Research Center, 2010)! And many of these "baby boomers" (individuals born between 1946 and 1964) want more input and should have more say in their own end-of-life care and planning, as discussed in the next section, as the next trend (PBS, 2014).

Compassionate End-of-Life Care and the Need for Improvement

Much has been written about end-of-life care in the United States. Sadly, the medical model of treating through death, sometimes even when not wanted by the patient or family and/or when it's not appropriate or effective, continues. This has been eloquently addressed by Atul Gawande in an article called "Overkill" as well as in the book *Being Mortal:*

Medicine and What Matters in the End. This is a topic many do not wish to discuss or address, but we know the worst time to have these conversations is in the emergency department or the intensive care unit (ICU). This is also not the time to guess what someone's specific wishes would be.

The good news is that the use of hospice and more compassionate care models toward the end of life is expanding, and the total number of hospice patients served has increased every year over the past 5 years (National Hospice and Palliative Care Organization [NHPCO], 2015). At the same time, "7 out of 10 Americans say they would prefer to die at home while only 25% actually die at home" (PBS, n.d.).

In a *Lancet* article, Harvard researchers identified that of 1.8 million Medicare beneficiaries who died in 2008, almost one in three had surgery in the last year of their life, so clearly a lot of surgery is performed at the end of life (Kwok et al., 2011). In addition, almost 1 in 10 had surgery in the last week of life (Kwok et al., 2011). As one non-medical friend said to me when he saw his father in the hospital, "Why are we torturing old people?"

We can and must do better in the management of pain, depression, anxiety, and other symptoms that older adults and the oldest old experience. We still have much to learn about the very old. Home care nurses are on the front lines and are able to identify the special needs of this population, such as frailty, nutritional impairment, barriers to care, and other areas to improve care. It is very good news that Medicare now reimburses physicians and other healthcare professionals for having conversations about wishes and choices related to end-of-life care and related care planning.

Complexity and Safety in Healthcare

Because of the complexity of healthcare and the many moving and faceted parts that must align and work together, especially in hospitals, safety is an identified and very important driver for change. According to a study by the Centers for Disease Control & Prevention (CDC), "common medical errors total more than $4.5 billion in additional health spending a year" (Centers for Medicare & Medicaid Services [CMS], 2008, p. 1). Safety is a significant enough issue that there was a hearing held before the Subcommittee on Primary Health and Aging in the 113th Congress on July 17, 2014, titled "More than 1,000 Preventable Deaths a Day is Too Many: The Need to Improve Patient Safety." This hearing can be viewed at http://www.c-span.org/video/?320495-1/hearing-patient-safety.

The Health and Medicine Division (HMD) of The National Academies of Sciences, Engineering, and Medicine (formerly the Institute of Medicine or IOM) published a seminal report in 1999 titled "To Err is Human: Building A Safer Health System" and presented a "strategy by which government, health care providers, industry, and consumers can reduce preventable medical errors" (p. 2). This was an eye-opening glimpse into the world of errors and other complex problems that impact patients and their families. You can read it here: https://iom.nationalacademies.org/~/media/Files/Report%20Files/1999/To-Err-is-Human/To%20Err%20is%20Human%201999%20%20report%20brief.pdf.

The Health and Medicine Division is a nonprofit, nongovernmental organization that provides and publishes evidence-based research with corresponding recommendations. Since the publication of that 1999 report, the government has initiated the concept of "never events," initially introduced in hospitals. Simply put, these are events that should be prevented and/or avoided. They include:

- Falls and trauma
- Pressure ulcers
- Surgical site infections
- Vascular-catheter associated infections

- Administration of incompatible blood

- Air embolism

- Foreign objects unintentionally retained after surgery

- Wrong-site surgeries

- Surgery on the wrong patient

- Wrong surgeries performed

- And others

What this means operationally is that if this is a hospital-acquired never event, the hospital is not reimbursed for treatment related to the event. This is another way the government is working to realign incentives and effectively link payment to value, which helps ensure the prudent use of limited Medicare, Medicaid, and other resources.

Regulatory and Structural Changes

Many parts of healthcare are starting to come together to truly make healthcare become a "system" with better and more effective coordination and continuity. Some of these efforts at coordination and continuity include an emphasis on the "harmonization" of healthcare, which means terms and goals are aligned across care settings.

One example of harmonization is using the same terms or glossary across all care sites. This includes such things as patients being asked about their influenza or pneumococcal vaccines in all care settings. For example, whether the patient is in a nursing home, a hospital, a home health agency, or a doctor's office, they are asked about these same health indicators/data points. At the same time, Medicare is looking at payer models that are value-based, and it is projected that Medicare will be using a value-based reimbursement models in the not too distant future.

We know more surgery does not always mean better care—in fact, many reports have noted the costs of unnecessary services and surgeries performed in the United States. Add to this that we have a system that "slices and dices" many components of care (think of all the providers involved in a patient's care for a fall and then hip surgery and rehabilitation) and the fact that often the more interventions that are used, the more providers get paid (assuming covered care, of course). Sadly, we hear stories about surgeons or organizations purposefully providing unnecessary care and see convictions for overbilling or fraudulent practices for unnecessary procedures or care.

 We may be learning that more is not better in healthcare, and some countries have demonstrated better healthcare outcomes with fewer interventions than the United States. This may be particularly true for some older adult populations, and the Hippocratic mantra "first do no harm" comes to mind. In this patient population in particular, effective care coordination and communications across care sites is very important for safety.

One initiative Medicare has chosen to pilot is a program for some kinds of surgeries where all the related components of care are "bundled" together. One example is for people needing joint replacements, including hips and knee replacements. Under the pilot program, all providers involved in care must work together to help the patient and the organization meet agreed-upon goals. The hospital where the surgery is performed will be responsible for the quality and the costs of care from surgery through 90 days after discharge. This model is being piloted in approximately 800 hospitals throughout various geographic areas across the country. It is a model of carefully planned and truly managed care that can only mean better care for patients. It should put all the parties on a more unified team and should ensure more effective coordination and communications—which is a challenging area across all care settings.

Another structural/regulatory change is that Medicare, which sets the standards for many payers, pays for some preventative and well older adult care, which was unheard of some years ago. Pursuant to the Affordable Care Act (ACA), Medicare covers many preventative services, usually at no cost (no co-pay) to the patients. These "preventative services" can include:

- A first annual wellness visit (when first on Medicare)
- Cardiovascular risk screening
- Colorectal cancer screenings
- Depression screenings
- Diabetes screenings
- Prostate cancer screenings
- And more, usually based on the person's history, findings, and risks

These efforts are helping to shape/reshape the healthcare system into a more preventive-focused model that puts the spotlight more on health than disease. True health is not just the absence of disease or pathology but also the entire constellation of health factors, choices, access, and environment. When we review that holistic definition of home care at the beginning of this chapter, it is easy to understand why home care nurses and leaders are ahead of the learning curve in this movement toward true health—community-focused home care while integrating prevention and promotion—because we have always been focused on this model!

Efforts Related to Decreasing Hospital Admissions and Readmissions

Hospitalizations and rehospitalizations are very costly to Medicare and other payers. *Pay for performance* or *value-based* are the terms used to explain this model, which is tied to positive and improved outcomes for patients. For some years, Medicare has initiated what is called the Hospital Readmission Reductions Program (HRRP), which was begun in 2012 to address costly hospital readmission rates.

One study found that up to one-fifth of Medicare beneficiaries who were hospitalized were readmitted within 30 days of being discharged from the hospital (Jencks, Williams, & Coleman, 2009). Under the HRRP program, Medicare hospital revenue is reduced up to a certain percentage of the hospital's total Medicare revenue, based on a number of factors and certain patient problems, starting with patients with acute myocardial infarction, heart failure, and pneumonia (CMS, 2015a).

Simply put, if certain patients come back into the hospital for the same problem within 30 days, the hospital will not be reimbursed for this care. Of course, the thought is that if hospitals provide the care needed while in the hospital, then part of that care will include an effective discharge plan, appropriate patient/caregiver education, and more overall effort taken to prevent such rehospitalizations. Medicare, the largest payer of healthcare services, identified some years ago that the problem of readmissions was very costly. According to AHRQ, "hospitals spent $41.3 billion between January and November 2011 to treat patients readmitted within 30 days of discharge" (Shinkman, 2014, para. 1).

Readers who are practicing and leading in home care can clearly see the rationale for the emphasis of decreasing hospitalizations from the home care perspective as well. This is another example of the harmonization of healthcare—working to make the entire system and related processes make sense and be congruent across all care settings—with the overall goals of decreasing costs and improving patient safety and quality.

Redefining and Strengthening Nursing Roles

We are seeing the emergence of new roles in healthcare with many being created, clarified, and/or strengthened. For example, not that many years ago there were no "scribes," people who document in real-time for other clinicians, such as physicians, in various healthcare settings, including the emergency department, outpatient clinics, and offices. The goal is to increase efficiencies while allowing the primary clinicians to be able to spend more time with the patient. Other roles undergoing significant shift include programs whereby some states and communities are teaching emergency medical technicians or emergency medical service providers to make home visits and assess when the patient does not require emergent care, but can better and more safely be cared for at home.

Think of older adults who fall frequently and their frail spouse cannot move or lift them, or other examples where there is not a need for a higher level of care but the patient can be assessed or cared for at home. Pharmacists are also taking on larger roles as the go-to person not only for the safe dispensing of medications but also for related medication management. Some pharmacists are a significant part of the home care team and make home visits to try to decrease rehospitalizations by identifying early on the risk factors with certain medications or types of higher-risk medications. Others manage high-risk heart failure patients.

Nursing as a profession is undergoing change to help the larger healthcare system improve the nation's health. In the seminal report *The Future of Nursing: Leading Change, Advancing Health*, the HMD recognized the important role or nurses in healthcare. Released in 2011, the initiative made four main recommendations (IOM, 2011):

- Nurses should practice using their "education and training"
- Nurses should seek out higher education
- Nurses should help redesign healthcare
- More data collection is needed to improve workforce planning

The full report can be accessed at http://www.nap.edu/read/12956/chapter/1, and you can learn more about the subsequent Robert Wood Johnson Foundation and AARP partnership that established the "Future of Nursing: Campaign for Action" at http://campaignforaction.org/.

The Drive Toward Patient-Centered Care

The longer term goal is directed toward implementing truly patient-centered care. About patient-centered care, do you also find it interesting that many services are provided only on Monday through Friday at set hours? Obviously the best patient care is a 24-hour-a-day commitment for access to needed services. Another example that occurs in hospitals is that blood draws/venipunctures are scheduled *very* early in the morning. As boomers and others see what healthcare "looks like," they know from other industries that some things can be improved upon or benchmarked with and against. Such discussions are a great opportunity for quality improvement and should be embraced.

For example, I was at the bedside of a 96-year-old who was visited daily at 4:30 a.m. for a blood draw. Of course, we know that is not the best way to be woken up for a test that was not a stat or an emergency. I asked that this be done after 7 a.m. if possible, and it was. This is just one example of many things that occur "because that is how they have always been done," even though they do not support the intent of true patient-centered care (nor the tenets of customer service and the patient experience).

This is especially true for the patient population in hospitals, which includes many older adults and the "oldest" old—those over age 85 (National Institute on Aging [NIA], 2011). This age group particularly needs their sleep, especially while in the hospital, since sleep deprivation and disruption can lead to increased confusion or delirium and increased risk of falls in a new/changed environment. Using available science-based data, evidence-based resources, and common sense with patient input needs to drive us toward a more personal and gentle care model.

We still have a long way to go with some very fundamental operational changes to move toward the healthcare setting of the future—one that is truly designed around patient and family needs. We all have a role in moving the best healthcare forward by identifying such operations or areas for improvement and respectfully pointing them out when asked about the patient experience. This new approach of patient-centered care, emphasized by the government and now by many leaders in healthcare, means that the patient makes the decisions, and to accomplish this means that the patient/family needs to be more prepared with information to implement this effectively and feel comfortable about it.

Technology and Related Innovations

There was a time when patients and consumers could not just "Google" something to find out about a medication or a disease. Now we take this gift of access and communication for granted, and many patients and families are very educated consumers—and this is a good thing and should be embraced. The more we as clinicians and leaders can empower and help patients on their self-management and healthcare journey the better.

But we must note that not all care providers embrace this theory and/or change. So this is another change or shift in thinking—that patients and family members are truly equal partners in care and care planning. This begins at/on admission/assessment and continues through the care planning or scientific process, through to the determination of goals and discharge. This also includes goals/choices about when to stop painful or futile treatment(s) and when to move toward other goals, such as hospice or other end-of-life care models, with the limited time a person has left.

We may be moving from a paternalistic model—where the healthcare professional "knows best"—to the patient-, family-, and consumer-driven decision based on the data they collected and where the patient and family seek validation or counsel about decision-making from physicians and others on the team of professionals caring for them. Put another way, we are moving toward partnerships, where consumers research and make treatment decisions based on science and gathered data.

Technology is also critical to the communication and coordination of patient care across care sites, in what are called *transition points*. This is the time that patients are most at risk for an untoward event or problem. This could be, for example, when an older adult man moves to an assisted living center and falls the second night there because he was alone, in a new space, or because of other factors related to an older adult in a changed environment like furniture placement or different floor surfaces.

These transitions of care must be carefully planned, and risks need to be identified and addressed to improve safety and quality. Effective data management and systems can also help patient safety as patients traverse these risk points of change across settings. This is because some data (for instance, in this example, his allergies, medications, the fact that he says he can walk without a cane even though he cannot, his history of two falls, and numerous other facts) need to come "with" the patient. In this way, team members in all care settings are apprised of critical information needed for a safe transition when data is accurate, timely, shared, and known.

The Move to Value-Based Care

For some years we have heard the term *value-based care*. What does this mean exactly, and what are the real-world operational implications for home care and other providers? According to CMS, in a fact sheet released in 2015, the ACA "law gives us the opportunity to shape the way health care is delivered to patients and to improve the quality of care system-wide while helping to reduce the growth of health care costs" (2015b, para. 1).

Simply put, CMS wants to "reward value and care coordination—rather than volume and care duplication" (2015b, para. 2). To this end, and with public–private sector partnerships, they are testing and expanding new care models that can "improve the quality and reduce the cost of health care" (CMS, 2015b, para. 1).

What this means from a practical perspective is that CMS (and other payers) may not pay for duplicative care or care that does not improve patient outcomes. Examples include unnecessary surgeries, duplicative tests or exams because the system is inefficient or cannot (re)locate original tests, patients getting treatments and therapies that are not effective, and others. What this means to us in home care is that we need to ask questions like:

- Does the care, visit, shift, and/or call I made to a patient and family support quality and help improve outcomes toward the patient's predetermined goals?

- Does the care planned support the evidence known and used for this care?

- Does the care meet the standards of a skilled nursing or other visit?

- From a data perspective, do I add value to the care provided from a data perspective, where measurable outcomes have occurred and are attributable to my care/intervention/ management?

Skillful Caring for Patients in Poor Socioeconomic Conditions

An emerging and known body of science and research relates to poor health and living situations. Those of us that have been visiting nurses for many years learned early that patients who have no or very poor socioeconomic supports or resources generally fared poorly in response to care compared to patients with adequate support and resources.

One particular patient comes to mind. I will call her Mrs. Smith. Mrs. Smith was in her late 70s, and whenever the summer heat in Baltimore reached the 90s, she would start wheezing and sometimes develop bronchitis. There were no organized efforts or programs to decrease rehospitalizations back then, but after seeing this pattern of bronchitis and then hospitalization over many months and seasons, it was easy to see that she needed an air conditioner to help keep her out the hospital. She did get an air conditioner and that made all the difference for her. She was able to breathe because she could stay comfortable, cool, and out of the humidity and heat that affected her so many times before. This was an "aha" moment for me as a young nurse.

When people do not have reliable transportation, they can miss appointments. If fast food is all that's accessible to them, they may also suffer from obesity and/or poor nutrition. They may have no phone, so it may be hard to reach them and remind them about medications, appointments, and other factors that positively impact health. The home care nurse has an important role to play in the identification and referral of these underserved and at-risk patients and families.

Health systems will continue to be affected by these sometimes complex patients who often are very well known to emergency departments because the patients do not have insurance and therefore do not have access to preventative or primary care. This causes them to go to the emergency department more often and means they often need higher levels of care and/or higher-cost care. These challenges require more comprehensive care planning, as well as performance improvement, and they will remain an important focus for healthcare leadership and organizations.

Transitional Care

For some years, it has been apparent that the greatest risk areas for patients, especially older adults and the oldest old, is between *transitions* in care. Transitions can be from the hospital back to home, from the hospital to a skilled nursing facility, or to a family member's home after inpatient care. It is for this reason that a number of transitional care models have emerged.

One of the most studied and known is actually called the *Transitional Care Model,* and it was designed by Mary Naylor, a nurse and scientist. The innovative model she developed has 10 elements including specially trained nurses who help patients through the care from hospital and into the home (Transitional Care Model, n.d.). Those practicing or managing in home care hear the (sad) story too many times of the older adult who goes into the hospital, comes back out "fine," and goes back home or to a family member's home and has problems like a fall, an issue with her medication(s), or other safety-related problem(s) necessitating the next readmission, and the cycle continues.

The Houses of Yesterday

The house of yesterday, often a two-story home, may not meet the safety needs of the older (and getting older) population. As visiting nurses, we see sometimes that houses have no master (or any) bedrooms downstairs. This is a problem for a number of reasons since the stairs will continue to be a safety concern for "aging in place." This is where the nursing and therapy team members can bring a specialized skillset to help make a home environment safer and try to address identified safety concerns.

Prescription and Other Medications and Their Costs

According to the Henry J. Kaiser Family Foundation, approximately 24% of people taking prescription drugs report they have difficulty affording their medications (2015). At the same time, if you have patients needing insulin for their diabetes, you are seeing these costs rising. This is due to a number of factors, and spending on medication prices continues to grow. Some drug companies have even defended some incredible prices, even for drugs already in the marketplace (the price of one such drug was recently increased 5,000%). This is appropriately engendering pushback against this trend from consumers and payers. In fact, the Medicare Payment Advisory Commission (MedPAC, see p. 27) recently endorsed that mechanisms to address spiraling drug costs be initiated (Seidman, 2015).

The Number of People Involved in Care

Having too many people involved in a patient's care is a trend that may contribute to errors and other problems in care coordination and communications. Let's look at one example to see how many people might be involved in a sample patients' care across the continuum.

An older adult, Mr. Sam, falls on the front steps of his home while sweeping off leaves. A neighbor sees this fall and calls 911. The EMS takes Mr. Sam to the local hospital's emergency department (ED). At the hospital, it is noted that Mr. Sam's hip is fractured, and he has hypertension. A blood test shows some level of renal failure. At this point, the EMS, the nurses in the ED, the ED physician, the orthopedic surgeon, and a nephrologist are all involved, and Mr. Sam needs a cardiac workup before he can have his hip repaired and the surgery scheduled.

Next, he gets to the pre-operative room and then the operating room, and there is a whole other team and the care coordination and (sometimes mis) communication continues. Postoperatively, there are the recovery room nurses and then the inpatient unit where he goes after the recovery room stay. Now a hospitalist, inpatient nurses, therapists, a dietitian, and others are involved, depending on his trajectory while in the hospital. Because Mr. Sam is very old and that brings its own frailties, he develops a catheter-associated urinary tract infection (CAUTI), postoperative pneumonia, wheezing, and pulmonary edema confirmed by radiology. Mr. Sam now also has respiratory therapy for breathing treatments, a urologist for the UTI, and so on.

No wonder there is so much complexity in healthcare! In the past, there would have been a patient's doctor who would have followed him into the hospital and truly "knew" him as an individual and his unique care history needs. I would like to think we are beginning to understand that "More is not better," and "First, do no harm," should be our mantras. This complexity has created the need for skillful case management.

Skillful Case Management

Case management means different things in different settings. Insurers/payers have case managers, hospitals have them, and home care uses the term also. Whatever the term, home care patients—especially the oldest old, infants, children, those with complex and debilitating diseases, or other patients requiring specialized care—need this level of oversight and careful, detailed management. It is the coordination and communication that can sometimes make all the difference.

Healthcare is easy to "turn on," but sometimes very hard to slow down when it is appropriate and patients make individualized choices. This role of advocacy and the need for a care/case conference or a discussion with the patient and family, physician, and others to revisit goals and patient wishes is very important. Case management is a skill that includes listening and advocating for the unique needs of the patient and family. As one patient's family member said to me about her family member, "Can we just bring him back home and let him spend what time he has left with us at home?"

The Growth of Care in the Home

When asked, most people report that they wish to stay at home through illness and death when possible. For example, in Florida, growth in home care and all kinds of related services have emerged to help people remain at home or "age in place." Be they "non-medical" services, personal care, pet services, or anything in between, all of these have emerged to help people remain at home. This choice or self-determination to remain at home can sometimes be difficult to understand and accept. Sometimes, it's hard to see how some patients stay at home (and sometimes alone) given their health status, frailty, or other problems.

This balance of patient choice, self-determination, and safety is sometimes hard to watch—but as I have been told by my very old neighbors and friends, "It is my choice to make." I agree. In addition to these "non-medical services," there are home health agencies, which may be reimbursed by Medicare and Medicaid, private duty skilled nursing services, registries, and other models of care that place patients with caregivers. The complexity of the definitions and the services and licensure (if any and for what services) varies by states.

Caregiver Considerations

Family, friends, adult children, and others can all be caregivers. This is probably the largest group of untapped people resources for the patient and the healthcare system at large. Caregivers are very important team members who know more about the patient than the provider can ever know. This is the reason experienced nurses and other clinicians listen when a patient's caregiver says something like "I have never seen him like this before," "His breathing has changed," "Something is different—this is not her usual color," or any number of similar statements based on their observation of the person for which they are they are caring. Trust this knowledge!

It is this thoughtful listening and then critical thinking and further assessment that makes for compassionate and skillful care. In home care, we must depend on our family or friend caregivers—they are the communicators and observers, truly valued eyes and ears. Numerous studies and surveys report that when asked where one wishes to receive care, a person's home is overwhelmingly the answer. There truly is no place like home!

Summary

The issues in this chapter represent only some of the multifaceted and complex trends that contribute to healthcare undergoing cataclysmic change. The upheaval is huge and if you work as a nurse, therapist, pharmacist, or leader in home care, hospice, or a hospital, it is more than a feeling. Putting these changes together with timely and effective daily operations, while also complying with numerous regulatory requirements, takes a lot of energy, skill, and know-how.

The next chapter addresses home care specifically—in all its complexity. All these changes, it could be argued, are getting us realigned to where healthcare as a "system" needs to be. This is not to say it will be easy. Rest assured that home care will have an important part to play. What it "looks like" may be very different from some traditional models of home care. And while it may look very different in the future, many of the fundamentals will remain the same!

Questions for Further Consideration and Discussion

1. Out of the drivers listed in this chapter that impact change in healthcare, which are the most important and why?

2. Identify three pros and three cons of the Affordable Care Act.

3. Define value-based healthcare and explain what this means in practical terms for organizations and patients and their families.

4. List three types of technology that enhance care for patients and their caregivers.

5. Imagine the healthcare world with home as the preferred setting for healthcare. What do you envision this to "look like" from a nursing and organizational perspective? Be as specific as possible.

For Further Reading

- Self Directed Services from Medicaid.gov: https://www. medicaid.gov/Medicaid-CHIP-Program-Information/By-Topics/ Delivery-Systems/Self-Directed-Services.html

- *Teaching IOM: Implications of the Institute of Medicine Reports for Nursing Education*, 3rd Edition, by Anita Finkelman and Carole Kenner

- *To Comfort Always: A Nurse's Guide to End-of-Life Care*, 2nd Edition, by Linda Norlander

- *Being Present: A Nurse's Resource for End-of-Life Communication*, by Linda Norlander and Marjorie Schaffer

- *Handbook of Home Health Standards: Quality, Documentation, and Reimbursement*, 5th Edition, by Tina M. Marrelli

- *Clinical Case Studies in Home Health Care*, by Leslie Neal-Boylan

- The Role of Post-Acute Care in New Care Delivery Models: http://www.aha.org/research/reports/tw/15dec-tw-postacute.pdf
- Home Health Value-Based Purchasing Model: https://innovation.cms.gov/initiatives/Home-Health-Value-Based-Purchasing-Model/index.html

References

Agency for Healthcare Research and Quality (AHRQ). (2014a). *2014 national healthcare quality and disparities report chartbook on rural health care.* Retrieved from http://www.ahrq.gov/sites/default/files/wysiwyg/research/findings/nhqrdr/2014chartbooks/ruralhealth/2014nhqdr-ruralhealth.pdf

Centers for Medicare & Medicaid Services (CMS). (2008). SMDL #08-004. Retrieved from https://downloads.cms.gov/cmsgov/archived-downloads/SMDL/downloads/smd073108.pdf

Centers for Medicare & Medicaid Services (CMS). (2015a). Readmissions reduction program. Retrieved from https://www.cms.gov/medicare/medicare-fee-for-service-payment/acuteinpatientpps/readmissions-reduction-program.html

Centers for Medicare & Medicaid Services (CMS). (2015b). Better care. Smarter spending. Healthier people: Paying providers for value, not volume. Retrieved from https://www.cms.gov/Newsroom/MediaReleaseDatabase/Fact-sheets/2015-Fact-sheets-items/2015-01-26-3.html

The Commonwealth Fund. (2014). Mirror, mirror on the wall, 2014 update: How the U.S. health care system compares internationally. Retrieved from http://www.commonwealthfund.org/publications/fund-reports/2014/jun/mirror-mirror

The Henry J. Kaiser Family Foundation. (2015). Kaiser health tracking poll: August 2015. Retrieved from http://kff.org/health-costs/poll-finding/kaiser-health-tracking-poll-august-2015/

Institute of Medicine (IOM). (1999). *To err is human: Building a safer health system.* Retrieved from https://iom.nationalacademies.org/~/media/Files/Report%20Files/1999/To-Err-is-Human/To%20Err%20is%20Human%201999%20%20report%20brief.pdf

Institute of Medicine (IOM). (2011). *The future of nursing: Leading change, advancing health.* Retrieved from http://www.nap.edu/read/12956/chapter/1

Jencks, S. F., Williams, M. V., & Coleman, E. A. (2009). Rehospitalizations among patients in the Medicare fee-for-service program. *New England Journal of Medicine, 360,* 1418–1428.

Kowk, A. C., Semel, M. E., Lipsitz, S. R., Bader, A. M., Barnato, A. E., Gawande, A. A., & Jha, A. K. (2011). The intensity and variation of surgical care at the end of life: A retrospective cohort study. *Lancet, 378*(9800), 1408–13.

National Hospice and Palliative Care Organization (NHPCO). (2015). NHPCO's facts and figures: Hospice care in America. Retrieved from http://www.nhpco.org/sites/default/files/public/Statistics_Research/2015_Facts_Figures.pdf

National Institute on Aging (NIA). (2011). Why population aging matters: A global perspective—Trend 3: Rising numbers of the oldest old. Retrieved from https://www.nia.nih.gov/publication/why-population-aging-matters-global-perspective/trend-3-rising-numbers-oldest-old

PBS. (n.d.). Facing death: Facts & figures. Retrieved from http://www.pbs.org/wgbh/pages/frontline/facing-death/facts-and-figures/

PBS. (2014). *The boomer list: Timeline of a generation.* Retrieved from http://www.pbs.org/wnet/americanmasters/the-boomer-list-timeline-of-a-generation/3153/

PBS NewsHour. (2012). *Health costs: How the U.S. compares with other countries.* Retrieved from http://www.pbs.org/newshour/rundown/health-costs-how-the-us-compares-with-other-countries/

Pew Research Center. (2010). Baby boomers retire. Retrieved from http://www.pewresearch.org/daily-number/baby-boomers-retire/

Seidman, B. (2015, September 22). Drug price increases 5,000 percent overnight. *CBS News.* Retrieved from http://www.cbsnews.com/news/generic-drug-price-increases-5000-percent-overnight/

Shinkman, R. (2014, April 20). Readmissions lead to $41.3B in additional hospital costs. *Fierce Health Finance.* Retrieved from http://www.fiercehealthfinance.com/story/readmissions-lead-413b-additional-hospital-costs/2014-04-20

Transitional Care Model. (n.d.). About TCM. Retrieved from http://www.transitionalcare.info/about-tcm

Warhola, C. (1980). *Planning for home health services: A resource handbook*, DHHS Publication No. (HRA) 80-14017. Part One. Washington, D.C.: U.S. Public Health Service, Department of Health and Human Resources.

2

What Is Home Healthcare and Home Care Comprised of Exactly?

This chapter provides an overview of what home care "looks like" in the home. As you read this section, it is easy to see that varying kinds of programs, services, and models can all be under the umbrella of these seemingly two simple words: "home care." Home care and home healthcare can mean many things. In the United States, the addition of the word *health* is often used in relation to Medicare and other insurance-covered care—meaning the medically focused care model.

Yes, many people need this model and its level of expertise and care. However, it is important to understand the scope of services that are being provided, and to keep in mind that many social and personal care models are very appropriate for some patient populations. These might be people who need personal care, assistance with activities of daily living (ADLs), meal preparation, and other important tasks that make the difference in remaining safely at home.

The care and models discussed in this chapter can range from someone coming into a home to assist with this needed personal care, such as helping patients take a bath or providing assistance with dressing, to very skilled levels of care with credentialed, licensed nurses where the patient's home looks like a room in an ICU, complete with a ventilator, oxygen, monitors, alarms, intravenous "drips," complex medication regimens, and more.

This wide and sometimes confusing variation can be difficult for consumers of home care, such as family members seeking care for a loved one, to understand and navigate. This is part of the reason that "home care" does not mean just one thing and may be viewed as having more than one voice. There are many voices and models. For purposes of this book, the broadest definition of home care (and most understandable for clarity) will be used: "Any kind of healthcare provided at home." This definition then includes the myriad and far-reaching types of services provided in a patient's home. It may also work for care models and innovations that we do not even have right now! Let's see what some of these home care services "look" like.

Medicare—The Basics Only!

This chapter starts by covering Medicare only because of the sheer volume of care provided and the dollars spent there. Some readers may know that after I had been a visiting nurse and a home care and hospice manager for some years, I also worked for four years at the Health Care Financing Administration (HCFA) central office, which became the Centers for Medicare & Medicaid Services (CMS).

Medicare is the largest health insurance program in the United States (and one of the largest in the world). As such, it is also the largest payer of home care and hospice services in the United States (Leonard, 2015). As with all medical insurance programs, Medicare has specific parameters for coverage and exclusions to care. If you are working or managing in the Medicare environment, you are strongly encouraged to read and understand the rules.

The CMS estimates there are over 55 million Medicare "beneficiaries," or those people who qualify for and have their medical insurance coverage through Medicare (CMS, 2014). Generally, this includes those over age 65, those who are disabled, people of all ages with end-stage renal disease, and the blind. Medicare pays for home healthcare (HHC) through what are called "Medicare-certified" home health agencies (HHAs). Because the government is the payer for these services, we have access to data and numbers that can be aggregated and reported. Keep in mind that this data reporting and data compilation reporting mechanism is lacking in some other kinds of home care. However, because Medicare is the largest payer, they have also set many of the standards and rules for other payers. This is important to note since this can add to the complexity, even when the agency is not Medicare certified.

According to Medicare Payment Advisory Commission (MedPAC), there were approximately 12,613 home health agencies in the United States in 2013 (the latest data) providing care to approximately 3.5 million patients (2015a). Of course, these are only the Medicare-certified organizations. As this chapter explains, there are numerous other models of what is all called "home care."

There are very specific requirements for the provision of Medicare home care services. This is because there are both statutory and other regulations that must be adhered to when admitting patients, throughout the care and through to discharge and related processes such as billing. Medicare is divided into various "parts." Medicare home care and hospice services and many other services are provided under Medicare "Part A" benefits. Other services under Part A include care provided at acute hospitals and skilled nursing facilities (SNFs).

 An in-depth discussion of what Medicare services may specifically be covered by Medicare Parts A, B, C, and D is outside the scope of this book. For more information, refer to https://www.medicare.gov/what-medicare-covers/.

The Medicare Conditions of Participation—What Are They?

It is important for readers to understand that Medicare Part A providers must work under/within the defined structure of the Medicare Conditions of Participation (CoPs) that are written specifically for the type of services provided; in this case, we will be focusing on home health agencies. The CMS states that the CoPs are developed as "health and safety standards" that are "the foundation for improving quality and protecting the health and safety of beneficiaries" (CMS, 2013, para. 1).

Organizations must meet these defined standards "in order to begin and continue participating in the Medicare and Medicaid programs"; CMS also "ensures that the standards of accrediting organizations recognized by the CMS (through a process called "deeming") meet or exceed the Medicare standards set forth in the CoPs" (CMS, 2013, para. 1). This means that the home care CoPs are very different from the SNF and the hospice CoPs, although there may be some commonality in the language used, as mentioned in Chapter 1 as "harmonization."

Harmonization is one way to standardize terminology across care providers and settings. For example, some harmonized terms are seen both in home care and also in other settings. This includes patients being asked about immunizations and vaccines, such as for influenza or pneumonia. The best part of this, from a provider and user perspective, is that as electronic health records (EHR) become more the norm, the patient's data will move with them as they move across care settings, such as the doctor's office or the emergency department at the hospital.

Part A providers, such as hospices, also have their own specific CoPs. Some of the home care CoPs include patient rights, plan of care, conformance with physician orders, and many more. Also, the Medicare home care CoPs are being revised, and these new CoPs are anticipated to be released in late 2016. Readers are referred to the Medicare and Medicaid Program: Conditions of Participation for Home Health Agencies; Proposed Rule (CMS 42 CFR Parts 409, 410, 418, et al.): http://www.gpo.gov/fdsys/pkg/FR-2014-10-09/pdf/2014-23895.pdf.

An HHA becomes "Medicare certified" through a standardized, rigorous process of an onsite visit to the HHA's office by a surveyor from the state department of health or, in some cases, by an accreditation body surveyor who reviews documents, interviews staff, visits patients, and works to ensure that patients would be cared for safely and that the organization meets the requisite intent of the CoPs. To receive this certification, the agency must be "deficiency free" (that is, meet all of the requirements, with no areas of deficient practice or documentation). These surveyors are usually experienced home care nurses or managers. Issues about home care regulatory fundamentals that must be understood and operationalized are further addressed in Chapter 6, "The Fundamentals: The Interface of Law, Regulation, and Quality."

How Medicare Defines Home Care

Many of the services provided under the scope of Medicare (and Medicaid) more fully support a true healthcare-specific definition of home care, which the U.S. Public Health defines as:

> *"that component of a continuum of comprehensive healthcare whereby health services are provided to individuals and families in their places of residence for the purpose of promoting, maintaining, or restoring health, or maximizing the level of independence, while minimizing the effects of disability and illness, including terminal illness. Services appropriate to the needs of the individual patient and family are planned, coordinated, and made available by providers organized for the delivery of home care."* (Warhola, 1980).

This government definition supports a holistic, broad-based vision of home care that the best home care organizations and team members strive to provide.

Specific disciplines and services may be covered if numerous other requirements, such as eligibility and qualifying criteria, are met. Of course, all clinical managers who practice or lead in any aspect of Medicare home care must become proficient team members in and have an operational understanding of Medicare home care and its benefit "package." A Medicare beneficiary must meet all of the numerous "qualifying criteria" to be covered under the Medicare home health benefit. These include:

- The patient is eligible for Medicare
- The services are provided by a Medicare-certified home health agency

- The patient is homebound as defined by Medicare
- The services are provided as defined in Chapter 7 of the *Medicare Benefit Policy Manual*
- The services meet the specific coverage rules related to the six services, which are nursing care, physical therapy (PT), occupational therapy (OT), speech/language pathology (SLP), medical social services (MSS), and home health aide services
- The care to be provided must also be "medically reasonable and necessary services," and the patient must have received physician certification and oversight of the HHA patient's plan of care

This certifying physician must attest to five things:

- That the patient needs intermittent SN care, PT, and/or SLP services.
- That the patient is confined to the home (for example, homebound as per Medicare's specific definition).
- That a plan of care has been established and will be periodically reviewed by a physician.
- That services will be furnished while the individual was or is under the care of a physician.
- That a "face-to-face" encounter occurred. The face-to-face encounter must have occurred no more than 90 days prior to the home health start of care (SOC) date or within 30 days of the start of the home care services; the face-to-face must be related to the primary reason that the patient requires home care services; it must have been performed by a physician or allowed non-physician practitioner; and the certifying physician must also document the date of the face-to-face encounter.

It is only when all these conditions are met that Medicare can pay for any part-time or intermittent skilled nursing, PT, OT, SLP, MSS, and/or home health aide visits. It is recommended that readers stay apprised of Medicare and Medicaid changes and other regulatory requirements. This is particularly true since some components of the face-to-face requirement continue to be a discussion point. For more information, see the *Medicare Benefit Policy Manual* "Chapter 7, Home Health Services" (https://www.cms.gov/Regulations-and-Guidance/Guidance/Manuals/downloads/bp102c07.pdf), which is reprinted in Appendix D, beginning on page 304.

What Kind of Organizations Provide Home Care?

As discussed in Chapter 1, healthcare generally and home care specifically is undergoing significant, never-before-seen changes and increases in complexity. Historically, HHAs were classified as "freestanding," hospital- or systems-based, or "voluntary." There are also designations and differences depending on whether the home care organization is a for-profit or a non-profit entity. Examples of non-profit and voluntary organizations are the visiting nurse associations (VNAs) or organizations. Then national chain or franchised organizations that are for-profit and freestanding. In addition, you have mergers and other relationships, such as a voluntary organization providing or being the home care organization for a system or hospital. Many of the differences have evolved with the industry, and the organizations providing home care have developed over time. The visiting nurse organizations enjoy a long history of nursing and care in their communities.

Though outside the purview of this book, this history is a very important topic to better understand how home care evolved to what it is today. Readers are referred to the classic work *No Place Like Home: A History of Nursing and Home Care in the United States,* authored by Karen Buhler-Wilkerson.

Generally, a number of different organizations provide home care or healthcare at home. In addition to the Medicare and/or Medicaid-certified HHA described previously that meets the framework of the Conditions of Participation, other models include the "hospital at home" model, faith-based models, and other programs providing care at home.

If you define home care in the broadest sense, you could include the medical equipment and supplies including the provision of pharmaceuticals and infusion services that may also be delivered to a patient's home. This model of care is where the products and medications are delivered for infusion services, and oversight from the physician, a pharmacist, and infusion nurses keeps the services functioning properly and safely in the home.

Similarly, insurance models of home care are used where the insurance company provides oversight, nurses, geriatricians, nurse practitioners, or others to provide care to a member of their insured group, called a *beneficiary*.

The following sections discuss in more detail organizations or models that provide some kind of home care. Please note: This list is not all-inclusive and varying states have some different care models as do payers and other organizations.

Hospice Programs

Hospice programs also provide care at home. Though they are clearly different programs with very different missions and CoPs, the majority of hospice care is provided at home. In fact, according to the National Hospice and Palliative Care Organization (NHPCO), in 2014 in 6,100 hospice agencies, 1,200,000 patients died while under the care of hospice; of those, 35.7% died at their home (2015). According to MedPAC, 97.6% of hospice care that was paid for by Medicare in 2013 was provided as routine home care (2015b).

Private Duty Agencies

There are also "private duty" agencies. The National Private Duty Association (NPDA) represents more than 1,200 member companies (Committee on Ways and Means, U.S. House of Representatives, 2011).

Also, many thousands of home care organizations may have a private duty business as well as a Medicare/Medicaid "skilled" side of the business that provides private duty services. These agencies may be a part of a chain, may be freestanding, and/or may be one agency in a specific community. These agencies usually do not get reimbursed by Medicare since the patients may pay privately or have another insurance that may pay for care. A private duty agency may provide aides and care oversight for aide- or companion-level care or provide 24-hour "skilled" care depending on the patient's needs, the organization, and the state rules and definitions for this level of care.

Area Agencies Specializing in Aging

Some area agencies on aging also provide home care services. This is an example of a usually non-profit, freestanding organization providing home care. They may also provide home health aide services, meals on wheels, or support congregate lunches or dinners, which can be a very important community-based service that sometimes makes the difference between if an older adult can remain at home or must move to another level of care.

Home Community-Based Programs

There are also what are called "home community-based services" programs. These are usually state-based and administered through Medicaid. The programs and their services may vary across the country. Medicaid, as a state-based payer, has eligibility criteria based primarily on financial indicators, such as income. In addition, states may have other criteria, such as being disabled or having "aged out" (such as a child reaching 18 or 21 and losing needed healthcare services) from other programs. These programs can include home visits for new mothers and infants, children, and people with developmental disabilities and disorders such as autism, and others.

The states have different programs and names for these programs, such as those directed toward healthy pregnancies and infants, the frail elderly, those who would otherwise be institutionalized, and others. These all depend on the state and the populations they serve. According to Medicaid.gov, "the 1915(c) waivers are one of many options available to states to allow the provision of long term care services in home and community based settings under the Medicaid Program" (n.d-a, para. 1). These "services may assist in diverting and/or transitioning individuals from intuitional settings into their homes and community" (Medicaid.gov, n.d-a, para. 1).

Programs can include a combination of standard medical services and non-medical services. "Standard services include but are not limited to: case management (i.e. supports and service coordination), homemaker, home health aide, personal care, adult day health services, habilitation (both day and residential), and respite care" (Medicaid.gov, n.d-a, para. 1).

Program of All-Inclusive Care for the Elderly (PACE)

The Program of All-Inclusive Care for the Elderly (PACE) is another program that can provide home care services. PACE "provides comprehensive medical and social services to certain frail, community-dwelling elderly individuals, most of whom are dually eligible for Medicare and Medicaid benefits. An interdisciplinary team of health professionals provides PACE participants with coordinated care. For most participants, the comprehensive service package enables them to remain in the community rather than receive care in a nursing home" (Medicaid.gov, n.d-c, para. 1). Like all payer programs, there are eligibility criteria for PACE participants.

Hospital-Based Home Care

Hospital-based home care, whether through a Medicare- and Medicaid-certified organization or through a mechanism such as a transitional care model where hospital team members follow the patient back home, is also an option.

It is well-documented that some of the riskiest times, especially for older adults, to be (re)hospitalized are periods known as "transitions." This is when patients move/transition from one care setting or site to another. Examples include being discharged from the hospital back to home or (even riskier!) from the hospital to a skilled nursing facility or other site not known to the patient. These transition points, where the patient may not know the staff and the staff does not know the patient well, and where the patient does not know the new space and physical layout so may become disoriented, can contribute to an untoward event, such as a fall and fracture.

To help support patients through this transition time, managed care organizations and some hospitals have nurses, physicians, social work-ers, specialized aides, or others who visit and follow the patient through transition points. Some of these programs may be age-specific or disease management-specific, such as a palliative care program, a congestive heart failure management program, or others, based on the organization and the patient's needs.

It is important to note that in some of these emerging models, the nurses and others may not be providing patient care or services *through* a hospital-based home care organization as we think of hospital-based home care per se. The nurse could be sent to the patient's home through the hospital case management or another follow-up program, such as a part of a heart failure protocol aimed at decreasing the risk of rehospitalizations. This is still "home care," but it is a different model with inpatient hospital team members providing the care in the home. Such information is also important for nurse or other team member to know when a home visit is made and a nurse from the hospital is also there—this is a part of "coordination of care," one of the Medicare CoPs, and knowing who else is visiting and providing some kind of healthcare, and what their roles and goals are for the patient, should be clearly documented.

This may also raise the concern of duplication of services, so clarity is needed about roles and care planning. The best care is provided when all team members are known and working toward common goals for the patient. Of course, always ask to see if other care team members are involved so you will know who will be providing what care, and with whom you need to communicate and coordinate care.

Case Manager Care

Case managers (CMs) are important to providing home care and oversight. CMs are credentialed nurses or social workers who "follow" patients for families. They may provide a detailed, comprehensive assessment, analyze the data and findings, and create a specialized care plan to support safety or continued care in the home. They are usually very knowledgeable about resources when needed since they practice in the local healthcare community.

More and more we are learning how important the socioeconomic status of patients is and how this can negatively impact their health, and CMs can help determine when help is needed based on these factors. Credentialed CMs follow the patients across care sites, coordinate care, and communicate with all involved. This is important given the complexity of care. They may also accompany the patient to healthcare provider visits, and more.

Readers can visit www.aginglifecare.org for a list of care managers by geographic area.

Physician Home Care Services

Physician home care services can also be used since some physicians and physician groups are now providing oversight and care and making home visits to people. This model may increase as it is very difficult and sometimes unsafe for very ill and/or technology-dependent patients to leave their homes. In addition, it may be difficult for the patient and takes considerable and taxing efforts. It is also difficult for the family and the nurse who might also have to accompany the patient with their customized wheelchair and bring back-up safety equipment (such as a tracheostomy tube, g-tube, etc.) in case their equipment has a problem, the ventilator becomes dislodged, a seizure occurs while en route, or myriad other reasons.

Also consider the challenges presented by patients living in very cold or snowy or hot areas of the country; this environment may compound safety issues. The humidity, temperature, and other health factors can also complicate travelling outside of the home.

Telecare or Telehealth

The innovations of telecare bring more care to patients needing oversight and monitoring; and home care associated with telehealth, interactive telecare, and monitoring technology is increasing. Of course, not all patients are in situations appropriate for this innovative technology, but it is one more tool in the toolkit to care for chronically ill patients and to help support population health initiatives. Home visits may also be a part of these services in conjunction with the technology or telehealth.

Gray Market Home Care

There has been some discussion about what is called the gray market in home care. A *gray market* has been defined as an unofficial market or trade in something, especially controlled or scarce goods (O'Brien, 2014). In home care, families sometimes hire people directly, in other words, not through a licensed, accredited, certified, or otherwise credentialed company. They may see an ad in the paper or place one for a caregiver. This presumes that the family understands the scope and care needs of their family member. In other words, the family or direct employer assumes all the related competency concerns of the caregiver—such as is this aide or nurse competent/proficient to care for my family member? In addition, there may or may not be background checks, health testing (such as for TB), and numerous other checks that help support quality home care. Because of the costs of home care, particularly when privately caring for older adults or needing skilled levels of care for a very sick child or adult, many families choose this option.

Community-Based Long-Term Living Services

One of the most interesting home care models that has an emphasis on bringing people back home from institutional settings is the Federal initiative called the "Money Follows the Person" (MFP) Rebalancing Demonstration. The MFP is an innovative program that provides assistance to people who live in institutions so they can return to their own communities and live independently.

This waiver is the largest single investment in Home and Community Based Long Term Living Services ever offered by CMS. The government is providing 450 million dollars per year to the states participating in this initiative (Medicaid.gov, n.d-b).

"Over 51,000 people with chronic conditions and disabilities have transitioned from institutions back into the community through MFP programs as of December 2014" (Medicaid.gov, n.d-b, para. 1).

The elderly, those with physical disabilities, those with mental or developmental disabilities, and those with mental illness may qualify for this program.

States participating in this program (Medicaid.gov, n.d-b) are:

1. AL	16. MA	31. OH
2. AR	17. MD	32. OK
3. CA	18. ME	33. PA
4. CO	19. MI	34. RI
5. CT	20. MN	35. SC
6. DE	21. MO	36. SD
7. GA	22. MS	37. TN
8. HI	23. MT	38. TX
9. IA	24. NC	39. VA
10. ID	25. ND	40. VT
11. IL	26. NE	41. WA
12. IN	27. NH	42. WI
13. KS	28. NJ	43. WV
14. KY	29. NV	44. District of
15. LA	30. NY	Columbia

This was a part of the Affordable Care Act (ACA), which strengthened and expanded this project. The ACA also expanded "the definition of who is eligible for the MFP Program to include people that live in an institution for more than 90 consecutive days" (Medicaid.gov, n.d-b, para. 10). For more information, visit https://www.medicaid.gov/medicaid-chip-program-information/by-topics/long-term-services-and-supports/balancing/money-follows-the-person.html.

The Veterans Health Administration's (VHA) Home Based Primary Care (HBPC) Program

The Veterans Health Administration's (VHA) Home Based Primary Care (HBPC) Program is a well-respected model that provides veterans with home care services. "Home-based primary care (HBPC) interventions have roots in the house call and community health outreach of the past. Today, HBPC is a model that combines home-based care for medical needs with intense management, care coordination, as well as long-term services and supports (LTSS) when needed. HBPC interventions have been proposed as an alternative way of organizing and delivering care that may better address the needs, values, and preferences of chronically ill, frail, and disabled patients who have difficulty accessing traditional office-based primary care or newer models of care that also require office visits" (Agency for Healthcare Research and Quality [AHRQ], 2014, para 2).

The HBPC program was:

> *"developed as a pilot model in the U.S. Department of Veterans Affairs (VA) more than three decades ago. While the details can vary across the many different VA medical centers, today's VA HBPC program includes an interdisciplinary team that provides care in the home to veterans with complex needs for whom clinic-based care is difficult due to function or disease. The VA model has expanded over time to include more mental health services and to facilitate collaboration with other services. In other environments, HBPC has developed based on elements of programs designed for people who are eligible for both Medicaid and Medicare (frequently referred to as dual-eligibles), home and community-based LTSS programs, and physician house call programs."* (AHRQ, 2014, para. 5)

Summary

It is clear that policy changes are being made to be more supportive of bringing care back into the community and into the home. As a mentor of mine at the CMS would say, there will be "intellectual violence" needed to get us where we need to go. I am heartened by these changes since they support that we are heading back the "right" way, to provide care where patients say they want to be—at home.

States also have rules and laws that impact home care. These include state licensure for home care or hospice, the nurse practice acts, and the state boards of nursing or other licensed disciplines professional practice acts, such as therapy or pharmacy. The state health authority employs state surveyors who make visits to review home care and hospice organizations, and others. For this reason it is imperative that home care and hospice organizations know about and be active participants in their home care organizations. There is a list of the home care and hospice/palliative care associations listed in Appendix A. The state-based home care initiatives and models can be complex, and knowing the "rules" will help protect you and your organization as well as help you advocate for patient and family care needs.

The complexity of home care and hospice at home demands accountability and a grounded knowledge of the framework and coverage aspects of care. What this means practically and operationally is that home care as we know it may be eclipsed or otherwise changed by new entrants and forces. We must bend, stretch, and diversify to succeed and thrive.

Now that the environment of coverage and varying care models have been introduced, the next chapter moves to the environment of care—the patient's home—and the implications for the provision of safe and effective care and practice in that most unique and variable care setting!

Questions for Further Consideration and Discussion

1. Identify three kinds of "home care" services.

2. Discuss what Medicare certification means for organizations and for patients receiving care.

3. List three kinds of programs that provide care in the home.

4. Support the statement that "home care nursing has a long and important place in healthcare in the United States." Research and report on that history.

5. What is healthcare policy and why should nurses in any practice setting be involved in its development?

For Further Reading

• The Future of Home Health Care: A Workshop: http://iom. nationalacademies.org/Activities/Aging/ FutureHomeHealthCare/2014-SEP-30.aspx

• Evidence-based Practice Center Systematic Review Protocol Project Title: Home-Based Primary Care Interventions Systematic Review: http://effectivehealthcare.ahrq.gov/ehc/ products/590/2003/home-based-care-protocol-141119.pdf

• *No Place Like Home: A History of Nursing and Home Care in the United States,* by Buhler-Wilkerson

• *Handbook of Home Health Standards: Quality, Documentation, and Reimbursement, 5th Edition,* by Tina M. Marrelli

• Home-Based Primary Care Interventions from the Agency for Healthcare Research and Quality's Effective Health Care Program: http://www.effectivehealthcare.ahrq.gov/search-for-guides-reviews-and-reports/?pageaction=displayproduct&productID=2183

References

Agency for Healthcare Research and Quality (AHRQ). (2014). Home-based primary care interventions systematic review. Retrieved from http://effectivehealthcare.ahrq.gov/index.cfm/search-for-guides-reviews-and-reports/?pageaction=displayproduct&productid=2003

Centers for Medicare & Medicaid Services (CMS). (2013). Conditions for Coverage (CfCs) and Conditions of Participations (CoPs). Retrieved from https://www.cms.gov/Regulations-and-Guidance/Legislation/CFCsAndCoPs/index.html?redirect=/cfcsandcops/16_asc.asp

Centers for Medicare & Medicaid Services (CMS). (2014). Data analysis brief: Medicare-Medicaid dual enrollment from 2006 through 2013. Retrieved from https://www.cms.gov/Medicare-Medicaid-Coordination/Medicare-and-Medicaid-Coordination/Medicare-Medicaid-Coordination-Office/Downloads/DualEnrollment20062013.pdf

Committee on Ways and Means U.S. House of Representatives. (2011). National Private Duty Association, Statement for the record. Retrieved from http://waysandmeans.house.gov/national-private-duty-association/

Leonard, K. (2015, July 30). America's health care elixir. *U.S. News & World Report.* (2015). Retrieved from http://www.usnews.com/news/the-report/articles/2015/07/30/medicare-changed-health-care-in-america-for-the-better

Medicaid.gov. (n.d-a). 1915(c) home & community-based waivers. Retrieved from https://www.medicaid.gov/medicaid-chip-program-information/by-topics/waivers/home-and-community-based-1915-c-waivers.html

Medicaid.gov. (n.d-b). Money Follows the Person (MFP). Retrieved from https://www.medicaid.gov/medicaid-chip-program-information/by-topics/long-term-services-and-supports/balancing/money-follows-the-person.html

Medicaid.gov. (n.d-c). Program of All-Inclusive Care for the Elderly (PACE). Retrieved from https://www.medicaid.gov/medicaid-chip-program-information/by-topics/long-term-services-and-supports/integrating-care/program-of-all-inclusive-care-for-the-elderly-pace/program-of-all-inclusive-care-for-the-elderly-pace.html

Medicare Payment Advisory Commission (MedPAC). (2015a). Home health care services. Retrieved from http://www.medpac.gov/documents/reports/chapter-9-home-health-care-services-(march-2015-report).pdf?sfvrsn=0

Medicare Payment Advisory Commission (MedPAC). (2015b). Hospice services. Retrieved from http://medpac.gov/documents/reports/chapter-12-hospice-services-(march-2015-report).pdf

National Hospice and Palliative Care Organization (NHPCO). (2015). NHPCO's facts and figures: Hospice care in America. Retrieved from http://www.nhpco.org/sites/default/files/public/Statistics_Research/2015_Facts_Figures.pdf

O'Brien, J. (2014). *Supplier relationship management: Unlocking the hidden value in your supply base.* Kogan Page: Philadelphia, PA.

Warhola, C. (1980). *Planning for home health services: A resource handbook,* DHHS Publication No. (HRA) 80-14017. U.S. Public Health Service, Department of Health and Human Resources: Washington, D.C.

3

What Makes Home Care the Most Unique Practice Setting?

The first two chapters addressed some of the structural and other changes that are making "home" the preferred, and desired, setting for care. This chapter explores the practice setting itself, the setting of home as the place where care is being provided. The home environment brings with it some unique dynamics that must be fundamentally understood for success. In fact, it is important to note that the environment itself may change throughout the day when a clinician makes visits or fills a shift—all while caring for different patients and families in their various homes. Let's explore some of the reasons that make home care the most unique practice setting.

Generally, and outside the realm of home care, when we are invited into and go into someone's home, we already "know" them. They are comfortable inviting us inside, thus providing entry into their personal, and some would say sacred, space. But in home care, we are invited in as "strangers" when we first meet a new patient and family. This is an honor, and those in home care embrace and value this dynamic. In home care, we must honor and respect this home place and space.

I believe that the best home care is the opposite of care provided in the hospital or other inpatient settings. Let's explore why. Inpatient settings seek to provide generally high intensity and safe care to large groups of people or patients. With this model comes some intrinsic challenges. Of course, there must be mechanisms to provide care while housing, feeding, and otherwise caring for a large population in a building developed for that goal. For sheer economy-of-scale reasons, this includes some basic structures and processes that are standardized, so that patients tend to be treated generally the same—even with all the new focus on patient-centered care. There must be organized processes to get the work of the organization accomplished while still meeting patient needs. Examples include mealtimes, which must be generally at the same times, and patients wearing the same matching hospital gowns, as well as many others. These measures are all intended to provide safe care to a diverse population in one space at the convenience of the staff.

Home care can be viewed as the antithesis of this structure. Home care is the most unique practice setting because the nurse or other team member must fit into and function effectively in the patient space, and their most beloved place often times, rather than the patient fitting into the hospital or other setting. Think of it this way: When entering an inpatient setting, such as a hospital, patients must conform to that structure; conversely, when entering a patient's home/space, it is the visiting clinician or other team member who must adapt and be flexible. This seemingly simple fact changes the dynamic in many ways. Being in and on the patient's turf makes it clear that we are guests in patient and family homes, and we must conduct ourselves differently as a result.

I believe and have seen that coming into the patient's home to provide care changes the typical patient–clinician construct and expectations in numerous ways. The following discussion addresses some of these ways and the implications for this unique and dynamic practice setting.

First, home care is truly where patients and clinicians are equal partners in care, care planning, and numerous components related to care, including goals, desired outcomes, and much, much more. For example, in healthcare we call to make an appointment at a physician's office, and the assumption is sometimes that we are not working full time and that we have to adjust our schedules or "fit into" the physician's office schedule. In home care, the exact opposite occurs. In fact, patients and families are called prior to scheduling the first visit or for any care; this courtesy and standard practice occurs whether for intermittent care visits, shifts, or other home care. In this way, home care behaviorally demonstrates respect for patient and family time. We truly are guests in another person's home!

With this understanding comes an incredible shift in power and responsibility.

 Home care clinicians visit patients at the best of times and sometimes the worst times in their lives. The range across the lifespan includes everything from newborn assessment "wellness" visits to compassionate, supportive care at end of life and includes emotions from very happy to very sad. Home care clinicians are honored to witness and support people in the setting they value most—their homes.

Let's step back and think about this and how truly individualized the setting can be. Patients wear what they want (there are no hospital gowns), and they have no restrictions on visiting hours, the age of visitors, or the number of visitors. Meal planning, food choices, and eating times are up to the patient. I could cite many more examples of how patients choose to set up their own homes and schedules as well. Family, friends, and/or other caregivers are valued as the unit of care and as such are included in education and health coaching. In fact, they are viewed as very important members of the home care team, when permitted by the patient.

The mindset change—that we are guests in a patient's home—can be difficult for some clinicians or those new to home care. This special dynamic helps ensure that patients have input into all aspects of care, care delivery, and related decisions. In their home, patients truly have all the rights; they wear what they want, go to bed when they want, wake up when they want, have "pets" (some are animals that most would not think of as pets!), and eat whatever and whenever they want. With no imposed restrictions, home care is truly patient-centered care and all about unique lifestyles and choices.

The following sections provide information about these differences from both the nurse/clinician perspective and from the patient/family perspective, supporting what makes home the most unique practice setting from each perspective. Each of these topics is explored in detail from both perspectives—first the clinician's and then the patient/family's:

- Physicians and orders
- Patient assessment and/or initial visit
- Care environment
- Care or case management environment
- Communications and care coordination

- Home care team
- Planning ahead and problem-solving

Physicians and Orders: The Clinician's Perspective

Just as in the hospital setting, home care is not usually provided without oversight for that care. Depending on the program and payer, there are usually verbal or signed physician orders. In home care, these orders may be called the plan of care (what used to be called the CMS Form 485, referring to the government form number), interim orders, verbal orders, or telephone orders. This is the form or data elements required by Medicare and Medicaid. Other programs and payers may also use this form and information. What forms are called depends on the organization, their policies, and related requirements. Patients are usually "certified" or "recertified" on a regularly recurring basis/timeline, and it is the physician who does this certifying. Because of this, the plan of care is sometimes called the certification form. It is important to note that Medicare and Medicaid are medical insurance programs, and, as such, they have medical necessity parameters that must be met for eligibility, coverage, and payment. This information is more fully addressed in Chapter 6, "The Fundamentals: The Interface of Law, Regulation, and Quality."

The best home care is a team effort, and the physician can be seen as the quarterback of the team. The physician signs the plan of care/certification and, therefore, certifies and clarifies such items as the patient's ordered medications, functional limitations, activities permitted, allergies, safety measures, the patient's nutritional requirements, durable or medical equipment, needed supplies, and more. The required plan of care also comprises such data elements as specific goals of care for the patient, the specific care to be provided, the services/disciplines to be providing that care, and the frequency and duration of those services. In addition, for Medicare, and in some states Medicaid, home care, physicians must

49

have a face-to-face encounter with their patients to ensure the need or continuing need for home care services. Readers are encouraged to stay apprised of changing requirements.

Physicians and Orders: The Patient/ Family Perspective

The case manager manages the complexity of many moving parts that occur with providing care to patients at home. There can be changes to medications, services, and any other of the elements of care. One example of a change of service is when the patient goes to the physician's office and the physician tells the family caregiver and patient that the patient is ready for therapy services. In this example, the family member calls the home care nurse to say this is what the doctor said at the office visit. The nurse would then confirm the information, obtain an order as it is a change to the physician-ordered plan of care, and make a referral to home care therapy for the initiation of services. Family and other "lay" caregivers are valued members of the care team and are instrumental in helping patients meet goals and in assisting nurses and other interprofessional clinicians and team members in care coordination and communications.

Patient Assessment and/or Initial Visit: The Clinician's Perspective

The first visit is a lengthy and comprehensive one. This is particularly true if the patient's insurance is Medicare or Medicaid. Because of the environment of care—the home—components of an effective comprehensive assessment are related to that unique and personalized environment. Those components include elements of the home space itself, including assessing factors related to home safety, and also a detailed history and physical assessment. A standardized data collection tool called the OASIS (Outcome and ASsessment Information Set) is used to gather data that is a part of a quality improvement process as the government seeks to improve care and related processes. This tool is undergoing change, and, like other Medicare or government reimbursed programs, will continue to be modified as needed.

It is important to note that the OASIS and its data collection is just a part of what is considered a "comprehensive" assessment. These visits range from 1.5 hours to 2 hours (or more) and can be provided only by a registered nurse or therapist because of the assessment and other components. These assessment visits may also require hands-on care. In other words, the patient is initially assessed to be sure they meet the organization's admission criteria per their policy, as well as the qualifying or other requirements for insurers such as Medicare, Medicaid, and others. Patients may also need physician-ordered care on that first visit, such as, for example, a wound assessment, teaching and training related to the wound and infection control, and related education and hands-on care of that wound, per the specific physician orders.

The case manager (or admitting clinician) at these visits is also the admission expert, the expert clinician providing skilled hands-on care, the explainer of insurance benefits, and much more. The best part of orientation, an important step to becoming a competent and effective home care nurse, is to accompany and listen to experienced home care nurses ask questions, listen quietly, reflect on gathered information, and generally begin the care planning process.

 Of course, safety and other concerns, such as dangerous pets or hoarding, may also be identified on the first visit or encounter. Notify your manager of these findings or concerns. For more information, Chapter 5, "The Environment of Care: The Home and Community Interface," addresses community and personal safety concerns and Chapter 7, "The Home Visit: The Important Unit of Care," illustrates an initial visit with a case study about Mr. Hinckley.

I have had nurses ask, "How did you get so much information from this one patient in that period of time?" The answer is we must truly observe and "hear" and not assume or rush the answers. Otherwise, we only get a piece of the picture, and the picture is always more complex than a list of data items to complete. I try to think of it as 1) content and 2) intent. The latter is harder to discern, but sometimes it makes all the difference in meeting the patient's prioritized care goals. We just have to be open to seeing and hearing it. These initial visits are quite lengthy and comprehensive and are addressed in more depth in Chapter 7, "The Home Visit: The Important Unit of Care."

Patient Assessment and/or Initial Visit: The Patient/Family Perspective

The first visit and/or admission visit with the completed documentation requirements is a lengthy process. Often, patients have been discharged from hospitals or rehabilitation centers, so these visits may be very tiring for patients and families. Because of patient fatigue or other reasons, sometimes not all of the data is collected and assessed on that first home visit, particularly when the patient has complex assessment findings with associated critical thinking or clinical reasoning and then related hands-on care needs.

Often, calls are made from the patient's home to confirm orders with the physician, such as which wound care products are to be used or a medication found in the home needing clarification for the medication regimen and reconciliation process. From customer service and patient-centered care perspectives, always tell the patient the projected length of time of the visit and, of course, the time of expected arrival for the visit. Patients and their families should also be notified when the nurse or other scheduled clinician is running late and the new projected time for arrival.

Care Environment: The Clinician's Perspective

Organizations providing care at home have specific policies related to admissions. It is recommended that readers review these policies prior to assessment visits. It is for this reason that "assessment visits" are called just that—not admission visits. Not all assessed patients become admitted patients. Patients who do not meet the organization's admission criteria or where there are safety or other concerns should be discussed with the supervisor. For those who are new to home care, this review of the agency's policies and procedures should be a fundamental part of a comprehensive orientation and onboarding information.

The patient's home and environment are key to effectively meeting the goals on the developed plan of care. For example, suppose the patient is on a complex medication regimen, some part of which requires that the medication be refrigerated. What does the nurse do when the patient does not have a refrigerator? Similarly, for patients requiring infusions when there's not a cool place for storage as required by the medication or fluid policy, what does the nurse do? When the patient does not have a phone and is on some complex technology, what is the procedure to follow? These and other questions must be discussed with your supervisor to have a holistic understanding of the policy and the intent of the organization related to safe care and acceptance of patients onto service.

The Care Environment: The Patient/ Family Perspective

Patients should not simply be told that they do not meet admission criteria. Otherwise, the hospital, physician, or other referring entity would not have thought of home care in the first place. These patients usually do have some problem necessitating some kind of intervention. Usually these patients still need some level of care, even if it's not appropriate for this particular organization. This is where a local knowledge of community resources and linkages is very important.

 Patients should be referred to other services if the referring organization cannot adequately care for them and meet their needs or admit them per the organization's admission criteria. Organizations should also keep track of these patients/families who are referred but not admitted for care, and why. This data can be reviewed, analyzed, and trended. This data may be a part of the agency's quality assurance and performance improvement (QAPI) process. It may help in identifying the need for new services or specialty clinicians, such as WOCNs (wound, ostomy, and continence nurses) or infusion-certified nurses.

Should a patient not meet admission policies for whatever reason, talk with your supervisor for direction. Usually someone at the organization communicates back to the referral source to relay the information found on the home visit, which includes the reason that the patient is not appropriate for the organization. Patients are often referred from an inpatient setting, and of course, the hospital may have no information on how the patient truly lives and what their daily health and lifestyle "looks like" on a daily basis in their unique home environment.

Care or Case Management Environment: The Clinician's Perspective

Patient care and patient care assignments in home care may be organized along specialty lines, geographic or catchment areas, and/or a combination of factors. For example, your organization might provide specialized infusion services and employ certified infusion nurses, or provide skilled wound care with nurses certified as wound, ostomy, and continence nurses (WOCNs). Whatever model your organization uses, there is usually a care or case manager, what may also be called a primary nurse, assigned to that patient and family. This provides the patient and family with one person who knows them, their history, and their unique needs.

One of the most important roles of the case manager is to be an advocate for your patient and your patient's needs. As population health truly becomes integrated into healthcare in the United States, I believe home care will be at the forefront of these changes. Readers are referred to the section entitled "Skillful Caring for Patients in Poor Socioeconomic Conditions" in Chapter 1.

In home care, the clinician sees the unique needs of these patients and, with ongoing assessment and analysis, tries to intervene where possible with whatever tools or interventions may best help a certain patient and family meet their goals. With experience, home care—nurses using well-honed critical thinking, assessment, communication, sometimes thinking "out of the box," and other skills gained over time working in home care—can have a huge impact on people's lives. This is especially true once a relationship is initiated, nurtured, and sustained.

As is true in all relationships, you have an opportunity at every home care interaction, visit, and phone call to either improve that relationship or not. Positive and constructive negotiations can occur. I have found that patients and families are usually open to new ideas when things have not "worked" or they are tired of feeling "sick and tired." The home care nurse can have a great and positive impact because of these communications and interactions and this earned trust.

Care or Case Management Environment: The Patient/Family Perspective

Having one nurse or case manager to contact when a question arises helps patients and families get their questions answered and needs met. In this way, they have one person to call and develop an ongoing therapeutic relationship with over time. When patients are asked what is important, they note this ability to have someone who knows them and have someone call them back promptly is important and are contributors to quality from a customer service and patient/family experience perspective.

Communications and Care Coordination: The Clinician's Perspective

Communications and care coordination go hand-in-hand and are key to helping patients achieve goals. Of course, these are very different in home care than in the inpatient setting, where everyone is in the same building and can more easily meet to talk about a patient or have face-to-face care coordination meetings. Though there may be face-to-face meetings in home care related to care coordination, often numerous and multiple phone calls to different team members are what keep everyone apprised of what is happening with a patient. Electronic medical or health records (EMR or EHR) and information systems have helped greatly in this quest to literally have everyone on the same page about what is happening with the patient and family.

Communications and Care Coordination: The Patient/Family Perspective

Phone calls from the nurse or other team members between visits can be effective ways to update them on what is happening with patients and families. Sometimes the family picks one "point" person for communications. This person or representative may be the primary caregiver or not. This is just one example of how the family can participate in care coordination and communications. These communications are key to safely maintaining patients at home and to keeping the nurse apprised of any changes, such as a re-hospitalization, a new or worsening symptom, or a new need emerging.

These communications may help prevent the need for a higher level of care, such as an emergency department visit. They also help empower patients to understand the nurse's information when they have a question. In this way patients have their questions answered and can continue on their health journey with the right information, and an understanding of that information. Encouraging patients and family members to call when they observe a change in a patient's status helps the team stay informed. Some examples might include an increased weight; a change in the patient's clinical condition, such as a fever; or other information.

Home Care Team: The Clinician's Perspective

Home care historically has used an interdisciplinary or interprofessional team approach. Here is an explanation of the differences between these terms:

> *"Interdisciplinary means that two or more disciplines work or learn together to solve a problem or gather information. Interprofessional describes the relationship*

between various disciplines as they purposely interact to
work and learn together to achieve a common goal." (St.
Joseph's Care Group, n.d., para. 1)

Although the term *interprofessional* is relatively new, the team approach
has been the essence of home care and hospice since its inception. All
work in home care and home care operations gets done through the
team. This includes the important clerical and administrative team
members, leaders in the organization, and peer nurses or clinicians;
the work all gets done through the team. This is even more important
in home care since one cannot always "see" the patient or "run down
the hall" when there is a question. In the hospital setting, someone is
coming in for the next shift to relieve the earlier shift; in home care,
the entire team may be on that next shift. In other words, there are not
those institutional supports to rely on, or they cannot be relied upon
in the same way. This is particularly true for "intermittent" patients
or patients receiving "visits." In private duty or 24-hour care at home,
there may in fact be another shift coming in.

The home care team may include the physician; the nurse; therapists,
including physical and occupational therapists; and speech language
pathologists. There may also be a home health aide; a dietitian or
nutritionist; and, of course, the physician who is involved in the patient
care. In the case of more complex patients, a number of physicians who
are authorized to write orders for patients to safely meet their unique
specialty care needs.

The patient's home care team revolves around the patient and
information, continually communicated to or handed over to other
team members, particularly when different services are involved, such as
in a more complex patient's care. For this reason, many organizations
leave a calendar for the patient to know which service is coming in, the
team member's name, on what day/date, and projected time for arrival.

With this calendar, patient visits are coordinated and not scheduled all on the same day or afternoon. It's truly patient-centered care, and the visits are staggered and planned appropriately by the team to meet patient needs. This also may help with better decision-making since decisions are then based on the most relevant and up-to-date information. The best home care is based on extensive and up-to-date fact finding. Then the detailed information is collected, processed, analyzed, acted upon, documented, and shared among team members.

Home Care Team: The Patient/Family Perspective

A simple calendar in the home helps with planning and scheduling for patients and families. In this way, patients can try not to get overtired or exhausted with many services on one day. In addition, families need to plan their days. Calling when one is running late is a must! Having someone come into the home, particularly on a regular basis, is like having someone invade your personal space. Think about just wanting to sleep in some mornings or enjoying a quiet cup of coffee alone, but being unable to do that since the nurse comes at 7:00 a.m. to care for an adult with complex care needs. Or think of wanting to have some private time with your spouse, but having a child with 24-hour-care needs necessitating shifts of nurses coming in at all hours.

Privacy is very important and, therefore, sticking to a schedule and respecting the home, the things in the home, the space, and family time is paramount to quality of life for families. Having the experience of first finding caregivers and then having people who start out literally as "strangers" coming in to your personal space can be a jarring and exhausting experience. Families may also be unnerved by the nurse needing to provide intimate and personal care on that very first encounter or visit.

From personal experience, whenever possible, consider what it would feel like for you to have people in your home while also trying to work, raise children, maintain a household, and do all of your day-to-day activities. Be empathetic and act accordingly.

Planning Ahead and Problem-Solving: The Clinician's Perspective

Home as the patient care environment is as variable as the people and populations served in the organization's geographic or catchment area. In some places, this can be a few ZIP codes, which can include a few large counties. In rural areas, it may be many miles of counties and sometimes stretch across state lines. It all depends on licensure, state laws, and other requirements. Keep this in mind, because your environment is not like the hospital where you can run down the hall if a forgotten supply is needed or a urinary catheter is dropped. In the home, you generally have no back up onsite. The nurse or other clinician must function independently and autonomously; this can be a very good thing for some or very uncomfortable for others who are used to more structure. This is not to say it is good or bad. It just depends on the person and their experience.

In home care, one of the best ways to avoid problems is called the Noah's Ark philosophy: Always take two of any needed supply for visits. Similarly, this is also a good model for the nursing bag and its supply contents. (For a listing of general supplies needed for a nurse visit bag, see "Sample Visit Bag Contents" on page 173 in Chapter 7, "The Home Visit: The Important Unit of Care.") Being prepared also may necessitate communications with the hospital prior to patient discharge to ensure that the supplies needed for the visit are at the home or are sent home with the patient from the hospital, for example, specifically ordered wound care supplies, an extra tracheostomy tube, or whatever that patient must have in the home for quality and safety.

From personal experience, especially in some areas of the country, you would be hard-pressed to find an extra indwelling urinary catheter of a particular size or type. I've been in that position and had to drive to a hospital about an hour and a half away. One of the lessons learned here is from a practical perspective—always bring more than you think you might need, because if you don't have it with you, you will need it!

Planning Ahead and Problem-Solving: The Patient/Family Perspective

It can be frightening to a family and the patient when they have been waiting for the nurse visit since being discharged from the hospital and they realize the nurse did not bring what is needed for their care. The patient and family are usually already somewhat anxious after being discharged. They are only referred to home care because they have some specific medical problem necessitating the specialized skills of a home care organization and nurse. Many times they are very excited you are coming there and that you—the nurse—can answer the myriad questions that have arisen since pulling back into the driveway.

Always communicate with the patient/family before the visit to help ensure that what is needed will be brought and that you will be able to answer any questions that they are very concerned about asking. Things may have changed since discharge, and as a nurse, it is better to know earlier than later about these changes. Changes might include a new wound or a new symptom or finding that becomes a priority and makes your "planned" visit placed on the back burner or otherwise reprioritized appropriately. Communication is the key to avoiding preventable problems and to assist in effective problem solving when necessary.

Summary

This chapter provides an overview with some examples of why home care is so different from any other practice setting in healthcare. The specialty of home care demands additional skills. Not only is the nurse who conducts the assessment visit the admissions expert, she also acts as the expert clinician, listener for data collection and interpreter of its nuanced implication for the care plan, and patient and family "go-to" person for care once they are back in the community.

The nurse is also the care or case manager, the scheduler who considers numerous factors for the next visits(s), the clarifier for confusing or non-congruent orders with the physician(s), the coordinator of care with the team, and more. One of the most important roles the nurse plays in the home care environment is explaining the glossary of healthcare to people in understandable terms. The healthcare model has become so "medicalized" that common sense and terms are hard to find or understand. Home care nurses have a huge role to play in "flattening" the language of healthcare and making it truly understandable and accessible for all. They do that daily in patient living rooms or bedrooms!

The tables are truly turned in home care because of the power shift, and we must sometimes negotiate and care for patients with varying lifestyles, beliefs, houses and environments, relationships, values, and myriad other variables. From visiting the most economically disadvantaged to caring for those who are very well-to-do, home care is a diverse and exciting practice setting. Home care is a reflection of the community, and, as such, home care clinicians are often experts about their communities and geographic areas. In this way, they can know of, and offer to help with, community linkages and resources that may help patients and families find better health and care in their homes.

This overview leads to further discussion in the next chapter about the important skills and competencies needed should you wish to practice in the primary healthcare setting of the future—the patient's home.

Questions for Further Consideration and Discussion

1. List the main reasons why care provided in one's home is so different from that provided in an inpatient building.

2. Who are the members of the home care "team" and what are their roles?

3. Discuss the difference between the terms *interdisciplinary* and *interprofessional*.

4. Identify five factors that make the care environment of the home key to helping patients meet goals.

5. Brainstorm and list three reasons why electronic medical, health records, and information systems can assist in communications and care coordination in home care. Specifically, how are they helpful to nurses and other clinicians? How are they helpful to patients and families?

For Further Reading

- *From Novice to Expert: Excellence and Power in Clinical Nursing Practice,* by Patricia Benner

- Framework for Action on Interprofessional Education & Collaborative Practice from the World Health Organization: http://apps.who.int/iris/bitstream/10665/70185/1/WHO_HRH_HPN_10.3_eng.pdf

- Core Competencies for Interprofessional Collaborative Practice (Report of an Expert Panel): http://www.aacn.nche.edu/education-resources/ipecreport.pdf

- *Handbook of Home Health Standards: Quality, Documentation, and Reimbursement,* by Tina M. Marrelli at http://marrelli.com/, Mosby, 2012, 5th Edition

References

St. Joseph's Care Group. (n.d.). FAQ for education. Retrieved from http://www.sjcg.net/departments/education/faq.aspx#ipid

4

Becoming a Home Care Clinician or Manager: Information Needed for Success

Home care, like any specialized area of knowledge and practice, demands a person have a set of defined skills and competencies in order to be effective. Of course, if one is seeking or moving to a defined management position, one must also have an understanding of the foundations of home care and home care operations and regulations. This chapter will address these unique roles and the important, grounded knowledge needed to succeed.

If one is new to home care or considering moving from the inpatient practice setting to home care, this chapter will also provide a broad-based view of home care and the orientation needed. This information may help determine if home care may be a "good fit." Not all nurses and managers can be successful in home care because it is a truly multifaceted role, one in which every day can be so different. Let's face it—some people do not want to drive to different places every day, such as when providing intermittent "visits," when they can instead drive, stay, and practice in one place, such as a hospital, inpatient hospice, or nursing facility.

The practice itself can be lonely for some and incredibly fulfilling for others—it all depends on the person and the skills developed and brought to the role. This chapter addresses some of the most important of these skills and the knowledge areas needed for success in home care. Of course, managers need the preliminary and fundamental information presented as well! It is important to note at the onset that, by definition, nurses in home care are/become managers. They manage a group of patients, care plans, and sometimes other team members, such as home care or hospice aides. They also perform "supervisory" visits that are a part of regulatory and oversight responsibilities. In any home care role, a broad base of clinical, administrative, and business-operation skills and knowledge is needed for success.

HOME CARE NURSING
HOME CARE IS A GROWTH AREA

It is estimated that many nurses and other clinicians will be moving into home care as the shift to home care and community-based healthcare models continue. The American Nurses Association (ANA) estimates that about 140,000 nurses work in home health nursing, and this practice setting is projected to outpace the growth in other settings in the coming decades (ANA, 2014). By now, no doubt you have an understanding that "home care" is not solely healthcare being provided in another venue—the home—but it is an entire constellation of factors and nuance that supports the larger picture of what home care is and how it encompasses its own specialty area. As home care and other community-based care models become more formally entrenched in health and the healthcare system, more nurses, other clinicians, managers, and administrative team members will be moving into this realm.

Throughout this book, the term *home care* is used to describe the varying types and models of care provided in the home. *Home healthcare* is used to describe the traditional medical model of care in the home and generally refers to insurance-reimbursed—such as Medicare or Medicaid—home care, in the United States. For purposes of clarity, *home care* is the umbrella term that will be used to encompass all kinds of home care and health-related care provided at home.

The ANA has published specific standards and competencies for home health nursing and home health nurses (HHNs), which are meant to "define, direct and guide the practice of home health nurses" (ANA, 2014, p. 3). They define home health nursing as "a specialty area of nursing practice that promotes optimal health and well-being for patients, their families, and caregiver within their homes and communities. Home health nurses use a holistic approach aimed at empowering patients, families, and caregivers to achieve their highest levels of functional, spiritual, and psychosocial health. Home health nurses provide nursing services to patients of all ages and cultures and at all stages of health and illness, including at end of life" (ANA, 2014, p. 7).

In *Home Health Nursing: Scope and Standards of Practice*, the ANA notes six standards of practice and ten standards of professional performance. You are encouraged to review these standards for a holistic view and better understanding of home health nursing and nursing practice. For clarity, the term *home care* will be used throughout the book to encompass all kinds of home care practice, operations, and care models provided in patient homes.

Before Making the Leap to Home Care: A Checklist of Considerations

To assist with the initial exploration and decision-making processes and help determine if home care is a viable option for those considering a change, this section contains a checklist of considerations for self-assessment.

These questions are directed toward nurses, therapists, other clinicians, and managers who are considering making the change to home care. They are phrased as yes or no questions, and there are no right or wrong answers! These questions are framed to encourage thoughtful consideration about the care setting: the patient's home. Other important and practical environmental or community-based factors are also included. Of course, there are always more questions to be asked; these are just enough to get started on the journey.

❏ *Are you an excellent and experienced clinician with strong and detailed physical and other assessment skills?*

In home care or hospice at home, you are one clinician in the home—alone. As a result, you alone must be able to identify a change in condition, such as a new symptom or something else that must be further assessed and communicated to the physician and team. This is very different from the inpatient setting, where you can run down the hall and find another nurse to have a "consult" or have the other clinician look at the patient for another opinion. Of course, in the case of home care, you have a supervisor or manager to call, but this is different mindset. It can be a big change when you're not used to this. This is why a background of medical/surgical care or other areas of practice are required prior to working in home care at many organizations.

❏ *Are you proficient with computers and information systems?*

Home care clinicians are dependent on the notes of other clinicians
involved in the patient's care to aid in subsequent and important care
decisions. Documentation is an important responsibility. Home care
clinicians are encouraged to complete their documentation while at the
patient's home, when it's safe to do so. Effective clinical information
systems help support this goal. Documentation plays a critical role in
reimbursement and in that way, nurses in home care are in a unique
position. Their documentation of the patient's status and other findings
communicated through this documentation can either help support
or not support Medicare, Medicaid, or other coverage for payment as
discussed in other parts of this text. Effective documentation has ties
to numerous regulatory compliance components, and clinicians must
understand this basic responsibility and adhere to these standards.

❏ *Are you comfortable driving, even at night or in sometimes stormy, very cold, or otherwise inclement weather?*

Like the proverbial postman who delivers mail no matter what the
weather is like, home care nurses and other clinicians make visits 365
days a year, sometimes at night, such as for on-call or other reasons.
This is not the usual 7:00 a.m.–3:00 p.m. or 9:00 a.m.–5:00 p.m.
work schedule seen in other healthcare settings. The schedule revolves
around the patient's schedule and care needs. This may mean providing
infusions at certain times per the physician's orders or twice a day
dressing changes for a wound. In fact, patients often need home care
more on snowy or other poor weather days because Meals on Wheels or
other volunteer support systems may not be available. Because of this,
emergency preparedness and its management also play an important
role in home care practice.

❐ *Are you an effective, positive, and collaborative team member?*

The important work of home care gets accomplished through the inter-professional or interdisciplinary team. Though varying team members, such as therapists and others, have unique practice acts, there may be some overlap and interface for the best care for the patient. This will depend on the patient and state practice acts and other factors; examples may include medication management, wound care, and other sometimes overlapping practice areas. Whoever does what, it is very important to value all team members' contributions to the patient care that supports desired patient outcomes.

❐ *Will you be comfortable working alone or by yourself most days?*

This particular question is sometimes a "rule out" question for who will be successful in (and who might not be suited for) home care. When it all works, home care nurses become proficient over time in knowing where the coffee shops with the best wifi are located, who will let them use the phone when there is no cell phone service, what local fast food manager provides the best directions, and more. They become experts on which apps help them find an address, where to get a cost-effective, good lunch, and numerous other important community resources.

❐ *Do you have effective time management and organizational skills?*

In home care, some days a nurse may visit and care for anywhere from one (usually a single shift) to seven (or more) patients for visits, depending on the geographical location, the caseload, emergent needs, and numerous other factors. Of course, a visit is never just that; it's also travel time, assessments, hands-on ordered care, critical thinking, required documentation, follow-up, unexpected phone calls to physicians for clarification of new or changed orders, a call to the office related to concerns identified in the home, care-coordination calls, and more. Setting up the schedule for patients, confirming the schedule for these patients, obtaining and bringing needed supplies, and many other details are all important components and examples that support the need for effective time management and organizational skills.

❏ *Do you believe that all team members in the interdisciplinary or interprofessional group make equally important contributions to patients and outcomes?*

This belief is key to collegial, respectful communications and care coordination for patient safety and to achieve desired patient outcomes. In fact, no member of the team is any more important than another member—*we all need each other to meet patient goals.*

❏ *Can you generally talk to anyone about almost anything?*

When patients are referred to home care or hospice at home, they are generally very ill or may be at the end of life. With this in mind, patients and their families may be stressed, tired, and otherwise preoccupied. They have been discharged from the hospital or may have been ill for some time and now (sometimes finally) visiting nurses are becoming involved. Most families and patients look forward to the nurse visit, particularly as the patient might no longer be able to get out of the home. The nurse's interpersonal and social skills and an ability to talk about anything like sports, weather, and other appropriate topics sometimes takes patients' and family members' minds off the illness and serves as a welcome relief. Usually patients and their families look forward to the nurse or other clinician's visits. This interface and communication also helps to initiate and maintain the therapeutic relationship.

❏ *Do you understand what professional boundaries are and how important they are in home and community-based care settings for privacy and other concerns?*

Because home care nurses are in the special and personal space where the patient and families live, they may know very personal aspects of a person's life. Your opportunities for crossing boundaries are more plentiful in home care and your risk for crossing them is higher because of this fact. Boundaries should be clear and clarified if the patient or family unknowingly or knowingly cross these boundaries. The employing home care organization should have policies about boundaries that clarify this important area in home care. Contact your manager if there are boundaries crossed, such as the patient or family member calling your home or sending/giving you gifts. This topic of boundaries should be a part of your organization's orientation/onboarding process.

❏ *Do you have an awareness of your personal safety and general environment?*

Home care nurses and hospice nurses caring for patients at home may visit patients in various communities where patients live. This visit may take place in what are considered very nice neighborhoods and also in areas that are sometimes socioeconomically disadvantaged and/or are known to be not as safe. Whenever you are in the community, such as driving to a home or visiting in a home, and when you are in the office area, always be aware of your surroundings.

❏ *Do you have a passion for lifelong learning?*

Home care is continually changing. Practice changes, policies may change, and new technology to help the office operations or to assist in or improve patient care may be introduced. Because of this, you will always have new things to learn and incorporate into the repertoire of home care. Such ongoing learning is also a key component of quality assurance and performance improvement.

❏ *Would peers describe you as flexible?*

Flexibility is an important attribute in home care (and life). Just as soon as you think that your schedule is "set" for a given day, one patient might have to go to the emergency department, or you might get a call notifying you that a certain road is closed or that a patient's family member has a doctor's appointment and your visit schedule must change accordingly. Make it okay to know that the projected schedule is just that, only a projection that may change at any time. Knowing this may help better frame your outlook and days.

❏ *What is your likability factor?*

The best home care is truly a team effort, and the work revolves around patients and families and their unique needs. So, it is understandable that people who like people generally excel in this multifaceted specialty. Everything gets done through people, and home care is truly a customer service business and practice. This ranges from calling a pharmacist to clarify a question about a patient prescription to speaking with staff at the doctors' offices to calling the medical equipment company about a missing supply and numerous other interfaces. Home care truly involves relationship building over time and across many different professions.

❏ *Do you value and understand the importance of documentation in home care?*

Documentation in home care must be valued because it is where the care provided, quality, and payment perspectives all intersect. The documentation must be detailed and must clearly paint the picture of the patient. This documentation includes the care planning that is developed based on the assessment and findings and other information that helps paint a picture of the patient, the care plan, the movement toward goals (or not and why), the adherence to the plan of care, and numerous other factors. For example, in home care and hospice, payment is predicated on documentation that supports medical necessity and other coverage requirements and meets documentation requirements as specified by insurer, law, and regulation.

❏ *Are you interested in or seeking certification in a specialty area?*

The specialty of home care also employs clinical and other specialists supporting the generalist home care nurse. In home care, there may also be wound ostomy continence nurses (WOCNs), infusion-certified nurses (such as through the Infusion Nurses Society), cardiovascular specialists, educational clinical specialists, certified diabetes educators, hospice and palliative care nurses, pediatric specialists, quality-improvement credentialed nurses, and more. Other specialties include psychiatric nurses, oncology-certified nurses, maternal child specialists, infection control specialists, and informatics systems specialists. You also find specialty credentials for administrators and managers in home care and hospice. Bringing such skills to the organization helps raise the level of quality provided to patients at bedside and is important to the education of other team members.

You may be wondering why home healthcare nursing certification was not mentioned in this list. Sadly, the final certification exam was held in 2005. At this time, there is no specialty certification for home care nurses. There are some nurses who maintained their certification. As so eloquently phrased by Rea in 2003, "Certification has been linked to increased confidence, increased clinical knowledge, and increased job satisfaction. Increasingly, agencies and accreditation bodies are encouraging and rewarding staff for certification as evidence of continued professional development ... Although original licensure represents a basic knowledge level, certification represents current practice standards and expertise. This is especially true in home health nursing with its unique set of practice requirements" (Rea, 2003, p. 761).

As readers continue to review the material in this chapter and through the end of this text, it is easy to clearly understand and envision why there is a need for this specialty certification. The practice of home health nursing is multifaceted and complex. In fact, a group of home care nursing leaders is spearheading this important effort. If you have a passion or interest in this topic, please email me at news@marrelli.com.

❐ *Do you like to teach and consider yourself a proficient teacher?*

One of the most important roles in home care is teaching and coaching patients and family members about their disease process, which usually includes more than one disease process, particularly in older adult patients with chronic disease. This could include diabetes, heart failure, and a need for wound care all in the same patient. In this example, the nurse would teach about the processes of these diseases and complications; the medications and their management; the wound care, which would include the actual hands-on care of the wound and surrounding skin, infection control measures (including disposal of used dressings and observation and assessment for signs of infection); and more. It all depends on the patient and the assessment findings. In this example, a knowledge of teach-back, assessing baseline knowledge, and other educational skills to transfer knowledge that impacts and changes behavior and aids in reaching goals would need to be used and specifically documented.

The other side of being a good teacher is having an openness to learn about the patient and his illness from the patient and family, who often know more about the specifics of the patient's status and condition than the healthcare professionals do. Family members possess different and valuable information than the healthcare professionals. Teaching and learning are truly a two-way street.

❏ *Are you a role model for health and healthy behaviors?*

Patients and families will look to the home care team for modeling of health and other behaviors. A well-groomed, neat, professional appearance and an organized presentation of any paperwork or other information to be discussed with patients and families are examples. Patients and caregivers must also keep the record organized for doctor visits and other care continuity. They will look to your system if it looks like it works! In addition, patients and families will watch your hand hygiene, exactly how you wash your hands, and any ordered care activities, such as changing gloves, etc. In this way, the nurses and others coming into the home are role models.

❏ *Are you seen/described as being approachable by aides and others?*

Aides, caregivers, and other home care workers are sometimes hired by the family or sometimes through an insurance program or benefit, such as the Veterans Administration's Aid & Attendance program. Aides and other caregivers truly are the "eyes and ears" and can notice and report important changes or findings to the nurse or therapist. In addition, these private or other caregivers sometimes have been with the patient/family for a long time before Medicare or another program for "skilled" care was needed or initiated—they know their patients well and, as such, must be valued as key team members, which they are!

❏ *Are you interested in performance improvement that is integrated into daily care practice and operations?*

Quality assurance and performance improvement (QAPI) is an important part of home care. You will have new things to learn and processes to emulate as you grow in knowledge about home care. For example, how are infections identified, reported, tracked, analyzed, and trended?

Who is the point person for infection control and prevention-related processes? There is always more to learn, which frequently translates into improved quality when data is collected and reviewed and then helps to create better processes and systems.

You will formulate other questions as you learn more about the practice and setting of home care. Once you make a decision to join a home care organization and become a member of the home care team, a comprehensive orientation needs to be a part of the onboarding process. Always ask about the organization's orientation or onboarding process and program. This includes how long it is, if there is a formalized mentoring or "buddy" system, how many visits you will make with the preceptor or "buddy," "shadowing" opportunities, and more.

Other questions you should ask include the orientation related to the organization-specific policies and procedures; whether the organization is accredited and, if so, what are the implications for a new nurse or manager; and more. The accreditation bodies have standards related to onboarding and orientation. The following list includes some of the information that must be absorbed for success. Of course, it depends on the agency and the "kind" of home care provided, such as intermittent visits or shifts or other models of care, as described in Chapter 2, "Home Care: What Is Home Healthcare and Home Care Comprised of Exactly?"

Twenty Skills and Knowledge Areas Needed in Home Care

Welcome to home care! As explained in Chapter 1, "Healthcare: Overview of Change and Complexity," changes in the healthcare environment make home care a challenging practice and management field for both experienced and novice healthcare professionals. The clinician and patient/family interactions, the range and diversity of clinical and other skills employed, and the satisfaction that accompanies caring for patients in situations in which they are truly equal partners in care and outcome achievement are appealing to many. The following information outlines some of the characteristics common to team members who are successful in home care.

Knowledge of the Basic "Rules" of Home Care

Consisting of both administrative and clinical information, these "rules" are important to effective operations. For clinicians employed by Medicare-certified home health agencies, in addition to knowledge of the state nurse or therapy practice acts applicable to your organization, knowledge of the following is required:

- The Medicare Conditions of Participation (CoPs)

- The Medicare Program Integrity Manual provisions related to home care coverage and documentation requirements

- The Medicare Manual section that addresses the correct completion of the Centers for Medicare & Medicaid Services (CMS) plan of care (POC)

- The CMS OASIS-C/ICD-10 Guidance Manual that addresses the OASIS-C data set requirements

- State-specific rules and regulations, such as licensure requirements. Because Medicare and Medicaid and many states set numerous standards and licensure requirements for home care, being familiar and up-to-date with these rules is important.

Other insurers may use Medicare's criteria for qualifying for coverage, the coverage itself, and the payment mechanism(s). In addition, many insurers, such as state Medicaid programs and private insurers, use the CMS POC (what used to be called the HCFA/CMS 485 Form) data elements for the required physician POC or plan of treatment (POT).

Whatever name it is called at the organization, there must also be physician orders for reimbursable and quality care.

Repertoire of Service-Driven and Patient/Family-Oriented Interpersonal Skills

Effective interpersonal skills, including community liaison and public relations activities, are an integral part of being a home care clinician. These interpersonal skills represent your organization in the community!

Ability to Pay Incredible Attention to Detail and Enjoy It

This is true both in addressing complex patient needs and in documenting the care and services provided. Both are equally important and go hand-in-hand. For example, the initial comprehensive assessment, including the OASIS data elements, must be completed within mandated time frames. The comprehensive assessment must be accurate and reflect the patient's true state of health and function, because home health agency reimbursement and care planning are based on this assessment and the continued documentation of care.

Possession of Multifaceted Skills Accompanied by Flexibility

The home care clinician is the one who must "bend" or renegotiate to meet patient needs and achieve patient-centered goals. This flexibility usually includes managing visiting times, scheduling of supervisory visits, and other aspects that center on accommodating patient and caregiver needs and schedules.

Possession of a Reliable Car and Safe, Effective Driving Skills

The home care clinician must like—or at least not mind—driving, have a good sense of direction (and a navigation system or good map), be willing to drive in heavy traffic and/or inclement weather, and possess a spirit of adventure!

Ability to Undertake Full Responsibility for the Patient and the Patient's POC

True case management is possible in home care and essential to the optimal achievement of outcomes. From the initial comprehensive assessment visit through the identification of needs and desired outcomes, the home care clinician assists the patient and coordinates with other team members regarding the planning and follow-through for patient care.

Because of these factors, the nurse or other team member in the community setting can directly affect the care and impact the results of that care. Communications may be required between the home care organization and the payer/insurer's case manager. This holistic and "big picture" patient management function, with its associated priority-setting, critical-thinking, and complex decision-making skills and its related resource-utilization decisions, makes home care unique. This aspect also allows team members to receive personal satisfaction and positive feedback from patients and their families, friends, and caregivers.

Up-to-Date and Proficient Clinical Practice Skills, Including the Ability to Function as a Generalist and a Specialist

Home care is provided to patients from all age groups—from infancy to the "oldest old" adults. In addition, the diagnoses and care needs of patients can vary from day to day, visit to visit, or shift to shift—all depending on the patient. In home care, although the clinician may have to address a wide range of clinical problems, interventions, and desired outcomes, having an area of expertise is helpful for both the individual clinician and the organization. These special skills (e.g., certification or advanced practice credentials) are also useful when teaching, acting as a resource, case managing, or orienting clinicians new to home care. For patients with special needs, such as high-risk obstetric care, medically complex child care, and some infusion or wound therapy, staff must sometimes have specialized training and experience to support safety, competent practice, and other standards.

Self-Direction

This includes the ability to function autonomously, establish priorities, and manage diverse tasks and responsibilities while adhering to organizational policies, clinical paths, and other standardized protocols.

Self-direction also encompasses well-honed and effective time-management skills to address the many aspects of home care, including scheduling visits; completing documentation; and detail-oriented administrative duties, such as making phone calls, entering required data, and completing POCs and OASIS assessments timely and accurately. The best clinicians in home care are well organized and use organizational skills in their daily routines, such as creating detailed schedules, documenting at the patient's home (unless safety concerns preclude this standard), and generally seeking to do things right the first time. Day scheduling calendars, cell phones, voice/e-mail, and other technology assist in this important endeavor, of course, all while being HIPAA-compliant per the organization's policies.

Desire to Continue Learning and Being Open to New Information, Knowledge, and Skills

This desire especially applies as new kinds of technologies are introduced into the home setting. Complex heart failure management, apnea monitoring, telehealth technology, innovative pain and symptom management, and ventilator care are just some of the kinds of patient care problems addressed daily by home care clinicians. As new technology moves into the home, such as new ventilator models or software applications, nurses in home care must continue to learn.

Sincere Appreciation of/for People

Home care is a people business! This includes interacting positively with and being empathetic to physicians and patients and their families/caregivers who are often in the midst of crises. Because many traditional family caregivers work outside the home, team members use observation and assessment findings, teaching and training skills, and patient-education tools to maintain patients safely in their homes. This teaching or consulting role also provides job satisfaction to home care staff and comfort and security to the patients and their families.

Ability to Be Open and Sincerely Accepting of People's Unique Personalities and Lifestyles and of the Effects These Lifestyles Have on Health

Sometimes these patient choices can be difficult for the clinician. The classic example is the patient who has a tracheostomy and continues to smoke. Ethical dilemmas must be identified, acknowledged, and addressed within the framework of the home care organization.

Awareness and Acceptance that a Constant Balance Must Be Maintained Between Clinical and Administrative Demands

The home care clinician knows and respects that both demands are equally important but in different ways and for different reasons. The regulatory environment mandates many processes, such as timelines for physician orders and OASIS transmission. Regulations are also promulgated by Occupational Safety and Health Administration (OSHA), CMS, Centers for Disease Control and Prevention, state law, professional practice acts, or other entities, such as accreditation bodies. For Medicare-certified agencies, note that one of the CoPs is adherence to applicable regulations and law. It is the organization's and staff's responsibility to be aware of and compliant with these regulations—and to be aware and cooperate with changes as they occur.

Ability to Function Independently

The home care work environment does not include the structure and "down the hall" camaraderie, supervision, and peer consultation that is available in other healthcare settings, such as hospitals. Home care clinicians must be able to function independently with input from supervisors and peers, just in a different manner or structure.

A Kind Sense of Humor to Help Patients, Families, and Peers Overcome Challenges

This sense of humor conveys a healing power when used appropriately and is sensitive to the patient's needs.

Knowledge of the Economics of Healthcare and of the Larger Environment that Impacts Home Care

Knowledge of reimbursement mechanisms in home care, including differences among payer sources, utilization, and payment mechanisms, is critical for the nurse or therapist clinician who must function as an admission and insurance specialist on the initial visit. For Medicare/Medicaid patients (and some insurance patients), the OASIS may be the basis for determining reimbursement; thus, it is imperative that clinicians have a solid understanding of the assessment process and impeccable assessment skills. As the role of case manager/care coordinator continues to evolve, it is this person who makes complex decisions authorizing limited resources based on patient needs, and a specific rationale for the increased use of resources must be clearly stated.

Practical Wisdom of Home Care Practice

This is information that comes with education, practice, and usually experience. It may be called understanding "the best way to do things" and may also be "best practices." Much of this knowledge comes from watching and learning from experienced home care clinicians, which may include learning practical tips, such as always having two sets of supplies with you (the "Noah's Ark" approach to home care)—because inevitably when you do not have a second set, you will need it! Other examples include organizing paperwork, setting up schedules, and tracking physician orders. Successful agencies support their home care clinicians with these processes, providing laptops, tablets, or other technology to facilitate effectiveness and timely documentation, coordination, and communication. As more agencies implement better clinical technologies, clinicians should embrace these innovative technologies that can help improve efficiency and provide better patient care.

Knowledge of Case Management Skills and Models

Certain growing patient populations in home care, such as the chronically ill or frail older adult, may not need "skilled care" but do need another level of care, such as case management services. These services may be geriatric case management or other services. As health insurers see the cost savings realized by effective case management models, home care has become more integrated with prevention efforts and community health initiatives. Telehealth, personal emergency response systems, and other technologies assist in caring for certain high-risk patient populations to keep them stable and out of high-cost hospital centers.

This is the time for care providers and managers to think "outside the box" and to be able to provide varying levels of care through innovative efforts. Case-managed care service programs may be Medicaid and other "waiver" programs for which patients do not have to meet stringent criteria for admission but are maintained in the home with the goal of keeping them safe, stable, and out of an institution. As Medicaid continues to administer increased amounts and types of home care, depending on the state, an increased number of older adult service providers can be seen linking with state programs to authorize and provide "personal care" and other kinds of important, needed support services. These programs can be either medical or social models or a combination of both, depending on the patient populations served. These programs to support "aging in place" will only increase.

Impeccable Assessment, Documentation, and Critical-Thinking or Clinical-Reasoning Skills

These skills go hand in hand. The assessment information is one main component that drives the care and reimbursement; the documentation of the comprehensive assessment must be thorough, accurate, and timely (within the defined time frames for the POC or recertification and the corresponding OASIS) because it ultimately determines reimbursement for that care. Continuing documentation of care and services needed by the patient must be determined in subsequent visits throughout the care. Some organizations have admitting clinicians (nurses and therapists) who possess a high level of assessment skills and validated credentials or a specialty certification (e.g., cardiac nurse for cardiovascular patients). This practice may not be feasible for many organizations, depending on finances, geography, staffing and availability, and the size of the organization.

Broad-Based Knowledge of Infection Prevention and Control (IPC)

This knowledge includes the fundamentals of infection prevention and control strategies, such as hand hygiene and effective handwashing and the appropriate use of alcohol-based gels/hand sanitizers. There is also personal protective equipment (PPE) (such as gloves, etc.) that the organization furnishes for patient care. Many organizations also have specific policies related to nursing "bag technique" and use. There may be a policy about the use of a "barrier" and cleaning and disinfecting equipment after each patient use. It is important to remember that many patients have compromised immune systems that may be due to illness, treatments, advanced age, or other reasons. Because of this compromised system, they may not have the ability to "fight" off infections like healthy people. In addition, germs can live for hours/days on surfaces, such as doorknobs, tables, and equipment. Like other care settings, "standard precautions" are the method used to help protect patients and team members from microscopic germs and organisms. When wearing gloves, always wash your hands immediately after removing the gloves. There are many stories about "super" bugs and drug-resistance, and home care and hospice nurses have an important role to play in IPC.

Organisms can be spread in several ways including:

- *Airborne and droplet*—Like the flu, a cold, or measles (e.g., spread through coughing or sneezing).

- *Bloodborne*—Like hepatitis B and HIV.

- *Oral*—This means through the ingestion of organisms from the hands or other sources, such as food. Mononucleosis is one example.

- *Foodborne*—Without proper hand hygiene, food preparation, food storage and handling, organisms can be spread that contribute to illness. *Escherichia coli* is common bacteria that can cause illness, hospitalizations, and, in some cases, death when food is improperly handled and exposed to the bacteria, which is then ingested with the food.

- *Insects*—Such as tick- and mosquito-borne illnesses—like Zika or malaria.

- *Direct and indirect contact with objects that are contaminated with disease producing organisms*—Of course, many home care and hospice patients are at further risk for this in particular because they have invasive devices, such as indwelling urinary catheters or venous access devices, or they may be home after being discharged from the hospital with pneumonia or a wound-related infection.

When you are sick, it is important that you do not see patients and stay up-to-date on your immunizations, as well as being aware of infections in your community and your own case load. Most organizations identify, track, and trend patients with infections, such as those with wounds or indwelling devices, as a part of their ongoing quality assurance and performance improvement (QAPI) initiatives. Infection prevention is a very important component of quality and safety in home care; when in doubt, ask your supervisor. You may wish to review infection prevention publications and resources specific to home care and hospice at www.HomeCareandHospice.com.

Enthusiastic and Successful Teaching Skills and a Knowledge of Evidence-Based Resources

Teaching skills are more important than ever! This includes a repertoire of evidence-based tools for patient and family teaching, including the organization's authorized and standardized teaching guides or booklets. These teaching skills are valued in the home care environment because education of the patient and family is a large part of clinical management in home care and because patients and their families usually want to, and should, achieve self-care and functioning, and as quickly as possible. See Appendix B, "Resources for Clinicians and Patient/Caregiver Education," for a list of helpful patient education and other information, beginning on page 277.

Adapted with permission from *Handbook of Home Health Standards: Quality, Documentation, and Reimbursement,* by Tina M. Marrelli (2012), 5th Edition.

Orientation: Three Components to Success

Numerous components go into an effective orientation. As in all specialties, you have new terms and abbreviations to learn. Ask your manager for this list at your organization. For safety reasons, you may also sometimes have a list of abbreviations that should not be used. When in doubt, always use the entire term so others are not guessing and everyone is on the same page for clarity and usage. Orientation can be divided into three discrete components:

- A general orientation to home care

- The organization-specific orientation

- The ongoing education that becomes continuing education (CE)

This book was designed to assist with all three components, but you will always have more to learn and know.

It is important to note, as with any new endeavor, that you cannot "know it all." It is at this point that the information in this book should be reviewed. In fact, one goal of an effective orientation might be that "you know enough to know who to ask what you do not know!"

There are no dumb questions in home care or healthcare—they are truly the ones that do not get asked. From a performance-improvement perspective, which the best organizations and operations demand, you can only increase knowledge and performance by asking questions. Asking questions and admitting you don't and can't know it all are important components you must understand to succeed in practice and daily operations. In addition, as mentioned previously, the employing organization may have their own list of terms and definitions. Do not hesitate to ask!

- *Home care orientation*—This orientation includes the fundamental information about onboarding at the organization and components of home care.

- *The organization-specific orientation*—This includes the home care orientation information plus any state nursing or therapy practice acts, the home care licensure for that state (if license for the kinds of home care provided is required), and specific regulations related to coverage for the state's Medicaid program or other payer or state-based programs. It is important to note that state programs for Medicaid (the state-based healthcare program for the economically disadvantaged) that meet state home care criteria may have names other than "Medicaid." These include MaineCare in Maine, Medi-Cal in California, SoonerCare in Oklahoma, TennCare in Tennessee, and others. Because of the complexity of payers and name similarities, it is important to clearly define terms and insurance/payer programs. This segment also includes all the organization's relevant clinical and administrative policies and procedures.

- *Ongoing education or continuing education in home care*— This CE includes any required education (such as by the state for nursing licensure renewal processes) and the changing external environment that must be understood across time for compliance and clinical practice. Once you are out of orientation and in practice or management, of course you must maintain your skills and refresh or reinforce information and education as needed. Because there are so many varying patients with numerous healthcare problems due to chronicity and complexity, CE may include those related to diabetes, aspects of transferring information and patient education, health maintenance, literacy, and more. These CE efforts are often related to helping patients achieve and maintain health and improve choices, thus moving from health "care" to holistic health through self-management. Other CEs may be more administrative, such as documentation, medical errors, and other topics.

As in all endeavors, improvement comes with effort and desire, continued practice, and time. In Patricia Benner's classic work *From Novice to Expert: Excellence and Power in Clinical Nursing Practice*, there is a statement that "a wealth of untapped knowledge is embedded in the practices and the 'know-how' of expert nurse clinicians, but this knowledge will not expand or fully develop unless nurses systematically record what they learn from their own experience" (2000, p. 11).

Because readers of this chapter may be new to home care, they have a special insight that experienced home care nurses or therapists may no longer be able to tap into or "see." We all become novices in new endeavors, and this is okay. As previously emphasized, you cannot know it all, especially when you're starting out in a new field/area. To this end, readers are encouraged to document their journeys as they enter home care. You can then revisit your notations and important "lessons learned" across time—while you are becoming proficient and experienced home care nurses. You may have much to share about with the next "class" or generation coming in, those new to home care and home care practice!

Summary

Welcome to home care—the practice setting of the future is here. An effective orientation with the foundational items listed in this chapter is essential for success. Though orientation and onboarding structures and related processes may vary across organizations, even experienced nurses new to the specialty of home care need a comprehensive and planned orientation.

Before making visits or providing shift care in a home, nurses and other clinician team members need to have a holistic understanding of what home care practice entails, demands, and "looks like" on a daily basis. The environment for home care, the patient's home and the community, represents the largest mindset change for those who are new to home care. Providing care in that unique space—the patient's home environment—is addressed in the following chapter.

Questions for Further Consideration and Discussion

1. Explain why you believe that the Bureau of Labor Statistics expects growth in the number of nurses in home care over the coming years.

2. What is the definition of home health? What is home care and why do we make the differentiation?

3. List three of the skills and knowledge areas needed in home care. Are there others that should be listed, and, if yes, what are they?

4. What comprises a comprehensive orientation to home care? Why would it be different from other care setting's orientations?

5. Benner's important book *Novice to Expert: Excellence and Power in Clinical Nursing Practice* about becoming or moving "from novice to expert" is a classic because certain levels of nursing practice are defined. These include five stages of skill acquisition starting with *novice* and achieving the highest level with *expert*. What do you think those terms mean from practical and operational perspectives in home care?

For Further Reading

- *A Nurse's Guide to Professional Boundaries,* from the National Council of State Boards of Nursing: https://www.ncsbn.org/ProfessionalBoundaries_Complete.pdf

- *Nurse Manager's Survival Guide: Practical Answers to Everyday Problems,* by Tina M. Marrelli

- "When Professional Kindness Is Misunderstood: Boundaries and Stalking Issues: A Case Study for the Home Health Clinician" by Cheryl Holz from *Home Healthcare Nurse* (Volume 27, Issue 7; pages 410–416)

- *Handbook of Home Health Standards: Quality, Documentation, and Reimbursement,* 5th Edition, by Tina M. Marrelli

- *From Novice to Expert: Excellence and Power in Clinical Nursing Practice, Commemorative Edition,* by Patricia Benner

- *Home Health Nursing: Scope and Standards of Practice,* from the American Nurses Association (ANA)

- "Implementing Home Health Standards in Clinical Practice" by Lisa Gorski from *Home Healthcare Now* (Volume 34, Issue 2; pps. 76-85.

References

American Nurses Association (ANA). (2014). *Home health nursing: Scope and standards of practice* (2nd ed.). Silver Spring, MD: American Nurses Association.

Benner, P. (2000). *From novice to expert: Excellence and power in clinical nursing practice, commemorative edition.* Upper Saddle River, NJ: Prentice Hall.

Marrelli, T. M. (2012). *Handbook of home health standards: Quality, documentation, and reimbursement* (5th ed.). St. Louis, MO: Mosby.

Rea, K. (2003). Home health certification: Recognition for specialty practice. *Home Healthcare Nurse, 21*(11), 761–768.

5

The Environment of Care: The Home and Community Interface

This chapter seeks to help both those who are new to home care and those with some experience in home care. In this way, you can either learn or refresh your information and understanding of the holistic nature of home care. Of course, a part of this holistic nature includes the patient's unique home and the community in which they live. Safety concerns may be impediments to care and achieving goals. This may also mean promoting the health, safety, and well-being of the patients in your care within their homes, and patients can be as unique as the home itself.

For purposes of this chapter, "home" can be an older adult high-rise apartment, a mobile home, a house in a neighborhood, and other locations. It can mean a number of places. I once visited and provided wound care to a homeless man who lived in a large cardboard box behind a convenience store. This was his home.

As home care transitions from the traditional medical model into more integrated, holistic, community-based models, home care nurses and managers can lead the way for this transformation. There has been much discussion about improving community health and creating healthier populations generally. It is generally accepted that socioeconomic factors and indicators impact health and healthcare, and may lead to poor health and lifestyle or other habits.

The first section of this chapter focuses on the community and how to conduct a windshield assessment and gather data about the neighborhood and geographic area that is in your purview or "catchment"/service area for patient care. Later sections address emergency preparedness and management and safety aspects when working in the home, as well as other hazards that nurses and visiting team members may encounter. Home and patient safety is also discussed, particularly in regards to how it may impact team members.

The Great News: Finally the Interface of Community and Health and Home Care

Healthy People initiatives have been creating national health-related objectives for three decades and their current initiative, Healthy People 2020, provides "science-based 10-year national objectives for improving the health of all Americans" (HealthyPeople.gov, n.d., para. 1). They establish benchmarks and monitor progress over time with aims to "encourage collaborations across communities and sectors," "empower individuals toward making informed health decisions," and "measure the impact of prevention activities" (HealthyPeople.gov, n.d., para. 2). The vision of Healthy People 2020, "a society in which all people live long, healthy lives," is very clear and is aligned with other programs and emerging care models (HealthyPeople.gov, n.d., para. 4).

As population health, faith-based initiatives, and other models change to bring people either back home to the community or help them stay in their homes and be cared for there—"age in place"—nurses and others practicing in home care need to understand this wide-ranging policy shift. This shift makes the community and home care settings more important than ever as practice settings. With this shift comes an awareness that must be developed in this unique practice setting. This awareness concerns the external and internal environments for practice and encompasses a broad and diverse set of attributes and considerations.

The Big Picture: Identifying the Most Common Hazards and Vulnerabilities in Your State

Emergency preparedness includes the roles of home care nurses when an emergency occurs, as well as the nurse's role in helping with the patient's emergency plan should such a plan be needed. Suffice it to say, all involved should plan for such events and revisit those plans on a regular basis. This is usually at least annually and includes the update of the patient-specific emergency plan. At a minimum, there should be an annual drill and an analysis of the "drill" followed by a summary of "what could have been done better or improved" and "lessons learned." This is why healthcare and other organizations practice fire drills, disaster drills, earthquake drills, and activities for other disasters depending on the risks identified in their area.

In a post-9/11 world, emergency preparedness and management is an important consideration requiring thoughtful awareness and analysis wherever one lives and practices. Natural and man-made disasters are frequently in the news. Sadly, oil spills, floods, tornadoes, contaminated water, and natural gas leakage are just some of the latest examples of events that have disrupted lives. Your organization-specific policies about this area should be a part of your orientation and must be reviewed and updated as needed.

No discussion of community and home care would be complete without an overview of the importance of identifying the most common hazards in a given city, region, or state. The first step in this identification is performing a hazard and vulnerability analysis. What drills are chosen for each organization should be congruent with that organization's geographic area. The U.S. Geological Survey lists Florida and North Dakota as the two states with the fewest earthquakes (2015a). Based on this, it might not make sense for those states to schedule regular earthquake drills. Drills and related processes need to be realistic for the area and based on data.

The cycle of disaster preparedness is defined by the Federal Emergency Management Agency (FEMA) as "a continuous cycle of planning, organizing, training, equipping, exercising, evaluating and taking corrective action in an effort to ensure effective coordination during incident response" (FEMA, 2015, para. 1). Being aware of disaster preparedness and the needed actions related to this preparedness must be initiated with a knowledge about the common hazards in your state or geographic area. These might include wildfires, floods, hurricanes, tornadoes, and other dangerous natural events.

By identifying what the most common "hazards" are based on topography, history, location, or other factors, those practicing in the community can have a realistic emergency disaster preparedness and management plan. This information should also be useful for one's own family plan and help patients/families make decisions such as whether they should leave or stay in the home, which is also called "sheltering in place." Of course, all states and communities have different risks that should be identified, and consideration should be given to the possibility of such risks.

For example, to return the earthquakes example, according to the U.S. Geographical Survey, the "Top Earthquake States" are as follows: 1) Alaska, 2) California, 3) Hawaii, 4) Nevada, 5) Washington, 6) Idaho, 7) Wyoming, 8) Montana, 9) Utah, and 10) Oregon (U.S. Geological Survey, 2015b). According to FloodSmart.gov, floods are the number one disaster in the United States (n.d.). The most recent data from 2014 shows that the following were the top ten states for flood claims: 1) Florida, 2) Alabama, 3) New York, 4) Texas, 5) Pennsylvania, 6) Louisiana, 7) Michigan, 8) Iowa, 9) Ohio, and 10) Illinois (n.d.).

By searching the state's name online, the most common "natural" hazard risk(s) for the area and information from the state or city can be located and reviewed. Many of the state sites also list www.ready.gov as a resource that provides emergency preparedness guidance including information about basic disaster supplies kit contents, how to build a kit, how to make a plan, FEMA for kids, natural disasters, information about hurricanes and earthquakes, and more. For example, by looking at information about Massachusetts, the city of Boston listed blackouts, cyber threats, earthquakes (where it stated that the state experiences an average of five earthquakes per year), extreme heat, fire, flood, hurricane, influenza pandemic, terrorism, thunderstorms and lightening, tornados, and winter storms and extreme cold as common hazards (CityofBoston.gov, n.d.). Of course, keep in mind that not all lists may include such events as active shooter incidents and terrorism that, sadly, are a part of life and culture and something you should remain aware of in your community wherever you live and work.

A sad, but true and poignant example of emergency preparedness and management that did not work is detailed in a book titled *Five Days at Memorial: Life and Death in a Storm-Ravaged Hospital* (by Sheri Fink, Crown Publishing). This is a hard-to-read and harder-to-put-down book about healthcare delivery, choices, ethical dilemmas, management, communication, and more during an emergency situation. This book can also be used as a basis for discussion about real-life emergency preparedness, management, coordination activities, and lessons learned through emergencies.

The bottom line is an awareness of the need for preparedness. Your organization will have specific policies related to emergency management and preparedness. When looking at these policies, two of the most important things to know are: 1) your role in an emergency; and 2) your role in helping with a patient's emergency plan, including determining if it is realistic and up-to-date.

Strategies for Conducting a "Windshield" Assessment

Once you know the big picture, the need to drill down to the community as the practice setting for care is next. This can best be accomplished using a "windshield survey." Those of us who practiced in community health when it was more integrated with home care remember this well. And you can make this as broad a view or as detailed as you like. A *windshield survey* or assessment is just that—driving around the neighborhood to get an overview of the community and recording or noting your observations and findings.

The following are some of the questions that can help you determine information about the community in the windshield assessment. Often the findings that come out of this assessment will help formulate a plan to improve the quality of the community and its neighborhood(s). This is harder to perform if you have lived in an area for some time; it is hard to "see" the neighborhood with new eyes. If that's the case, consider taking someone with you; then you will have four eyes and be able to gather more observations, notes, and information.

"Windshield" Assessment Questions

Questions related to the big picture questions include:

- What is the name of the town or neighborhood(s)?
- Overall, is the community primarily urban, rural, suburban, or a blend?
- How do you get there (e.g., is there an interstate or freeway)?
- Where is the biggest town/city nearby?
- What do the roads look/feel like while driving (are they smooth, pothole-ridden, or a blend of both?)
- Are the streets/roads clean or dotted with trash? Are they noisy?
- Are there sidewalks?
- Are there chain link fences segmenting certain parts or open green grassy areas?
- Where are the common areas in town (e.g., a "green" area or a community center)?
- Is there a town center? Is it crowded and thriving?
- Are there areas that are vacant and falling into disrepair?
- Is there a walkable downtown? Is it used? What businesses look busy? Are there a lot that are empty?
- Are there sport league signs, baseball diamonds, basketball courts, and/or tennis courts? Are they lit after dark?

- Are there walking trails, bicycle lanes, and parks or recreation areas?
- Are there areas for picnics or footpaths and trails noted along your drive?

Questions related to reading signage include:

- How many signs are there and what languages are they in?
- Are the signs well-maintained or peeling and unreadable?
- What are they advertising (e.g., new housing, concerts, cigarettes, liquor, etc.)?

Questions related to people watching include:

- Are there people gathered around churches, synagogues, or other religious or spiritual buildings?
- Are there people out on the street and/or "in town?"
- How are the people dressed?
- What are the people doing (e.g., taking a walk, smoking, playing outside)?
- Are there a lot of people riding bicycles?
- What are the approximate ages of the people you see (e.g., children, toddlers/infants in strollers, older youth playing basketball, adults, older adults, etc.)?

Questions related to educational opportunities include:

- How many schools are there?
- What kinds/levels of schools (e.g., kindergarten, grade schools, junior high, high schools, community colleges, extension schools, universities, etc.)?

- Are there libraries?

- Are there places offering ongoing education, such as yoga or exercise classes, or other classes?

- Are there buildings for local or regional newspapers or magazines?

Questions related to municipal administration include:

- Is there a town hall?

- Where are the public safety buildings, such as EMS, fire safety, and police/law enforcement, located?

- What is the model of government (e.g., a mayor, selectmen, county commissioners, city council, etc.)?

- What is the source of the town's water? Is it clean and safe (some assessments may perform testing)?

- Who runs the energy utilities and their management/maintenance (e.g., electrical cooperative)?

Questions related to commerce and business include:

- What businesses and kinds of business do you see as you drive by (e.g., factories, grocery stores, bars, taverns, nightclubs, convenience stores, etc.)?

- What are the most prominent business types (e.g., manufacturing, agricultural, technology, etc.)?

- Are there railroad tracks, and are there marked railroad crossings signs and gates?

- Are there airport signs?

- Are there a lot of bus stations/stops?

Questions related to general healthcare include:

- What hospital(s) are in the area?

- Are the hospitals community-based or part of a larger system?

- What levels of care do the hospitals provide (e.g., neonatal level of care, trauma, etc.)?

- How far is the medical center that can provide higher levels of care?

- Are there Health Resources and Services Administration (HRSA) care clinics/community health centers, veteran's centers, or primary care practitioners? (Check for HRSA clinics at http://findahealthcenter.hrsa.gov/index.html by entering the area's ZIP code.)

- How many pharmacies/drug stores are there? Where are they located? Are they open 24 hours a day?

- Are there any home health agencies?

- Are there any hospice(s), including inpatient hospice buildings?

- What is the availability of dialysis centers?

- Where are laboratories for blood and other testing?

- Are there veterinary services?

Questions related to housing include:

- What do the homes "look like" (e.g., new, old, dilapidated vacant, impeccably restored, historical, condos, row houses, huge single family, shared housing apartments, townhomes, etc.)?

- Are there mobile or manufactured homes?

- Are there prison(s) in the area?

- Is there a lot of construction happening (or none)?

Questions related to arts and entertainment include:

- Is there a theatre with active performances?
- Are there movie theaters?
- Is there a science center?
- Do you see signs for historical sites, such as lighthouses, museums, or historic buildings?
- Are there animal and animal conservation educational centers?
- Do you see any senior centers, adult day care centers, respite care centers, or other services?

Questions related to shopping venues include:

- Is there a mall/outlet mall?
- Are there individual stores in strip shopping centers?
- Are there a lot of pawnshops or secondhand stores?
- What kind of food and restaurants are available (sit down, fast, healthy, local, chain, etc.)?

Other Data to Be Collected

Other data that impacts health and healthcare can be collected online or by interview outside of the windshield assessment depending on the depth of the information sought. This could include the population numbers (and if the population is increasing or decreasing), the average age, and the average income of residents. Some environmental and health information might include smoking rates, leading causes of death in the county, amount spent on child per year at school (for benchmarking with national data amounts), number of high school students that go on to college, and more.

Other things to look into might include looking for known problems, such as contaminated or other water problems, oil spills, asbestos in buildings, superfund activities (large contamination cleanup), nuclear power sites, and more. All of these factors and observations help paint a picture of the community and its neighborhoods. After all of this data has been collected, it can be analyzed, and negatives and positives can be discussed along with a plan for improvement related to the findings and stakeholders involved.

The Community and Neighborhood— Safety Considerations

During home visits, you will see that homes often reflect the community. Of course, these homes can vary greatly. They can include very mean dogs, protective cats, bedbugs, rats (sometimes the size of cats), drug use, guns displayed in cabinets, and more. Some of the more unusual "pets" encountered in my visits include squirrels, snakes, and rats. All of these are examples of safety factors.

Personal safety is always an important component of orientation and an appropriate concern, in either the community or a patient home. The home environment and other safety issues are important in many aspects of home care practice and operations. They are also key components in quality, risk management, and accreditation standards. Safety may also influence other areas such as staff retention and satisfaction.

Personal safety begins with an awareness of your surroundings, such as when driving through a neighborhood and when you are entering, being in, and exiting a home, as well as during many other associated home care-related activities. Use the skills of observation and assessment that are essential to safety any time you are in the community. Speak with your manager if you have specific questions about safety and safety policies at your organization.

Safety begins before every home visit. If you are given certain geographic areas or ZIP code areas that identify the patient's home within your purview and catchment area, ask experienced team members and your supervisor for information about that area. Whenever you are going anywhere for the first time, confirm the address and try to get more information, such as landmarks, for confirmation of accuracy and "going the right way" along the way. Also ask if there is a house number on the home and/or on the mailbox or other location where you can readily see it. This may sound easy, but it may not be so easy after dusk or at night, or in communities with very similar street names, poor lighting, and/or no or very rare streetlamps.

Also confirm that you are to use/come in the front door. This would be very important if the front door is not used and the nurse is at the wrong door. I have made home visits to homes where the front door was "closed off" for years due to remodeling or the hospital bed (or other furniture such as large chest of drawers) was placed there so it could no longer be used. Some families use a garage, side, or other door as their usual entrance to the home instead of the front door. Ask questions and clarify information before you leave for the visit. There are no dumb questions—the clearer information can be before the visit, the better.

The good news is that your phone apps can give voice directions to you while driving, though sometimes they may not be as accurate or as direct as one might like. Some use the phone app and a GPS to be sure they will get to the correct address—and to have one as backup should there be a problem. Others still carry maps as a backup to online directions, such as those on the phone or other apps that can provide detailed driving information. Others prefer to have printed out directions, and these can be accessed on www.mapquest.com, www.randmcnally.com, and other sites of your choosing.

One of the helpful things about the apps for your phone is that many of them can reroute a driver when traffic or another problem like construction is impeding traffic and slowing the anticipated commute. Ask your preceptor or mentor questions about what works best in the geographic location where you practice, because some apps may work better in some geographic areas than others.

The following are tips about personal safety:

- Find out about and know your communities and neighborhoods.

- Carry your cell phone with you.

- When driving, always be aware of your surroundings. Keep maps out of sight and try to avoid looking lost or unfamiliar with the area if possible.

- Look for the landmarks that were reported and address numbers on the homes.

- Some team members call patients prior to leaving so that they are expected and can get specific help or information about parking. This way, the patient and family are also watching for the nurse's approach. Ask that they turn on outside lights; this is another way to easily identify the home. This is also the time to ask that any dogs or other pets (this can depend of course on the "pet") be placed out of the patient area. This can be problematic when the patient area is the living room when one walks in the door, but either way, dogs particularly can be very protective of their owners. I have known of dogs being described as "very sweet" and "all bark" and then someone is severely bitten by that same dog. Be careful around all animals.

- Communicate back to the office any details that were unclear about the address, the setup, the correct door to use, if the doorbell does not work so you need to call from the car, etc. This will help any other visiting team members that will follow and on-call staff who may also be making visits to that home.

- Lock the car doors and keep any valuables, such as a purse, out of sight. This might also include supplies, which should usually be locked in the trunk. Of course, no patient identifying information, such as file materials with names, should be visible in the car (or from outside the home either, such as through a window or door, etc.).

- Wear your seatbelt and lock your doors while driving.

- Try to park in an area that is well-lit. Some families are helpful with these kinds of details, such as telling the nurse "to park on the left side of the driveway where there is a 'flood' or garage light."

- Lock the car, reviewing your route to the front or other door, as directed.

- Keep emergency equipment or items in your trunk so you have them should they be needed. These might include (of course, depending on where you live) items needed for ice and snow, such as a shovel, snow/ice scraper for car windows, kitty litter and/or a small rug to get traction should that be needed. Other items could include a whistle, blankets, "yak tracks" for shoes or boots, emergency flares, flashlight, cellphone charger, scissors, water for drinking, and protein bars or other snacks. Sand or salt for icy areas or conditions and walkways may help prevent falls. It can be a dicey walk to the front door when the snow has not been shoveled! A full tank of gas is a very good idea in case you get stuck in traffic and must idle for some time and need to stay warm.

- When entering a large building with numerous apartments or homes, always be cautious when entering and exiting.

- Be careful about entering and exiting elevators. Some older adult community buildings have an entry hall with a vestibule, and a person controls the entrance and exit of the visiting nurse, who then gets "buzzed in." Sometimes the person who controls the entrance will ask for and keep your driver's license or identification when you are "signing in" so he or she knows who is coming in to care for the community's residents. Just make sure to pick up your driver's license or other identification on your way back out. This is also a reminder to carry some kind of identification with you for these kinds of reasons.

- Some home care patients live in hotels or motels. Again, safety is the watchword, and whenever you feel uncomfortable, it is okay to speak with your supervisor. The important thing is to trust your feelings. Home care nurses develop a sense that is all about safety. If you feel unsafe, your probably are—trust your feelings and instincts!

- When making evening or night visits, let your supervisor know when you are going and where. Also, let your family know (such as your spouse or a friend) before you leave if on call and what time you expect to return.

- When walking out to your car, have your keys out. Be aware that many car keys have "automatic" locks that unlock at the click of a button and some also have a "panic" button that makes a very loud noise.

- Before unlocking your car, check the car area and the back seat and floor areas.

- Leave an unsafe area/situation immediately and notify your supervisor.

- Be mindful of other aspects of personal safety, especially per specific policies and procedures at your organization.

Personal safety is an important aspect of home care practice and management. The following section is about the other aspect of home safety, that of the patient's unique environment, their home. These two components go together as the patient's environment can also impact the nurse as well as the patient and family.

The Interface of Safety and Patient Homes: Variable Environments of Care

Homes and the patient's physical environment impact the visiting team members in many ways. The number of nurses and aides expected to move into the home care and community-based sector will continue to increase as aging populations wish to remain at home and age in place. According to the Bureau of Labor Statistics (BLS), "employment of home health aides is projected to grow 38 percent from 2014 to 2024, much faster than the average for all occupations" (2015, para. 5). That projected change between 2014 and 2024 is estimated to require 348,400 new home health aides (BLS, 2015). Nurses and other clinicians practicing in home care are also expected to increase.

Those who make home visits are sometimes faced with a difficult environment in which they must provide care. According to Polivka et al., the "most often-reported hazards were trip/slip/lift hazards, biohazards, and hazards from poor air quality, allergens, pests and rodents, and fire and burns" (2015, p. 512). These are important data as this study used a questionnaire, focus groups, and individual interviews with 68 participants that included home care nurses, aides, therapists, and owners and managers from a broad geographically diverse areas and states. In addition, the hazards encountered were categorized room by room, such as the kitchen, bathroom, and so on.

Not surprisingly, "more kitchen hazards were mentioned by participants than hazards in any other room with trip/slip/lift hazards being the most frequently mentioned type of hazard" (Polivka et al., 2015, p. 515). The identification of hazards is very important for many reasons. We may know nurses or others who slipped on ice, were bitten by dogs, had a patient who refused the Hoyer lift (and then an aide "pulled something," seriously injuring her back, for instance), and more. When you are entering a new space in particular, use those "new" eyes to take in and critically look at and for safety hazards. What is identified can then be communicated to other caregivers and to the patient and family so they can try to address some of these problems and hazards. The interface of the home environment, the patient's unique home, and many safety factors all contribute to the environment of care in which home care nurses and other clinicians must practice.

See the form entitled "Home Environment Safety Evaluation" shown in Figure 5.1 for a sample form to help you evaluate home safety.

Structural problems can also be a challenge. I have made home visits to houses with huge holes in the floor where you could look down and see the basement. In one case, the patient was wheelchair-bound and had to maneuver around this hole in the floor, and they had for years according to her history. It wasn't until her husband died that she realized it was very unsafe because she was alone now and her husband was no longer directing her wheelchair around the holes.

HOME ENVIRONMENT SAFETY EVALUATION

Check Yes, No or N/A (Not Applicable) for each of the following items. For all "No" responses identify, in the space provided, item number, action plan to correct the problem and document the date the patient was instructed.

		YES	NO	N/A
1.	There is a working telephone and emergency numbers are accessible.			
2.	Electrical cords and outlets appear to be in good repair in the patient area (i.e., cords not frayed, outlets not overloaded, etc.).			
3.	There are functional smoke alarm(s).			
4.	Fire extinguisher is available and accessible.			
5.	Access to outside exits is free of obstruction.			
6.	Alternate exits are accessible in case of fire.			
7.	Walking pathways are level, uncluttered and have non-skid surfaces.			
8.	Stairs are in good repair, well lit, uncluttered and have non-skid surfaces. Handrails are present and secure.			
9.	Lighting is adequate for safe ambulation and ADL.			
10.	Temperature and ventilation are adequate.			
11.	Medicines and poisonous/toxic substances are clearly labeled and placed where patient can reach, if needed, yet not within reach of children.			
12.	Bathroom is safe for the provision of care (i.e., raised toilet seat, tub seat, grab bar, non-skid surface in tub, etc.).			
13.	Kitchen is safe for the provision of care (i.e., working appliances, hygienic area for food prep, etc.).			
14.	Environment is safe for effective oxygen use.			
15.	Overall environment is adequately sanitary for the provision of care.			
16.	Other			

FOR ALL ITEMS CHECKED "NO" ABOVE, SPECIFY ACTION PLAN AND DOCUMENT DATE PATIENT WAS INSTRUCTED

ITEM NO.	DATE INSTRUCTED	TEACHING MATERIALS PROVIDED	REVIEWED	ACTION PLAN

CHECK ANY OF THE FOLLOWING THAT NEED TO BE OBTAINED

❑ Raised toilet seat	❑ Plug covers	❑ Wheelchair	❑ Other____
❑ Tub seat	❑ Cabinet latches	❑ Lifeline or other PERS	❑ Other____
❑ Grab bar	❑ Window locks	❑ Car seat	❑ Other____
❑ Non-skid surface (bath)	❑ Ipecac syrup	❑ Seat/bed cushion	❑ Other____
❑ Infant tub	❑ Smoke alarm	❑ First aid kit	❑ Other____

Emergency preparedness plan discussed with/provided to patient? ❑ Yes ❑ No, explain: _____

SIGNATURE OF PERSON COMPLETING EVALUATION _____ DATE ___/___/___

CARE MANAGER SIGNATURE/TITLE _____ DATE ___/___/___

PART 1 – Clinical Record **PART 2 – Patient**

PATIENT NAME - Last, First, Middle Initial   ID#

Form 3542/2P 6/03 © 1994 BRIGGS, Des Moines, IA (800) 247-2343
Unauthorized copying or use violates copyright law. www.BriggsCorp.com PRINTED IN U.S.A.   **BRiGGS**Healthcare®   HOME ENVIRONMENT SAFETY EVALUATION

Figure 5.1 Home Environment Safety Evaluation

Copyright © 1994 Briggs Healthcare. Reprinted with permission.

Other patients had wooden steps up to the front door that cracked when pressure was applied in the "wrong" places. In one case, this important information was communicated to the nurse on intake; she was told not to step on the left side of the middle step. At this point, it is important to think about who could help rebuild these stairs to assist this patient with remaining in their home. Patients with poor/no resources or economic and social problems need to be referred to social services for assessment and possible intervention and follow-up with issues such as these.

Social work and medical social services are appropriate when the plan of care cannot be implemented because of an impediment like those mentioned. These impediments could be such basic things as the patient has diabetes and no food (and has no money or means to obtain food) or that the patient is on medications and lost his or her job, therefore preventing him or her from being able to afford medically necessary drugs per the physician plan of care. Other examples include when there is no heat (in the winter) and no or poor-functioning air conditioning in a chronic obstructive pulmonary disease (COPD) or heart failure (HF) patient (especially in the summer). Another situation requiring more care coordination and communication with the social worker might be if the patient cannot afford his or her needed equipment and/or supplies. This advocacy is an important role of the home care nurse.

 The role of *patient advocate* is very important when you're a home care nurse.

This role of patient advocate and advocacy is generally very important in these situations, particularly in patients where the system is not seamless and patients and their problems "fall through the cracks." Though such situations can be very challenging, the home care nurse and team can be problem solvers in such situations where the patient/family may not have a "voice." The best and most compassionate home care team members and organizations put themselves in the position of these sometimes powerless, voiceless people with very real medical, daily living, and other needs. At some point it will be the home care organization who may be held accountable (including financially) for that readmission that might have been prevented. This is particularly true as the paradigm changes and patients/people are cared for across their lifetimes and over many years. This alone is changing mindsets, and new innovative models are emerging to improve care for these patient populations. When you are in doubt about how to get your patient what is needed, talk with your supervisor.

Care coordination is a Medicare, Medicaid, and other home care standard and requirement. With this in mind, bring the team together, such as in a care or case conference, to talk about challenging patients. This can be a good time and place for thoughtful consideration and analysis of the situation—and of some "aha" moments that craft good ideas to try for possible solutions.

 HOME CARE NURSING
CASE STUDY: SAFETY IS THE WATCHWORD!

As home care nurses, we are aware of the (sometimes) glaring safety concerns upon crossing the threshold of a door in "Anywhere, USA." Upon entering one home, at first glance the nurse sees electrical outlets with extension cords going every which way and snaking under a throw rug toward the lamp on the other side of the living room. The nurse then notices that the wattage from that lamp is so poor it would be hard to see/read most anything, let alone to see enough to safely asses and observe a wound site prior to changing a dressing. This patient is also on oxygen, and there are no "No Smoking" signs posted on the front door per standard safety protocols. Looking further, the nurse notes that the clear oxygen tubing has 200 feet of "play" so that the patient can go either to the front door or the back door, be able to let the dogs out, or answer the phone in the kitchen, all while trailing that almost invisible clear oxygen tubing, which the nurse notices is sometimes getting snagged on a cocktail table's leg and on cluttered tabletops.

The nurse is also immediately greeted by the patient's pets. In this case, they are two small dogs that were, until the front door opened, sleeping on a loveseat; when the nurse enters, they scramble to get attention from the visitor, jumping off the couch, barking, and running! All the while, they are moving/jumping around this very old patient's painfully slow-moving slipper-clad feet (and there are no backs on the slippers).

This is a real-world example, and the nurse, once a positive and therapeutic relationship is established with the patient, may be able to impact some of the issues noticed in this first visit for the better.

Note: In this case study, the following areas for concern were noted: electrical outlets, extension cords, cords under rugs, low lighting, oxygen use without no smoking signage and with very long extension tubing (which can be a trip/fall hazard), clutter, two small dogs at the patient's feet, and the patient wearing slippers with open backs. This is just an example. Your patients will have less, more, or others. This is where the well-honed and used skills of observation and assessment are very important to support safety and aging in place.

The Joint Commission (TJC) has promulgated and updated/revised the National Patient Safety Goals (NPSGs) for some years. These NPSGs have stated specific goal areas that focus on problems in healthcare safety-related areas, and work to solve them. The "easy-to-read document" is a good resource in this application since patients, as well as family and other caregivers, can easily understand these goals and their intent.

In the 2016 home care NPSGs, there are five goals, and of these, two are directly related to the home as the environment for care:

- NPSG.09.02.01 recommends an assessment for finding out "which patients are most likely to fall" with questions like "is the patient taking any medicines that might make them weak, dizzy or sleepy?" (TJC, 2016, para. 5). Take actions to prevent falls in these patients.

- NPSG.15.02.01 recommends finding out "if there are any risks for patients who are getting oxygen. For example, fires in the patient's home" (TJC, 2016, para. 6). These are very simple, yet very important, questions to ask and information to determine to support safety.

Fire Safety

According to the American Burn Association (ABA), "more than 1,200 Americans aged 65 and older die each year as a result of fire.... Older adults between 65 and 75 years have twice the fire death rate of the national average. Those between 75 and 85 years have three times the national average and the rate for those above 85 is four times the national average.... Two thirds (2/3) of older persons that died in fires were in the rooms where the fire originated. This is usually associated with smoking materials, which injure or kill their victims by igniting their clothing, bedding or upholstery.... Scalds, electrical and chemical injuries also result in serious injuries to older adults" (ABA, n.d., p. 3).

Although it is hard to get a number related to injuries and deaths from smoking with oxygen specifically, it is a continuing and very dangerous problem. Given that home care patients are often older, have disabilities or other problems, and some are totally bedridden, the problem is magnified. It is for these reasons that home safety is taking a more dominant role in what home care will be and will "look like" in the future. If people are to "age in place" successfully (read: safely), structures and attributes have to be hardwired to make it safe and work properly—for all concerned.

Safety and Falls

Falls are a huge problem, particularly among the very young and older adults. According to the Centers for Disease Control and Prevention (CDC), "in 2013, direct medical costs for falls—what patients and insurance companies pay—totaled $34 billion" and "700,000 patients a year are hospitalized because of a fall injury, most often because of a broken hip or head injury" (CDC, 2015). Sadly, many people do not fully recover after such falls. Home care nurses and other team members are in a unique position to help identify those at risk and further assess what can be done to help prevent falls.

Older adults may be given a TUG (Timed Up and Go), Tinetti, or other objective measurement test as one way to determine fall risk. Nurses and therapists can perform these tests as necessary when they notice a fall risk. More tools can be viewed at http://geriatrictoolkit.missouri. edu. There are also other tests, as well as fall risk assessment tools, that organizations may use to better identify those at risk, and then use those assessments as a basis for further evaluation and intervention.

Interventions may include therapists for efforts to improve patient balance, strengthening, and gait training. The use of assistive devices, such as canes and walkers, may also be indicated. Sadly, patients some-times have these assistive devices but do not use them for a number of reasons. Orthostatic hypotension, medications, and numerous other variables and factors can all contribute to falls. In addition, we know that the greatest predictor of falls is the history of past falls, so these are the patients who must be watched and assessed for interventions and prevention most carefully.

Keep in mind that patients generally do not want you or their family to know they have fallen. It is a diplomatic dance of skill and concern, and sometimes humor and negotiation, that brings out the best for patients and home care nurses, too. These multifaceted skills can help in patient safety and in ensuring that you, as the nurse, have all the facts to give the patient the best care.

Summary

The environment in home care must be seen as an opportunity for improvement just like any other aspect of care and services. Common home health safety challenges include smoking, particularly with oxygen in the home; fall/trip hazards; a lack of ventilation and fresh air; dangerous heat sources (sometimes with fumes) and/or fire hazards; and pets and pet waste when the patient is unable to care for the pets(s). Home care nurses also must identify and address such problems as rodents, bedbugs, roach and flea infestations, and more. There are more medically specific safety-related considerations for patients, such as medications and bleeding precautions that will be addressed in the patient-specific care safety information in patient care and home visits in Chapter 7, "The Home Visit: The Important Unit of Care," beginning on p. 161.

Questions for Further Consideration and Discussion

1. What is a hazard and vulnerability analysis and why should one be done?

2. Define *disaster preparedness, emergency management,* and your role(s) in these.

3. List the three top "expected" disasters in your state/region/area.

4. Review two to three articles about safety in home care and compare and contrast findings and risk areas identified.

5. Identify five safety problems that a nurse or other team member might encounter in a patient's home and discuss/list how you would manage or address each of those five problems.

For Further Reading

- FEMA aims to "lead America to prepare for, prevent, respond to and recover from disasters": www.FEMA.gov

- Prepare for Natural Disasters: https://www.ready.gov/natural-disasters

- Safety Information from the National Fire Protection Association: www.nfpa.org/education

- Safety for Older Consumers—Home Safety Checklist: http://www.cpsc.gov/PageFiles/122038/701.pdf

- Preventing Falls: A Guide to Implementing Effective Community-Based Fall Prevention Programs: http://www.cdc.gov/homeandrecreationalsafety/falls/community_preventfalls.html

- Healthy People 2020: https://www.healthypeople.gov/sites/default/files/HP2020_brochure_with_LHI_508_FNL.pdf

- NOAA Weather Radio All Hazards (NWR): http://www.nws.noaa.gov/nwr/

- Emergency Preparedness and Response from the CDC: http://emergency.cdc.gov/

- *Handbook of Home Health Standards: Quality, Documentation, and Reimbursement,* by Tina M. Marrelli, 5th Edition

- *Five Days at Memorial: Life and Death in a Storm-Ravaged Hospital,* by Sheri Fink, 2013

- Oxygen safety by MedlinePlus: https://www.nlm.nih.gov/medlineplus/ency/patientinstructions/000049.htm

- In an emergency, remember not to leave your pet behind. Your pet also needs a plan and a good supply or food, water, and toys. Visit www.ready.gov/caring-animals for more information.

- "Learn How to Shelter in Place" from the CDC: http://emergency.cdc.gov/preparedness/shelter/

- "Preparedness for Natural Disasters Among Older US Adults: A Nationwide Survey" by Tala M. Al-rousan, Linda M. Rubenstein, and Robert B. Wallace (*American Journal of Public Health*)

- "Planning Resources by Setting: Long-term, Acute, and Chronic Care" from the CDC: http://www.cdc.gov/phpr/healthcare/planning2.htm

- American Burn Association (ABA). (n.d.). Fire and burn safety for older adults: Educator's guide. Retrieved from http://www.ameriburn.org/Preven/BurnSafetyOlderAdultsEducator'sGuide.pdf

- Grant, E. J. (2013). Preventing burns in the elderly: A guide for home healthcare professionals. *Home Healthcare Nurse, 31*(10), 561–573.

- Polivka, B. J., Wills, C. E., Darragh, A., Lavender, S., Sommerich, C., & Stredney, D. (2015). Environmental Health and Safety Hazards Experienced by Home Health Care Providers: A Room-by-Room Analysis. *Workplace Health and Safety, 63*(11), 512–522.

- Wills, C. E., Polivka, B. J., Darragh, A., Lavender, S., Sommerich, C., & Stredney, D. "Making Do" Decisions: How Home Healthcare Personnel Manage Their Exposure to Home Hazards. *Western Journal of Nursing Research, 38*(4), 411–26.

References

American Burn Association (ABA). (n.d.). Fire and burn safety for older adults: Educator's guide. Retrieved from http://www.ameriburn.org/Preven/BurnSafetyOlderAdultsEducator'sGuide.pdf

Bureau of Labor Statistics (BLS). (2015). Home health aides. Retrieved from http://www.bls.gov/ooh/healthcare/home-health-aides.htm

Centers for Disease Control and Prevention (CDC). (2015). Costs of falls among older adults. Retrieved from http://www.cdc.gov/homeandrecreationalsafety/falls/fallcost.html

CityofBoston.gov. (n.d.). Hazards. Retrieved from http://www.cityofboston.gov/ready_boston/hazards/

Federal Emergency Management Agency (FEMA). (2015). Plan & prepare: Preparedness cycle. Retrieved from http://www.fema.gov/plan-prepare

FloodSmart.gov. (n.d.). NFIP statistics. Retrieved from https://www.floodsmart.gov/floodsmart/pages/media_resources/stats.jsp

HealthyPeople.gov. (n.d.). About Healthy People. Retrieved from http://www.healthypeople.gov/2020/About-Healthy-People

Polivka, B. J., Wills, C. E., Darragh, A., Lavender, S., Sommerich, C., & Stredney, D. (2015). Environmental health and safety hazards experienced by home health care providers: A room-by-room analysis. *Workplace Health and Safety, 63*(11), 512–522.

The Joint Commission (TJC). (2016). Home care national patient safety goals. Retrieved from http://www.jointcommission.org/assets/1/6/2016_NPSG_OME_ER.pdf

U.S. Geological Survey. (2015a). Earthquake facts & earthquake fantasy. Retrieved from http://earthquake.usgs.gov/learn/topics/megaqk_facts_fantasy.php

U.S. Geological Survey. (2015b). Top earthquake states. Retrieved from http://earthquake.usgs.gov/earthquakes/states/top_states.php

6

The Fundamentals: The Interface of Law, Regulation, and Quality

This chapter seeks to provide a framework about the multifaceted and complex realm of home care since it intersects with regulatory requirements. Government-reimbursed home care, such as the Medicare and Medicaid programs, can be complicated, multilayered, and is continually undergoing change. There are interfacing and detailed regulatory requirements included. As this book goes to press, we are awaiting the new home care Conditions of Participation (CoPs) to be released.

Whatever the detail of the rules, such as the CoPs, whether for home care or hospice, as the government and other payers move to value-based care and care models, the key focus will be on value and outcomes, the intersection of cost and quality. We are starting to see value that is attributable to detailed and skillful care. In addition, home care is practiced differently in different states, and state practice laws and licensure laws may or may not exist or may vary from state to state. There may be different laws for varying kinds of home care, such as a certified home health agency, a registry, a hospice, an infusion organization, homemaker and companion services, home medical or durable equipment companies, and staffing. For home care–specific coverage, see Appendix D for the "Medicare Benefit Policy Manual Chapter 7— Home Health Services," beginning on p. 304. Of course, it is important to note that the Manual is sometimes updated and readers are advised to keep apprised of new updates.

The First Goal—Effective Daily Operations

Effective operations and processes can mean the difference between success and reactive problem-solving. These "problems" can span the scope from patient complaints to state regulators regarding care and services to the Office of the Inspector General (OIG) and the Federal Bureau of Investigation (FBI) involvement in suspected regulatory violations. For these and other reasons, it is imperative that home care and hospice organizations adhere to the "rules" and make effective daily operations and activities a hallmark of a well-functioning organization.

Like any business, there are missions, visions, and goals, as well as an organizational chart that should clearly designate the leadership and staff roles, functions, and responsibilities from the top down. Of course, in the home care business we serve patients, so the patient should also be listed on the organizational chart. This is also an accreditation standard that relates to all of this, and information about accreditation bodies with links for more information are listed later in this chapter.

Whether the home care program is freestanding; a part of a healthcare system, such as a hospital; or an integrated group of healthcare providers, such as part of a network or an accountable care organization (ACO), it must have the ability and functions of any successful business operation. This starts with human-resource capabilities, such as screening, interviewing, hiring, onboarding, and counseling. There are other very important fiscal functions, such as budget projections; capital expenditures (e.g., software and its support); report generation and analysis; accounts receivable (A/R) and accounts payable (A/P); payroll and taxes; health insurance and other benefits and their administration for employees; and more. Software systems support and track numerous "back office" functions, such as payroll, staffing, scheduling, quality improvement, infection control, and more. These systems may also assist in tracking and trending to support improvement of operations.

Because of its complexity, home care is one area where one "needs to know enough to know what they do not know." For this reason, it is important that new or "startup" organizations, those new to home care and/or hospice and without an extensive knowledge of the industry, work with experienced peers or consultants to learn the complexities they may not be aware of. Similarly, this is also true for existing organizations having challenges. The financial, operational, clinical, or other consultants should be credentialed and experienced in dealing with the regulations.

The daily operations must "work" to be effective, and the organization needs to have good leadership with quick and effective decision-making capabilities in order to address problems or glitches as they arise. And arise they will and do. Of course, great team members such as clerical, administrative, intake team members, sales representatives, business development specialists, receptionists, coders, medical records, clinical leaders, quality assurance and performance improvement (QAPI), human resource, billers, and more must work together to keep the functions up-to-date and on point. This is because home care and hospice at home are all about people and their care, and at some of the most vulnerable times in their lives. They may be very sick and (appropriately) very stressed, so it is not solely a people business but one of competent clinical excellence that incorporates relationship-building from the patient's perspective at their first call or contact and continues throughout the entire time the patient is cared for by the organization.

And we must think from that patient and family perspective. At this (usually) difficult time and circumstance, the patient is initially considering and then allowing home care or hospice at home to come into their world. Think again about the fact that we are usually "total" strangers at first, and they allow us into their sacred space: the place they call their home. This is one reason that home care is said to be a very "small" world, where reputation and references can make all the difference. All who choose to manage or practice in home care must do their best to value behaviorally this trust and honor the privilege of providing care in the patient's home.

Definition of Medicare Home Health Services

Along with the previously mentioned important daily operations of business comes the structure of law and relevant promulgated regulations related to home care services. Reading and understanding how regulators view home care and their expectations of home care organizations is foundational to success. Medicare was enacted in 1965 under President Lyndon B. Johnson. Title XVIII of the Social Security Act (SSA) is administered by CMS and the following information is from Title XVIII—Health Insurance for the Aged and Disabled (Section 1861).

The definition of *home health services* is: "(1) part-time or intermittent nursing care provided by or under the supervision of a registered professional nurse; (2) physical or occupational therapy or speech-language pathology services; (3) medical social services under the direction of a physician; (4) to the extent permitted in regulations, part-time or intermittent services of a home health aide who has successfully completed a training program approved by the Secretary; (5) medical supplies (including catheters, catheter supplies, ostomy bags, and supplies related to ostomy care, and a covered osteoporosis drug (as defined in subsection (kk)), but excluding other drugs and biologicals) and durable medical equipment while under such a plan; (6) in the case of a home health agency which is affiliated or under common control with a hospital, medical services provided by an intern or resident-in-training of such hospital, under a teaching program of such hospital approved as provided in the last sentence of subsection (b); and (7) any of the foregoing items and services which are provided on an outpatient basis, under arrangements made by the home health agency, at a hospital or skilled nursing facility, or at a rehabilitation center which meets such standards as may be prescribed in regulations, and—(A) the furnishing of which involves the use of equipment of such a nature that the items and services cannot readily be made available to the individual in such place of residence, or (B) which are furnished at such facility while he is there to receive any such item or service described in clause (A)" (SSA, n.d.).

They define "home health agency" as a "a public agency or private organization, or a subdivision of such an agency or organization" (SSA, n.d., para. 14). According to this same document, this organization "(1) is primarily engaged in providing skilled nursing services and other therapeutic services; (2) has policies, established by a group of professional personnel (associated with the agency or organization), including one or more physicians and one or more registered professional nurses, to govern the services (referred to in paragraph (1)) which it provides, and provides for supervision of such services by a physician or registered professional nurse; (3) maintains clinical records on all patients; (4) in the case of an agency or organization in any State in which State or applicable local law provides for the licensing of agencies or organizations of this nature, (A) is licensed pursuant to such law, or (B) is approved, by the agency of such State or locality responsible for licensing agencies or organizations of this nature, as meeting the standards established for such licensing; (5) has in effect an overall plan and budget that meets the requirements of subsection (z); (6) meets the conditions of participation specified in section 1891(a) and such other conditions of participation as the Secretary may find necessary in the interest of the health and safety of individuals who are furnished services by such agency or organization; (7) provides the Secretary with a surety bond—(A) effective for a period of 4 years (as specified by the Secretary) or in the case of a change in the ownership or control of the agency (as determined by the Secretary) during or after such 4-year period, an additional period of time that the Secretary determines appropriate, such additional period not to exceed 4 years from the date of such change in ownership or control; (B) in a form specified by the Secretary; and (C) for a year in the period described in subparagraph (A) in an amount that is equal to the lesser of $50,000 or 10 percent of the aggregate amount of payments to the agency under this title and title XIX for that year, as estimated by the Secretary that Secretary determines is commensurate with the volume of the billing of the supplier; and (8) meets such additional requirements (including conditions relating to bonding or establishing of escrow accounts as the Secretary finds necessary for the financial security of the program) as the Secretary finds necessary for the effective and efficient operation of the program; except that for purposes of Part A such term shall not include any agency or organization which is primarily for the care and treatment of mental diseases. The Secretary may waive the requirement of a surety bond under paragraph (7) in the case of an agency or organization that provides a comparable surety bond under State law" (SSA, n.d., para. 14).

In addition, "CMS periodically issues regulations to codify policies based on statutory provisions of the SSA. Regulations come in several forms, including the following:

- "Notice of Proposed Rulemaking (NPRM) that proposes policy approaches to implementing provisions of the statute and solicits public comment on the proposals.

- "Interim Final Rule with comments goes into effect when it is published, but will be open for public comment for a specific period of time and then potentially revised and issued as a Final Rule.

- "Final Rules take comments into consideration and formally codify policies that were proposed in the NPRM or IFC" (Medicaid.gov, n.d.).

It is important to note that later in this chapter in that definition of "Home Health Agency" there is link 1891(a) that brings one to the Medicare Conditions of Participation that an agency must understand and adhere to/practice in intent and content to be a participating agency with Medicare or Medicaid.

Home Health Services

(m) The term *home health services* means the following items and services furnished to an individual, who is under the care of a physician, by a home health agency or by others under arrangements with them made by such agency, under a plan (for furnishing such items and services to such individual) established and periodically reviewed by a physician, which items and services are, except as provided in paragraph (7), provided on a visiting basis in a place of residence used as such individual's home—

(1) Part-time or intermittent nursing care provided by or under the supervision of a registered professional nurse;

(2) Physical or occupational therapy or speech-language pathology services;

(3) Medical social services under the direction of a physician;

(4) To the extent permitted in regulations, part-time or intermittent services of a home health aide who has successfully completed a training program approved by the Secretary;

(5) Medical supplies (including catheters, catheter supplies, ostomy bags, and supplies related to ostomy care, and a covered osteoporosis drug (as defined in subsection (kk)), but excluding other drugs and biologicals) and durable medical equipment while under such a plan;

(6) In the case of a home health agency which is affiliated or under common control with a hospital, medical services provided by an intern or resident-in-training of such hospital, under a teaching program of such hospital approved as provided in the last sentence of subsection (b); and

(7) Any of the foregoing items and services which are provided on an outpatient basis, under arrangements made by the home health agency, at a hospital or skilled nursing facility, or at a rehabilitation center which meets such standards as may be prescribed in regulations, and:

(A) The furnishing of which involves the use of equipment of such a nature that the items and services cannot readily be made available to the individual in such place of residence, or

(B) Which are furnished at such facility while he is there to receive any such item or service described in clause (A), but not including transportation of the individual in connection with any such item or service; excluding, however, any item or service if it would not be included under subsection (b) if furnished to an inpatient of a hospital. For purposes of paragraphs (1) and (4), the term "part–time or intermittent services" means skilled nursing and home health aide services furnished any number of days per week as long as they are furnished (combined) less than 8 hours each day and 28 or fewer hours each week (or, subject to review on a case-by-case basis as to the need for care, less than 8 hours each day and 35 or fewer hours per week). For purposes of sections 1814(a)(2)(C) and 1835(a)(2)(A), "intermittent" means skilled nursing care that is either provided or needed on fewer than 7 days each week, or less than 8 hours of each day for periods of 21 days or less (with extensions in exceptional circumstances when the need for additional care is finite and predictable).

Home Health Agency

(o) The term *home health agency* means a public agency or private organization, or a subdivision of such an agency or organization, which:

(1) Is primarily engaged in providing skilled nursing services and other therapeutic services;

(2) Has policies, established by a group of professional personnel (associated with the agency or organization), including one or more physicians and one or more registered professional nurses, to govern the services (referred to in paragraph (1)) which it provides, and provides for supervision of such services by a physician or registered professional nurse;

(3) Maintains clinical records on all patients;

(4) In the case of an agency or organization in any State in which State or applicable local law provides for the licensing of agencies or organizations of this nature, (A) is licensed pursuant to such law, or

(B) is approved, by the agency of such State or locality responsible for licensing agencies or organizations of this nature, as meeting the standards established for such licensing;

(5) Has in effect an overall plan and budget that meets the requirements of subsection (z);

(6) Meets the conditions of participation specified in section 1891(a) and such other conditions of participation as the Secretary may find necessary in the interest of the health and safety of individuals who are furnished services by such agency or organization;

(7) Provides the Secretary with a surety bond:

(A) Effective for a period of 4 years (as specified by the Secretary) or in the case of a change in the ownership or control of the agency (as determined by the Secretary) during or after such 4-year period, an additional period of time that the Secretary determines appropriate, such additional period not to exceed 4 years from the date of such change in ownership or control;

(B) In a form specified by the Secretary; and

(C) For a year in the period described in subparagraph (A) in an amount that is equal to the lesser of $50,000 or 10 percent of the aggregate amount of payments to the agency under this title and title XIX for that year, as estimated by the Secretary that Secretary determines is commensurate with the volume of the billing of the supplier; and

(8) Meets such additional requirements (including conditions relating to bonding or establishing of escrow accounts as the Secretary finds necessary for the financial security of the program) as the Secretary finds necessary for the effective and efficient operation of the program; except that for purposes of Part A such term shall not include any agency or organization which is primarily for the care and treatment of mental diseases. The Secretary may waive

the requirement of a surety bond under paragraph (7) in the case of an agency or organization that provides a comparable surety bond under State law. (Social Security Administration [SSA], n.d.)

These definitions are the basis for the regulatory and other directives that come from CMS and their contractors, or Medicare Administrative Contractors (MACs) (See Appendix C, beginning on p. 301, for a map of the MAC areas). Some people still use the term fiscal intermediary (FI) or Regional Home Health Intermediaries (RHHI) from days when Medicare had specialty contractors who provided medical review and claims process for Medicare Part A home care and hospice providers that were defined by region. MAC is the correct and updated term. The overall purpose of MACs is to educate providers, process, and conduct billing-related activities, endeavor to correct inappropriate billing, and recover payments. However, there are also other entities that provide program integrity (PI) processes and activities to be sure that care and billing is appropriate and covered.

The Medicare monies and the trust fund belong to all of us. We should all have an interest in how these monies are allocated, spent, and/or misspent. The following sections address some of the initiatives that are occurring to identify fraud in healthcare. Sadly, these activities are sometimes reported about home care and hospice, as discussed next.

A Fundamental View of Additional Regulators in Home Care and Hospice Practice

Based on the previous section, it is clear that Medicare contracts with specialty businesses, such as insurance companies, MACs, or other contractors, to provide medical review, process claims, and handle other activities that the government outlines in specific scopes of work (SOW). Added to this can be specialty contractors such as Zone

Program Integrity Contractors (ZPICs). According to CMS, the primary mission of ZPICs is to "identify cases of suspected fraud, develop them thoroughly and in a timely manner, and take immediate action to ensure that the Medicare Trust Fund monies are not inappropriately paid out and that any mistaken payments are recouped" (American Health Care Association, n.d., para. 1). The CMS has a specific "Program Integrity Manual," which can be accessed at https://www.cms.gov/Regulations-and-Guidance/Guidance/Manuals/downloads/pim83c06.pdf.

Because CMS administers the Medicare program, this agency has many responsibilities, including management related to audits and/or overpayment prevention and recovery, as well as development and monitoring of payment safeguards. These safeguards are necessary to detect and respond to payment errors or abusive patterns of service delivery and to be sure that care is appropriate and covered. In addition, the Department of Justice and attorneys from the United States Attorney's office in the states have a criminal and civil authority to prosecute providers.

The Federal Bureau of Investigation (FBI) also investigates potential healthcare fraud under a special Memorandum of Understanding where the FBI has direct access to contractor data and other records to the same extent. "Fraud and abuse in the Medicaid program may occur in many different forms, including, but not limited to, the following: Medical identity theft; Billing for unnecessary services or items; Billing for services or items not rendered; Upcoding; Unbundling; Billing for non-covered services or items; Kickbacks; and Beneficiary fraud" (CMS, 2015b, p. 4).

The OIG summarizes its work twice a year in a report to Congress. Managers should review this information on an ongoing basis. In addition, an "OIG Work Plan" is released every fall for the following year. This is also important information on areas of concern and focus. A review of the "Criminal and Civil Enforcement" reports for January 2016 listed some of the following fraudulent actions related to Medicare and Medicaid services, including (OIG, n.d.-a):

- Not skilled, reasonable, or necessary services
- False and fraudulent claims
- Unnecessary treatment
- Undocumented services
- Miscoding claims
- Overbilling
- Conspiracy to defraud
- Kickbacks and bribes
- Not medically necessary
- False home healthcare certifications
- Services provided to patients who were not confined to their homes

Sadly, this list includes clinical directors, coders, therapists, physicians, recruiters, billers, and other roles and titles. It is obviously prudent to know the rules, and, if you do not know, find someone who does. For this reason there are numerous resources, especially the government website, where needed information can be found and reviewed with a few clicks. CMS and OIG websites are listed in the references and "For Further Reading" section at the end of this chapter.

In addition, the OIG investigates suspected fraud and abuse and performs audits and inspections of CMS programs. They may request information or assistance from CMS and its ZPICs, as well as the Quality Improvement Organizations (QIOs) at the state level.

> A Quality Improvement Organization (QIO) is a group of health quality experts, clinicians, and consumers organized to improve the care delivered to people with Medicare. (CMS, 2016, para. 1)

OIG has access to CMS files, records, and data as well as contractors. The OIG investigates suspected fraud and develops cases. The OIG has the authority to take action against individual healthcare providers, in the form of civil monetary payment (CMP) and program exclusion, and it can also refer cases to the Department of Justice (DOJ) for criminal or civil action. Readers are referred to the "Program Integrity Manual" and other manuals and government websites for more information and to review some of the specific areas of concern and interest:

- http://oig.hhs.gov/fraud/enforcement/criminal

- http://oig.hhs.gov/fraud/strike-force

- https://www.cms.gov/Regulations-and-Guidance/Guidance/ Manuals/Downloads/bp102c07.pdf

Because there were some areas of the country that seem to have overutilization, there is an FBI strike force addressing this concern and their offices are located in Los Angeles, Chicago, Dallas, South Texas, Detroit, South Louisiana, Tampa, Miami, and Brooklyn (OIG, n.d.-b).

Supportive Actions and Resources

Prudent providers are aware of regulatory requirements as well as the external environment in which one practices; it behooves all of us to know the rules and regulations and adhere to them. In addition, read the rules and become knowledgeable about them. If the organization provides services through Medicaid or other state-based care initiatives, understand the requirements and related information for all of those services. The OIG also offers helpful resources and information on their website. This includes information about "Compliance 101" at http:// oig.hhs.gov/compliance/101/.

Consider joining your state home care or hospice association; they will usually know the specific rules for their state's programs. State, national, and international associations and their executive directors and team members are very knowledgeable about home care, hospice, and the trends they are seeing in their states. Refer to Appendix A for a listing of the state, national, and international associations, the executive directors, and websites. Joining your state association and regularly checking their website can help you keep apprised of changes in the field and stay up-to-date.

Organizations should also develop and use compliance plans. Though outside the scope of this book, there are many resources related to compliance on the OIG and CMS websites. The OIG compliance guidelines are located at http://oig.hhs.gov/compliance/compliance-guidance/index. asp. Managers, clinicians, and other team members are encouraged to know the rules and do the right thing.

Other government agencies that are involved in home care and hospice at home are the Occupational Safety and Health Administration (OSHA); the Centers for Disease Control and Prevention (CDC); and the individual states' practice acts, such as for nurses, therapists, and others. There may also be state licensure and other state-based regulations. HIPAA laws, the Family Medical Leave Act (FMLA), civil rights laws, and other labor laws may also be involved. In addition, there are the state Medicaid programs, and these have their own rules and nuances as well as processes to determine overutilization, inappropriate billing, etc. Again, your associations and their executive directors are very knowledgeable about home care and the trends they are seeing.

CMS "maintains oversight for compliance with the Medicare health and safety standards" for numerous health-related organizations, including home health agencies and hospices (CMS, 2013, para. 1). "The survey (inspection) for this determination is done on behalf of CMS by the individual State Survey Agencies. The functions the States perform for CMS under the agreements in Section 1864 of the Social Security Act (the Act) are referred to collectively as the certification process. This includes but is not limited to:

1. **Identifying potential participants:** Payment for health services furnished in or by entities that meet stipulated requirements of the Act. Identification includes those laboratories seeking to participate in the CLIA program.

2. **Conducting investigations and fact-finding surveys:** Verifying how well the healthcare entities comply with the 'conditions of participation' (CoPs) or requirements. This is referred to as the 'survey process.'

3. **Certifying and recertifying:** Certifications are periodically sent to the appropriate Federal or State agencies regarding whether entities, including CLIA laboratories, are qualified to participate in the programs.

4. **Explaining requirements:** Advising providers and suppliers, and potential providers and suppliers in regard to applicable Federal regulations to enable them to qualify for participation in the programs and to maintain standards of healthcare consistent with the CoPs and Conditions for Coverage (CfCs) requirements." (CMS, 2013)

The states have "Bureaus of Health Facility Regulation," which, simply put, are state government entities that regulate and oversee various aspects of healthcare and the provision of care across a state. For example, in Florida this is the Agency for Health Care Administration (AHCA). AHCA employs state surveyors who are nurses experienced in the area for which they will survey organizations. For example, a nurse surveyor may come onsite and visit an organization that is seeking Medicare certification. Another example might be a nurse surveyor going onsite to an organization that has already been Medicare-certified when the state receives a call from a patient or family about a care-related problem.

These become complaints, and a "complaint survey" is initiated when the state receives them. A specialized nurse surveyor will arrive (unannounced) at the organization, and the state requirements and Medicare CoPs will be used as the benchmark against which the complaint will be investigated and addressed.

There are also specific state licensure laws for professionals and also may be state laws about varying aspects of home care, hospice, and other services provided at home. These requirements also vary by state, including who can do or provide what services and further information on state-specific rules. State laws might include the credentials of who can be an administrator in that specific state within home care or hospice, what qualifications and length and type of experience might be mandated to qualify to be a clinical director in home care, and other state-specific rules about credentials and qualifications for other positions. In some states, for nurses to practice or be hired in home care, they may be required to have worked a minimum number of years before going into home care, and they may also be required to have worked those years in a specific setting(s)—such as in a hospital or other inpatient setting. This experiential background makes sense given the autonomous role in home care, where one cannot ask questions of an experienced colleague onsite, as they can in the hospital. There are also state laws related to the professional scope of practice. Always check your state and the details of the state laws related to your practice in that state.

There are also accreditation bodies in home care and hospice. If Medicare certification is the first step for providing an initial or first level of standardized quality of care in home care and hospice, then accreditation is the next step. There are three main accreditation bodies in home care and hospice. These accreditation bodies are listed in alphabetical order:

- The Accreditation Commission for Health Care (ACHC) (www.achc.org)

- The Community Health Accreditation Program (CHAP) (www.chapinc.org)

- The Joint Commission (TJC) (https://www.jointcommission.org/)

The accreditation bodies have standards that must be met for an organization to become accredited. In addition, the accreditation bodies can "deem" home care and hospice organizations in states where this is allowed. For example, instead of the state surveyor coming onsite for the survey, the survey visit might be made by professionals from the accreditation body. "Deemed status may be requested by the HHA from an accreditation organization. The term 'deemed status' means that the HHA is found to meet the Medicare CoPs during an unannounced survey conducted by the accrediting organization. Check with your Home Health Agency's state governing body for specifics regarding deemed status for your state" (Allen, 2014, p. 25).

HOME CARE NURSING
HHQI [HOME HEALTH QUALITY IMPROVEMENT]: FREE QUALITY IMPROVEMENT RESOURCES FOR ALL

Since 2007, CMS's Home Health Quality Improvement (HHQI) National Campaign has been dedicated to improving the quality of care provided to America's home health patients. All HHQI resources are free, available for everyone, and include:

- **Education.** HHQI provides evidence-based multimedia resources covering a wide range of topics that include cardiovascular health, diabetes, immunization and infection prevention, patient self-management, acute care hospitalization, oral medication management, fall prevention, care transitions, underserved populations, and developing and implementing quality improvement programs and processes (including QAPI development). Many of these resources feature free Continuing Education credits.

- **Data.** The HHQI Data Access system ties home health provider actions to outcomes, all in a free, secure and easy-to-use online portal. Thousands of home health agencies are actively downloading individualized HHQI Data Access reports that show performance and trending related to acute care hospitalization, oral medication management, immunizations, cardiovascular prevention, and other measures.

- **Networking.** HHQI engages hundreds of local and national home health stakeholders to coordinate messaging related to home health quality improvement and connect the right people at the right time through strong partnerships. HHQI maintains these relationships through traditional grassroots means coupled with a wide array of social networking platforms, including LinkedIn, Facebook, Twitter, and Pinterest.

- **Assistance.** The HHQI team includes a deep pool of subject-matter experts and mechanisms to efficiently provide technical assistance to home health providers, both virtually and face-to-face. All HHQI assistance includes a key focus on underserved populations and small, non-profit home health agencies and those that serve a high proportion of health disparate patients.

HHQI's resources help home health agencies make a real difference in patients' health care and ultimately, their quality of life. Learn more at www.HomeHealthQuality.org or contact HHQI at HHQI@wvmi.org. Copyright Home Health Quality Improvement. Reprinted with permission.

Readers are encouraged to become familiar with accreditation, as it is another level of quality, and as the healthcare world moves toward value, it will be about quality and safety. In fact, TJC has promulgated "National Patient Safety Goals" (NPSGs) for some years, and some of these are very specific to home care and hospice at home. The nurse and other surveyors from these organizations are experienced and are great resources for questions about home care and practice and administration. I encourage you to learn all you can from these knowledgeable and committed colleagues. Remember to follow whichever rule is the highest or strictest standard to help meet all the numerous standards.

The Importance of Knowing the Rules: Medicare Requirements for Home Care

All home care team members must know and understand Medicare coverage. Other regulations governing care include the Medicare CoPs, the hospice CoPs, the state operations manual, and the Intermediary Manual.

There is a hospice-specific Medicare manual. The nuances of hospice care and coverage are outside of the purview of this book. The rules related to hospice care can be found in the Hospice section of the *Medicare Benefit Policy Manual*. For care and care planning purposes, readers are referred to *The Hospice and Palliative Care Handbook: Quality, Compliance, and Reimbursement* by Tina M. Marrelli.

A Medicare beneficiary must meet all of the following "qualifying" criteria to be covered under the Medicare home health benefit:

- Is eligible for Medicare;

- Is provided services by a Medicare-certified home health agency;

- Is homebound as defined by Medicare;

"Home Health Agency (HHA) services may only be ordered or referred by a Doctor of Medicine (M.D.), Doctor of Osteopathy (D.O.), or Doctor of Podiatric Medicine (DPM). Claims for HHA services ordered by any other practitioner specialty will be denied." (CMS, 2012, p. 4)

- Is provided services as defined in the "Home Health Agency Manual" and meets the specific coverage rules related to the six services (nursing, physical therapy [PT], occupational therapy [OT], speech/language pathology [SLP], medical social services [MSS], home health aide [HHA]);

- Is provided medically reasonable and necessary services; and

- Receives physician certification and oversight of the patient's POC.

About Physician Certification with Face-to-Face Encounters

Until April 2011, there were four longstanding physician certification requirements. As a result of federal legislation, these were expanded to include a fifth requirement mandating that a certifying physician attest that the patient had a face-to-face encounter with an approved physician or non-physician practitioner (NPP) 90 days prior to or within 30 days of any home health start of care.

Now, with this fifth requirement, the certifying physician must attest the following five things:

(1) "The patient needs intermittent skilled nursing (SN) care, physical therapy (PT), and/or speech-language pathology (SLP) services;

(2) "The patient is confined to the home (that is, homebound);

(3) "A HH POC has been established and will be periodically reviewed by a physician;

(4) "Services will be furnished while the individual was or is under the care of a physician; and

(5) "A face-to-face encounter:

   (a) Occurred no more than 90 days prior to the home health start of care date or within 30 days of the start of the home health care;

   (b) Was related to the primary reason the patient requires home health services; and

   (c) Was performed by a physician or allowed NPP." (CMS, 2015a, p. 4)

If all of these conditions are met, Medicare will pay for part-time or intermittent skilled nursing, physical, continuing occupational, and speech therapy; medical social services; and home health aide visits when patients qualify based on the need for skilled nursing or therapy. Beneficiaries are not liable for any co-insurance or deductibles for these services at this time and may receive an unlimited number of visits, provided the coverage criteria are met. Be aware that sometimes Medicare health maintenance organizations may restrict or otherwise change home care "rules." Readers are encouraged to stay up-to-date with Medicare and Medicaid changes and regulatory requirements, such as face-to-face encounter and other regulatory policies.

Detailed Certification Policy

The following information is important to note since medical review and audit initiatives have identified that the following area related to the community physician being identified is sometimes not clear in the documentation. There is a policy requirement that an in-patient physician identify the community physician who will be following the patient if that in-patient physician will be certifying the patient or home health.

30.5.1 - Physician Certification (Rev. 208, Issued: 04-22-15, Effective: 01-01-15, Implementation: 05-11-15)

"A certification (versus recertification) is considered to be anytime that a Start of Care OASIS is completed to initiate care. In such instances, a physician must certify (attest) that:

"1. The home health services are or were needed because the patient is or was confined to the home as defined in §30.1;

"2. The patient needs or needed skilled nursing services on an intermittent basis (other than solely venipuncture for the purposes of obtaining a blood sample), or physical therapy, or speech-language pathology services. Where a patient's sole skilled service need is for skilled oversight of unskilled services (management and evaluation of the care plan as defined in §40.1.2.2), the physician must include a brief narrative describing the clinical justification of this need as part of the certification, or as a signed addendum to the certification;

"3. A plan of care has been established and is periodically reviewed by a physician;

"4. The services are or were furnished while the patient is or was under the care of a physician;

"5. For episodes with starts of care beginning January 1, 2011 and later, in accordance with §30.5.1.1 below, a face-to-face encounter occurred no more than 90 days prior to or within 30 days after the start of the home health care, was related to the primary reason the patient requires home health services, and was performed by an allowed provider type. The certifying physician must also document the date of the encounter.

"If the patient is starting home health directly after discharge from an acute/post-acute care setting where the physician, with privileges, that cared for the patient in that setting is certifying the patient's eligibility for the home health benefit, but will not be following the patient after discharge, then the certifying physician must identify the community physician who will be following the patient after discharge. One of the criteria that must be met for a patient to be considered eligible for the home health benefit is that the patient must be under the care of a physician (number 4 listed above). Otherwise, the certification is not valid" (CMS, 2015c).

Homebound: A Major Qualifying Criterion

Homebound status is an essential qualifying requirement or criterion that must be met for Medicare coverage. The patient is either homebound and the POC is initiated, or the patient is identified as not being homebound or confined to the home as defined by Medicare and, therefore, cannot be admitted to the organization's home care program under the Medicare benefit. Thus, when performing the initial assessment, the clinician must identify the functional criteria that support the homebound status. The *"Medicare Homebound Policy"* as it appears in the *"Medicare Benefit Policy Manual"* is explained in the following section.

Medicare Homebound Policy

"30.1.1 - Patient Confined to the Home . . .

"For a patient to be eligible to receive covered home health that a physician certify in all cases that the patient is confined to his/her home. For purposes of the statute, an individual shall be considered 'confined to the home' (homebound) if the following two criteria are met:

"1. Criteria-One: "The patient must either:

- "Because of illness or injury, need the aid of supportive devices such as crutches, canes, wheelchairs, and walkers; the use of special transportation; or the assistance of another person in order to leave their place of residence

"OR

- "Have a condition such that leaving his or her home is medically contraindicated.

"If the patient meets one of the Criteria-One conditions, then the patient must ALSO meet two additional requirements defined in Criteria-Two below.

"2. Criteria-Two:

- "There must exist a normal inability to leave home;

"AND

- "Leaving home must require a considerable and taxing effort.

"If the patient does in fact leave the home, the patient may nevertheless be considered homebound if the absences from the home are infrequent or for periods of relatively short duration, or are attributable to the need to receive health care treatment. Absences attributable to the need to receive health care treatment include, but are not limited to:

- Attendance at adult day centers to receive medical care;

- Ongoing receipt of outpatient kidney dialysis; or

- The receipt of outpatient chemotherapy or radiation therapy."

"Any absence of an individual from the home attributable to the need to receive health care treatment, including regular absences for the purpose of participating in therapeutic, psychosocial, or medical treatment in an adult day-care program that is licensed or certified by a State, or accredited to furnish adult day-care services in a State, shall not disqualify an individual from being considered to be confined to his home. Any other absence of an individual from the home shall not so disqualify an individual if the absence is of an infrequent or of relatively short duration.

For purposes of the preceding sentence, any absence for the purpose of attending a religious service shall be deemed to be an absence of infrequent or short duration. It is expected that in most instances, absences from the home that occur will be for the purpose of receiving healthcare treatment. However, occasional absences from the home for nonmedical purposes, e.g., an occasional trip to the barber, a walk around the block or a drive, attendance at a family reunion, funeral, graduation, or other infrequent or unique event would not necessitate a finding that the patient is not homebound if the absences are undertaken on an infrequent basis or are of relatively short duration and do not indicate that the patient has the capacity to obtain the healthcare provided outside rather than in the home."

"Some examples of homebound patients that illustrate the factors used to determine whether a homebound condition exists are:

- "A patient paralyzed from a stroke who is confined to a wheelchair or requires the aid of crutches in order to walk.

- "A patient who is blind or senile and requires the assistance of another person in leaving their place of residence.

- "A patient who has lost the use of their upper extremities and, therefore, is unable to open doors, use handrails on stairways, etc., and requires the assistance of another individual to leave their place of residence.

- "A patient in the late stages of ALS or neurodegenerative disabilities. In determining whether the patient has the general inability to leave the home and leaves the home only infrequently or for periods of short duration, it is necessary (as is the case in determining whether skilled nursing services are intermittent) to look at the patient's condition over a period of time rather than for short periods within the home health stay. For example, a patient may leave the home *(meeting both criteria listed above)* more frequently during a short period when the *patient has multiple appointments with health care professionals and medical tests in 1 week*. So long as the patient's overall condition and experience is such that he or she meets these qualifications, he or she should be considered confined to the home.

- "A patient who has just returned from a hospital stay involving surgery, who may be suffering from resultant weakness and pain *because of the surgery* and; therefore, their actions may be restricted by their physician to certain specified and limited activities (such as getting out of bed only for a specified period of time, walking stairs only once a day, etc.).

- "A patient with arteriosclerotic heart disease of such severity that they must avoid all stress and physical activity.

- "A patient with a psychiatric illness that is manifested in part by a refusal to leave home or is of such a nature that it would not be considered safe for the patient to leave home unattended, even if they have no physical limitations.

- "The aged person who does not often travel from home because of feebleness and insecurity brought on by advanced age would not be considered confined to the home for purposes of receiving home health services unless they meet one of the above conditions.

"Although a patient must be confined to the home to be eligible for covered home health services, some services cannot be provided at the patient's residence because equipment is required that cannot be made available there. If the services required by an individual involve the use of such equipment, the HHA may make arrangements with a hospital, SNF, or a rehabilitation center to provide these services on an outpatient basis. (See §50.6.) However, even in these situations, for the services to be covered as home health services the patient must be considered confined to home *and meet both criteria listed above.*

"If a question is raised as to whether a patient is confined to the home, the HHA will be requested to furnish the *Medicare Contractor* with the information necessary to establish that the patient is homebound as defined above" (CMS, 2015c).

Information About Two Challenging Areas in Home Care

There are two areas in home care that can be particularly confusing. For this reason, here is information to better clarify (1) daily care and (2) management and evaluation of the plan of care (POC). When there are questions related to coverage, etc., refer them to your MAC for specific information.

Daily Care

A patient must receive nursing on an intermittent basis if that patient qualifies for home health based on their nursing needs. Medicare defines intermittent nursing as care delivered fewer than 7 days a week. However, Medicare will allow for part-time medically reasonable and necessary daily skilled nursing care (one or more times a day, 7 days a week) for a short period of time (two to three weeks), and will pay for daily nursing for longer periods of time if there is a realistic, finite, and predictable endpoint to the need for daily care. As soon as the patient's physician makes this judgment, which usually should be made before the end of the 3-week period, the HHA must forward medical documentation justifying the need for such additional services and include an estimate of how much longer daily skilled services will be required.

Physician orders must specify the need and the estimated endpoint whenever providing daily care (7 days a week) beyond 3 weeks, whether at admission or any other time during the course of care. The documentation in the record and on the plan of care, recertification or interim orders needs to support medical necessity and ensure the meeting of intermittent requirements. This endpoint must be finite and predictable. The estimated endpoint must be stated as a specific date or time period.

For example, "Daily RN visits until physician re-evaluates patient for further wound surgery on 2/22/16." Another example is "Daily for 3 months, or 02/01/16 to 05/01/16." The date that the 60-day certification period ends should not be randomly used as the endpoint for daily care. Rather, the date daily visits will no longer be necessary (end date) must be established by considering specific patient progress or patient/ caregiver behavior that will occur in order to reduce visits less often than daily. The estimated endpoint may be longer than 60 days if the physician believes that daily care will be needed for more than one certification period.

When establishing an endpoint to daily nursing with the physician, critically think/ask yourself the following:

- When will wound healing occur and/or care be less complex?
- When can the patient/caregiver be taught the procedure?
- What are the barriers to reducing care from daily to less often than daily?
- When/where can a willing and able caregiver be found?

When determining the projected date, it should be realistic based on the patient's unique medical condition—and that date is usually *not* the end of the episode. For example, if the patient has had a wound for 2 years and is referred to your HHA, it may not be realistic that the wound will now heal. In this case the patient may not be appropriate for home care because this patient may need a level of care (full time) that the Medicare program does not cover. Such cases need to be discussed with your manager.

If the initial orders were three-times-per-week skilled wound care and the physician increases these to daily, be sure to discuss and obtain a supplemental or telephone order with a projected endpoint in either a date format or a specific number of days or weeks. Be certain to include this updated order in the clinical record. Remember that it is only for daily visits and recertification that a finite, projected endpoint is needed.

Document progress or lack of progress and the specific clinical findings related to the wound and other problems having an impact on the care provided. For wound care patients, this includes accurate size, drainage, amount, character, presence of odor, etc.

If it is necessary to establish a new endpoint for daily visits when progress is not made as expected, document the patient's condition and provide the reason(s) why anticipated goals were not achieved. Establish, with the physician, a new endpoint for daily care and obtain revised orders. If orders are not changed, provide justification for continuing the original treatment plan.

Insulin administration is the only exception to daily intermittent care. Daily care to administer insulin does not require a specific endpoint. For unusual circumstances in which the patient is physically or mentally unable to self-inject and there is no available able and willing caregiver, the HHA can provide daily visits. The HHA must document efforts made to locate a caregiver. Of note, with the right equipment and circumstances, even blind persons with diabetes can be taught to give themselves insulin injections. (Adapted with permission from *Handbook of Home Health Standards: Quality, Documentation, and Reimbursement* by Tina M. Marrelli [2012]).

It is important to note that these cases usually trigger an in-depth medical review. This means that documentation must be specific and show efforts made to teach someone.

Management and Evaluation of the POC

According to the *Medicare Benefit Policy Manual,* skilled nursing visits for management and evaluation of the patient's care plan are considered to be reasonable and necessary where underlying conditions or complications require that only a registered nurse can ensure that essential *non-skilled* care is achieving its purpose. For skilled nursing care to be reasonable and necessary for management and evaluation of the patient's plan of care, the complexity of the *unskilled services* that are a necessary part of the medical treatment must require the involvement of skilled nursing personnel to promote the patient's recovery and medical safety in view of the patient's overall condition.

If Management and Evaluation (M&E) of unskilled services is the sole skilled nursing service being provided, an additional certification requirement must be met. The physician must certify that a patient's underlying condition or complication requires a registered nurse (RN) to ensure that essential *non-skilled care* is achieving its purpose, and the RN needs to be involved in the development, management, and evaluation of a patient's care plan. Further, the physician must include a brief narrative describing the clinical justification of this need. If the narrative is part of the certification, then the narrative must be located immediately prior to the physician's signature. If the narrative exists as an addendum to the certification, in addition to the physician's signature on the certification, the physician must sign immediately following the narrative in the addendum.

The following are typical issues that need to be addressed to determine that the patient is appropriate for M&E. In addition to the complexity of the unskilled care needs of the patient, the following evaluation of need and subsequent documentation may support M&E services:

- The patient's medical history
- Stability of the caregiver's support system
- Current or highly probable medical concerns based on past history

- Multiple medications listed on the POC indicating complex management issues

- Functional limitations that affect care

- Safety or other high-risk factors identified

- Unusual home and/or other environment

- Ordered disciplines and interventions

- Diagnoses and underlying pathologies that affect the POC

- Patient's and/or caregiver's mental status

- History of frequent hospitalizations

The clinician needs to assess and document the reason why nursing visits are required to observe and assess the effects of the non-skilled services being provided to treat the illness or injury until the patient recovers and to promote the patient's stabilization and/or (document evidence of movement toward patient goals) and ensure medical safety.

 Part Seven of the Medicare manual is located in the Medicare Benefit Policy Manual, Chapter 7, Section 30.1 (https://www.cms. gov/Regulations-and-Guidance/Guidance/Manuals/downloads/ bp102c07.pdf) for the Coverage section of the "Home Health Agency Manual" (see Appendix D). Readers are referred to this section for the specific services, skills, and information for care. Readers are also encouraged to review, understand, and operationalize care per the regulations.

Adapted with permission from *Handbook of Home Health Standards: Quality, Documentation, and Reimbursement* by Tina Marrelli (2012), 5th Edition.

Quality is being truly integrated into the process with the regulatory overview. OASIS, and the related information and outcomes, is another way to help home care team members interface with quality. Of course, documentation of care and related operational components supporting care are also reflections of the level of quality being provided by an organization. Documentation will be further addressed in Chapter 8, "Documentation of Care and Related Processes," beginning on p. 207. Quality is not "one thing" and should be integrated through all care and related processes, and this emphasis will continue. For example, in 2015, CMS released the first round of Home Health Compare quality of patient care star ratings to "show consumers how the performance of a home health agency compares to other agencies" (Medicare.gov, n.d.-b). These ratings are displayed on Home Care Compare and are another step toward home health value-based purchasing initiatives (https://www.medicare.gov/homehealthcompare/).

I was a home care nurse manager when I worked for the Health Care Financing Administration (now called CMS central office) for 4 years. This made me better understand the scope of the Medicare and Part A world. I hope this primer on the multifaceted and complex nature of home care helps you better understand home care and practice and manage within it. The next chapter helps to put that knowledge of Medicare and other coverage and rules in action through a discussion of home visits. This will help integrate the complex knowledge of care, coverage, and visits into everyday practice.

Summary

Home care is complex and will continue to change. Quality is a part of value, and as value-based care becomes the watchword and norm, Medicare and Medicaid providers must know the rules and work toward improved quality for patients. Effective daily operations are key to quality patient care—if those are not working, disorganization and problems ensue, taking limited time and people resources from other, more constructive and important initiatives, such as quality assurance and performance improvement.

Complying with the rules and regulations is a part of the responsibilities of any role in healthcare, particularly home care and hospice. Medicare has specific manuals for programs, such as home care and hospice, and also program integrity manuals to help professionals better understand the big picture.

Questions for Further Consideration and Discussion

1. Where is the Medicare definition of homebound and the coverage of skilled services found?

2. List three government entities/agencies that provide oversight to home care and hospice and may be involved in identifying overutilization, fraud, etc.

3. After a review of the coverage section of the online Medicare Manual, what are five of the skilled nursing services listed and explained?

4. Who are the accreditation bodies in home care and hospice and what is accreditation?

5. What is the law that started Medicare and when was it initiated?

For Further Reading

- *Survivor! Ten Practical Steps to Survey Survival,* by Nancy Allen

- *Handbook of Home Health Standards and Documentation Guidelines for Reimbursement,* 5th Edition, by Tina Marrelli

- "Chemotherapy in Home Care: One Team's Performance Improvement Journey Toward Reducing Medication Errors" by

Brenda Ewen, Rhonda Combs, Carl Popelas, and Gail Faraone in *Home Healthcare Nurse*

- "A Comprehensive Fall Prevention Program for Assessment, Intervention, and Referral" by Gale Bucher, Pamela Szczerba, and Patricia Curtin in *Home Healthcare Nurse*, March 2007, Vol 25(3): pp. 174–183

- "Root Cause Analysis: Responding to a Sentinel Event" by Brenda M. Ewen and Gale Bucher in *Home Healthcare Nurse*, September 2013, Vol 31(8), pp. 435–443

- "Status of Home Health Care: 2015 and Beyond" by Tina Marrelli in *Handbook of Home Health Care Administration* (6th ed.) by Marilyn Harris (2017)

- Survey & Certification - General Information from CMS: https://www.cms.gov/Medicare/Provider-Enrollment-and-Certification/SurveyCertificationGenInfo/

- Inappropriate and Questionable Billing by Medicare Home Health Agencies from the OIG: http://oig.hhs.gov/oei/reports/oei-04-11-00240.pdf

- Program Integrity: Hospice Care from CMS: https://www.cms.gov/Medicare-Medicaid-Coordination/Fraud-Prevention/Medicaid-Integrity-Education/hospice.html

- Health Care Compliance Program Tips from the OIG: http://oig.hhs.gov/compliance/provider-compliance-training/files/Compliance101tips508.pdf

- Compliance Education Materials from the OIG: http://oig.hhs.gov/compliance/101/index.asp

- Home Health Care data from the CDC: http://www.cdc.gov/nchs/fastats/home-health-care.htm

- Program Integrity: Fraud, Waste & Abuse Toolkit - Healthcare Fraud and Program Integrity from CMS: https://www.cms.gov/Medicare-Medicaid-Coordination/Fraud-Prevention/Medicaid-Integrity-Education/fwa.html

- *Medicare Benefit Policy Manual* Chapter 7 - Home Health Services from CMS: https://www.cms.gov/Regulations-and-Guidance/Guidance/Manuals/downloads/bp102c07.pdf

- CMS National Training Program: https://www.cms.gov/outreach-and-education/training/cmsnationaltrainingprogram/

- Prospective Payment System for Home Health Agencies from the Electronic Code of Federal Regulations: http://www.ecfr.gov/cgi-bin/text-idx?SID=fae2d7efac48c5bbcb0934abf0c86651&mc=true&node=sp42.5.484.e&rgn=div6

- Home Health Services Under Hospital Insurance from the Electronic Code of Federal Regulations: http://www.ecfr.gov/cgi-bin/text-idx?SID=fae2d7efac48c5bbcb0934abf0c86651&mc=true&node=sp42.2.409.e&rgn=div6

References

Allen, N. (2014). *Survivor! Ten practical steps to survey survival* (3rd ed.). Jacksonville, FL: Solutions for Care, Inc. and Marrelli and Associates, Inc.

American Health Care Association. (n.d.). Zone program integrity contractors. Retrieved from https://www.ahcancal.org/facility_operations/integrity/Pages/Zone-Program-Integrity-Contractors.aspx

Centers for Medicare & Medicaid Services (CMS). (2013). Survey & certification—General information. Retrieved from https://www.cms.gov/Medicare/Provider-Enrollment-and-Certification/SurveyCertificationGenInfo/

Centers for Medicare & Medicaid Services (CMS). (2015a). The Medicare home health benefit. Retrieved from https://www.cms.gov/Outreach-and-Education/Medicare-Learning-Network-MLN/MLNProducts/Downloads/Home-Health-Benefit-Fact-Sheet-ICN908143.pdf

Centers for Medicare & Medicaid Services (CMS). (2015b). Fraud, waste, and abuse toolkit—Health care fraud and program integrity: An overview for providers. Retrieved from https://www.cms.gov/Medicare-Medicaid-Coordination/Fraud-Prevention/Medicaid-Integrity-Education/Downloads/fwa-overview-booklet.pdf

Centers for Medicare & Medicaid Services (CMS). (2015c). *Medicare benefit policy manual*, Chapter 7 - Home health services. Retrieved from https://www.cms.gov/Regulations-and-Guidance/Guidance/Manuals/downloads/bp102c07.pdf

Centers for Medicare & Medicaid Services (CMS). (2016). Quality improvement organizations. Retrieved from https://www.cms.gov/Medicare/Quality-Initiatives-Patient-Assessment-Instruments/QualityImprovementOrgs/index.html?redirect=/qualityimprovementorgs

Medicaid.gov. (n.d.-a) Federal policy guidance. Retrieved from https://www.medicaid.gov/federal-policy-guidance/federal-policy-guidance.html

Medicare.gov. (n.d.-b). Quality of patient care star ratings. Retrieved from https://www.medicare.gov/homehealthcompare/About/Patient-Care-Star-Ratings.html

Office of Inspector General (OIG). (n.d.-a). Criminal and civil enforcement. Retrieved from http://oig.hhs.gov/fraud/enforcement/criminal/

Office of Inspector General (OIG). (n.d.-b). Medicare fraud strike force. Retrieved from http://oig.hhs.gov/fraud/strike-force/

Social Security Administration (SSA). (n.d.). Title XVIII—Health insurance for the aged and disabled, Part E—Miscellaneous provisions. Retrieved from https://www.ssa.gov/OP_Home/ssact/title18/1861.htm

7

The Home Visit: The Important Unit of Care

Home care service and practice are directed toward home visits—the unit of value in home care. This includes intermittent visits, shifts and staffing hours, hospice home visits, "well-baby" visits, or other therapeutic models and time spent in the patient's home. As explained in Chapter 2 ("What Is Home Healthcare and Home Care Comprised of Exactly?"), there are many kinds of visits and services provided in home care under the broad umbrella term of "home care."

This chapter provides exemplar practices that incorporate processes and important details to better frame home visits so you can understand their importance. For organizational, operational, and practice reasons, types of visits will be discussed as well as tips for the three distinct parts of a visit:

- The previsit activities

- The home visit

- The postvisit activities

It is important to note that a visit or a patient encounter comprises all three of these parts regardless of the type of discipline or service.

There are a few kinds of home visits in home care. These include the visits to perform the comprehensive assessment, a "revisit" for continuing care, supervisory visits of the aides (or other team members as promulgated by state or other regulation), on-call visits, and discharge visits. Of course, Medicare sets many of the standards, and as Medicaid and other insurers align more closely with Medicare, it is important to be aware of this trend and these standards as changes continue.

This chapter also addresses care and care planning and how the nursing or care-planning process becomes integrated into visits and across time. The case example presented in this chapter integrates some of the complex factors that illustrate home care and home care practice's unique value.

The Previsit Activities

The previsit activities include these steps: 1) obtaining physician orders, 2) obtaining permission(s), 3) eliciting patient information and status, 4) gathering supplies, and 5) knowing the community.

Planning is an important component seen in all kinds of visit activities. The previsit activities entail phone calls and other communications. Like all interactions, make these communications "set the stage" for success. These communications also begin the interface that becomes the basis of the "patient experience." Of course there must be positive patient satisfaction, but as the healthcare world shifts toward the patient "experience," all team members have a role in this holistic approach that generates patient and family perceptions of satisfaction.

It is also very important to "get off "on the "right foot." This begins with the referral source, such as the hospital discharge planner and the physician who will be signing the initial orders and/or following the patient once that patient is back at home. The physician is also the professional with whom the home care nurse interacts to obtain orders and (perhaps) subsequent certifications and other patient-related communications. The right start is also important for the seemingly simple call made to the patient and family for permission to come and visit their home for the initial visit and to explain services, obtain consent, and provide care.

Try to view all these communications and interactions from a long(er)-term perspective as the move is made toward population health and care. Populations will be followed across time or longitudinally. This is a "mindset" change from the traditional view of home care as a "certification" or "60-day" period. Try not to view care that way anymore, if possible, because many patients may have ongoing needs, particularly the older adults with chronic care problems. Even though home care may intervene only when/if there is an exacerbation of symptoms or other problems necessitating care, the patient may still need the ongoing expertise of the home care nurse. This may also be true for children and young adults with medically complex care needs, as well as other patient populations.

It is best to plan for the visit with the most information that can be collected and verified. Usually, a referral or request for an assessment or possible care may come from the hospital discharge planner. Some home care agencies and hospices have a centralized intake process for new patients and families seeking care based on specialty geography and/or other factors. Such standardized processes help ensure verification of insurance, physician information, addresses, eligibility, licensure, and numerous other important details needed for a patient admission and care.

HOME CARE NURSING
PATIENT EXEMPLAR—MR. HINCKLEY

The home care agency, which in this example will be called "St. Elsewhere Home Health," was initially called with referring information as hospital discharge was anticipated for Mr. Hinckley in the next few days. The information was primarily demographic and did not have much detail on the specific care ordered and needed. Because of this, the clinical director (CD), an RN, called the hospital discharge planner to find out additional details.

NOTE: Collecting more information is always better when done prior to scheduling the initial assessment or evaluation home visit.

The CD also contacted the nurse on the hospital unit where Mr. Hinckley, the CD was told, had been an inpatient for almost three weeks. During that time, his "stay" was characterized as problematic because of an open wound on his left lower leg with pain, two falls, a urinary tract infection necessitating an indwelling catheter for 5 days, and bacterial pneumonia. The antibiotics used caused frequent diarrhea, which distressed Mr. Hinckley a great deal. In addition, the CD called and spoke with the physician who was Mr. Hinckley's local medical doctor for many years. All this information helped provide the basis for the needed care and started "painting a picture" of Mr. Hinckley as an individual and his unique care needs. This "painting of the picture" is important since it becomes the basis for effective documentation, which is addressed in the next chapter.

Step 1: Obtaining the Physician's Orders

Physician orders are listed first in this list of previsit activities for a number of reasons. Of course physician "orders" are just that and must be obtained timely for the provision of care that meets statutory and other regulatory requirements. These orders are also needed for billing purposes, etc. It is important to note that Medicare, Medicaid, and most other insurers are "medical" models of care, and as such, they require physician-directed orders for care. These orders may be called *verbal orders* (such as when obtaining initial orders as in the following example of Mr. Hinckley), and they may also be called *interim* or *telephone orders*. Organizations may have their own terms of usage, so it is important if you are new to home care or to an organization that clarity be provided at the organization where you work.

Whatever the role and discipline, the home care clinician works collaboratively with the physician about the patient to create the "Home Health Certification and Plan of Care (POC)." This is also sometimes called the physician plan of treatment (POT) and was previously called the HCFA-Form 485. The POC contains the data elements that are required to meet the certification requirements. They are numbered #1 through #28. See the sample "Home Health Certification and Plan of Care" form shown in Figure 7.1 for an example of this documentation.

The following sidebar is the language from the *Medicare Benefit Policy Manual* that addresses the use of verbal orders. This process is what usually happens and begins with the call illustrated in the example of Mr. Hinckley and obtaining verbal orders prior to the first home visit.

HOME CARE NURSING

Save To Web

Department of Health and Human Services
Centers for Medicare & Medicaid Services

Form Approved
OMB No. 0938-0357

HOME HEALTH CERTIFICATION AND PLAN OF CARE

1. Patient's HI Claim No.	2. Start Of Care Date	3. Certification Period		4. Medical Record No.	5. Provider No.
		From:	To:		

6. Patient's Name and Address

7. Provider's Name, Address and Telephone Number

8. Date of Birth	9. Sex ☐M ☐F

10. Medications: Dose/Frequency/Route (N)ew (C)hanged

11. ICD-10-CM	Principal Diagnosis	Date
12. ICD-10-CM	Surgical Procedure	Date
13. ICD-10-CM	Other Pertinent Diagnoses	Date

14. DME and Supplies	15. Safety Measures:
16. Nutritional Req.	17. Allergies:

18.A. Functional Limitations

1 ☐ Amputation 5 ☐ Paralysis 9 ☐ Legally Blind
2 ☐ Bowel/Bladder (Incontinence) 6 ☐ Endurance A ☐ Dysnea With Minimal Exertion
3 ☐ Contracture 7 ☐ Ambulation B ☐ Other (Specify)
4 ☐ Hearing 8 ☐ Speech

18.B. Activities Permitted

1 ☐ Complete Bedrest 6 ☐ Partial Weight Bearing A ☐ Wheelchair
2 ☐ Bedrest BRP 7 ☐ Independent At Home B ☐ Walker
3 ☐ Up As Tolerated 8 ☐ Crutches C ☐ No Restrictions
4 ☐ Transfer Bed/Chair 9 ☐ Cane D ☐ Other (Specify)
5 ☐ Exercises Prescribed

19. Mental Status:

1 ☐ Oriented 3 ☐ Forgetful 5 ☐ Disoriented 7 ☐ Agitated
2 ☐ Comatose 4 ☐ Depressed 6 ☐ Lethargic 8 ☐ Other

20. Prognosis: 1 ☐ Poor 2 ☐ Guarded 3 ☐ Fair 4 ☐ Good 5 ☐ Excellent

21. Orders for Discipline and Treatments (Specify Amount/Frequency/Duration)

22. Goals/Rehabilitation Potential/Discharge Plans

23. Nurse's Signature and Date of Verbal SOC Where Applicable:	25. Date HHA Received Signed POT

24. Physician's Name and Address	26. I certify/recertify that this patient is confined to his/her home and needs intermittent skilled nursing care, physical therapy and/or speech therapy or continues to need occupational therapy. The patient is under my care, and I have authorized the services on this plan of care and will periodically review the plan.
27. Attending Physician's Signature and Date Signed	28. Anyone who misrepresents, falsifies, or conceals essential information required to payment of Federal funds may be subject to fine, imprisonment, or civil penalty under applicable Federal laws.

Form 3485R/4P BRIGGS, Des Moines, IA 50306 (800) 247-2343 R503 PRINTED IN U.S.A.

Form CMS-485 (C-3) (02-94)
(Formerly HCFA-485) (Print Aligned)

Figure 7.1 Home Health Certification and Plan of Care Form
Copyright © 2004 Briggs Healthcare. Reprinted with permission.

HOME CARE NURSING
MEDICARE BENEFIT POLICY MANUAL,
CHAPTER 7—HOME HEALTH SERVICES

"30.2.5 - Use of Oral (Verbal) Orders (Rev. 208, Issued: 04-22-15, Effective: 01-01-15, Implementation: 05-11-15) When services are furnished based on a physician's oral order, the orders may be accepted and put in writing by personnel authorized to do so by applicable State and Federal laws and regulations as well as by the HHA's internal policies. The orders must be signed and dated with the date of receipt by the registered nurse or qualified therapist (i.e., physical therapist, speech-language pathologist, occupational therapist, or medical social worker) responsible for furnishing or supervising the ordered services. The orders may be signed by the supervising registered nurse or qualified therapist after the services have been rendered, as long as HHA personnel who receive the oral orders notify that nurse or therapist before the service is rendered. Thus, the rendering of a service that is based on an oral order would not be delayed pending signature of the supervising nurse or therapist. Oral orders must be countersigned and dated by the physician before the HHA bills for the care in the same way as the plan of care.

"Services which are provided from the beginning of the 60-day episode certification period based on a request for anticipated payment and before the physician signs the plan of care are considered to be provided under a plan of care established and approved by the physician where there is an oral order for the care prior to rendering the services which is documented in the medical record and where the services are included in a signed plan of care"(CMS, 2015, p. 27).

Step 2: Obtaining Permission

There must be permission(s) from the patient and/or family, depending on the patient's age, mental status, etc., stating, in essence, that it is okay to visit and that they give permission or consent for the nurse or other team members to come to the home. This is an important part of patient rights, and patients can refuse care or any part of care at any time. Patients are equal partners in care and care planning, if not the most important partner, so their "buy-in" and "want-to" is key to successful care and improved outcomes. Of course, while at the first visit, a formal consent (and form) will be explained and signed prior to any hands-on care. (And again, assuming verbal or signed physician orders are obtained!)

This is also the time to ask about pets and ask that they be placed outside of the patient area, or where the nurse will be providing care, when the nurse is visiting. This aspect of home care is explained more fully in Chapter 5, "The Environment of Care: The Home and Community Interface," beginning on p. 95. Pets that are sometimes described as "sweet" or that "wouldn't hurt a fly" can be/become very aggressive when a stranger, such as a home care team member, comes into their "space" seeking to care for and touch their owners. Be careful.

Step 3: Eliciting Patient Information and Status

Once permission is obtained to visit the patient, it is very important to determine how the patient is feeling and doing once they are back at home. If all is okay, the visit is scheduled in a timely fashion. This is also the time to ask that all discharge papers, written instructions, and medications be gathered for the home visit. In home care and hospice at home, "medications," for purposes of a medication reconciliation and review processes, include prescriptions, over-the-counter medications, salves, herbs, vitamins, and more. This also includes PRN or as-needed items such as laxatives, pain remedies, sleeping aids, and others. Also check your organization's policy related to medications and medication safety. If the organization is accredited, there may also be a policy about and a list of "high-risk" medications.

Sometimes the patient may have been discharged and is waiting for the nurse to call. The patient may have distressing symptoms, such as being in pain or other problems, and be unsure of what to do, so they are waiting for that home care nurse call. While on the phone with patients or family members, ask for more information. Listening skills are a very important part of the effective and skillful home care and hospice nurse's toolkit. Did their prescriptions get filled? Are they being taken as directed? Is there food in the house if they live alone and are essentially bed- or chair-bound or if they are very frail or debilitated post-discharge? They may not be able to perform these important daily activities depending on their status (this may trigger consideration of the need for an aide to assist with personal care and activities of daily living [ADLs]).

As the home care nurse or therapist, it is important that such questions are asked respectfully and kindly. Sometimes symptoms must be probed further to help identify if the patient needs another level of care, such as to speak with or be evaluated by the physician. The best questioning leaves time for silences for the patient and family members to gather their thoughts and provide the best information. Remember, this is usually a stressful time for patients and families. They may be exhausted, especially as family members may have been at the hospital for days at a time. They may also be overwhelmed with the responsibilities that being a caregiver entails.

Though we try to keep patients at home and out of the emergency department or prevent a rehospitalization, sometimes when a patient is called, it is identified that there is "something going on" that should be further evaluated. This is another example of where good communication with the physician and office team is very helpful in "getting through" and being able to advocate for patients. This aspect of home care is ongoing and all about relationship-building and, sometimes, persistence.

Whoever talks to the patient or their friends or caregivers from the office, and whatever their title or role, it is very important that patients and family members are always treated with dignity and respect. Sometimes it helps to be empathetic, e.g., place ourselves in their "shoes" or place. Think how hard it might be to be dependent on care from someone else and have "strangers" (in essence, and especially at first) coming into your home and space every day, for example, in a patient with complex problems or in the case of shifts or hourly skilled care for a medically fragile child or young adult.

 From a personal perspective as a long-time home care nurse, it was even an adjustment for me to have caregivers come into our home to care for a very frail and ill 96-year-old who lived with us. Even though the team members were "great" (and they were very good), it can still be a difficult change—from privacy and other perspectives. There is someone in your home and in your personal spaces.

For this reason, it is a good idea for you to ask family members for any dos and don'ts on the first visit or care encounter. For example, the patient or family may want you to remove your shoes upon entering the home. Another example is that I never place my purse anywhere in the kitchen area for infection control and prevention reasons. I made that clear to the caregivers and made spaces elsewhere in the house that were solely for the caregivers and their things, such as purses and lunches/dinners/snacks. Keep in mind that there can sometimes be a negotiation as to where in the home the "visit" takes place. This is because the clinician needs a clean place to spread out the barrier and have a quiet space when talking to the patient and family. Such communications and clarity helps "set" the stage for a great relationship and clear communication, too.

When calling to set up an initial assessment/evaluation appointment, check in and ask how the patient is "doing" and feeling. The transition time back to home can be fraught with risk depending on the patient and circumstances. It is for this reason that the "timely initiation of care" is such an important process measure for quality and safety reasons. Of course, if onsite, the physician's office would be called for a concern or a change in condition, such as a fall, new fever, changing symptoms, etc., like in any other circumstance in home care.

Because of this, critical thinking, clinical reasoning, and ongoing evaluation and assessment are key components of the best home care and home care clinicians. It is for this reason that nurses in home care need experience prior to home care to be able to determine, identify, and communicate nuanced changes in patients. This requires impeccable and detailed assessment skills and is one of the areas where you have "to know enough to know" when you do not know something and need to reach out for help. Some organizations have very detailed orientation programs for "residencies" for nurses new to home care or entering a new specialty in home care.

Also, call your supervisor in these instances when the patient is "not okay" since being discharged back to home and whenever you are concerned. The supervisor can provide direction and guidance.

Step 4: Gathering Supplies

This step includes the forms for an admission or evaluation/assessment visit. Depending on the kind of home visit and payer/insurance, there may be varying forms and other paperwork. If Medicare or Medicaid (depending on the rules) is involved, there will be the OASIS-C tool, and this tool is often embedded into a comprehensive assessment form. This is important to note because the OASIS is just a part of a comprehensive assessment of a patient. Since the home care team is discussed later in this chapter, it is important to note that the other team members and disciplines also have their own unique discipline-specific assessment tools and visit records. Such tools are integrated into the following information for ease of understanding and to help explain the scope of these roles so that the admission nurse or therapist can identify a need for other team members when appropriate.

The nurse would usually also carry some standard supplies, such as a blood pressure cuff (sized appropriately for the patient), a stethoscope, and a thermometer with thermometer covers. Personal protective equipment (PPE), which is a foundation of infection control and prevention, should also be brought with you and includes gloves, soap, paper towels, alcohol-based hand cleanser, masks (when needed), and others. Hand cleansers, barrier shields, and other supplies would also usually be in the "visit bag."

Effective hand hygiene is a hallmark of effective home care visiting. Keep in mind that the nurse and other team members are role models for hand hygiene and numerous other aspects of care. The patient and caregivers will see the team as doing things "the way they should," so be great role models!

Review the patient's referral information carefully for what would be needed on this first visit. For example, if the patient has an indwelling catheter and insertion kit, or might need one given a history like Mr. Hinckley's, consider carrying one of those, too (hopefully, in the history and physical that was obtained from the referring hospital, it was specified the type and size of the catheter used while he was an inpatient). In that way, you would have the necessary equipment and would only need to call the physician for the order to use the catheter and the specific orders related to the catheter—including PRN orders, such as for pain, dislodgement, or other catheter-related problems. Because Mr. Hinckley had a wound on his leg, the dressing that was specified on the discharge plans and/or in the verification of the orders taken on the phone would also need to be brought along.

Always check when told that "everything was sent home for his first visit, including wound care supplies." Verify this before the visit by calling the patient/caregiver and asking if the needed supplies are there or if you need to bring them with you. Supplies are an important part of home care practice—especially when you do not have what is needed at the home! Like any orders, these are specified in the physician orders. The following is a list of supplies that may be in the visit bag. Your organization may also have a list of required supplies, so check with your supervisor.

HOME CARE NURSING
SAMPLE VISIT BAG CONTENTS

Every home health nurse should ensure that they have a fully equipped nursing bag in order to have the tools at hand needed to care for patients in the home. Routine contents of a visit bag may include:

- *Handbook of Home Health Standards: Quality, Documentation, and Reimbursement,* by Tina Marrelli
- Current, compact-sized drug reference book (this may also be downloaded as an app on your smartphone)
- Alcohol-based hand sanitizer
- Barrier (per policy)
- Disposable gloves
- Disposable masks
- Liquid hand soap and paper towels
- Scissors
- Forceps
- Thermometers (oral and rectal)
- Thermometer covers
- Plastic tape measure
- Stethoscope and sphygmomanometer
- Penlight
- Plastic aprons
- Sterile and non-sterile gloves
- Cotton balls

- Tape
- Tongue depressors
- Gauze (2x2 and 4x4)
- Alcohol wipes
- Disposable CPR mask
- Protective eyewear
- Disinfectant spray
- Disposable gowns
- Lab supplies for venipuncture
- Sharps container with labels
- Lubricant
- Other according to agency policy (e.g., pill organizer)

In addition, home care nurses might also carry a small supply of non-routine supplies in their cars, including:

- Hydrocolloid dressing 2
- Transparent dressing small 2
- Transparent dressing large 1
- Rolled gauze 3 inch 2
- Kerlix 2
- 4x4 sterile dressings 10
- Straight catheter 2
- #16 in-dwelling catheter 2
- Cotton tipped applicator 5
- Paper ruler 5
- Normal saline 2
- Sterile water 2

- Drainage bag 2
- Lab supplies and vacutainers

Other optional equipment includes:

- Pulse oximeter
- Glucose monitor
- Others per organization's policy

Step 5: Knowing the Community

Now that there is a verbal physician order authorizing the visit to Mr. Hinckley, Mr. Hinckley said on the phone call that it was okay to come to his home and visit, and you have the needed supplies organized and with you, the last step in the previsit list is to know the community or neighborhood. This knowledge can be gleaned from living in the area or from doing a "windshield assessment," as described in Chapter 5, beginning on page 95.

Patients and families may need services, supplies, or other assistance that cannot be obtained through Medicare or some other payers. Such socioeconomic factors or challenges can contribute to patient health problems. One study, published in the *Annals of Internal Medicine*, found that for Medicare patients who live "within the most disadvantaged 15% of neighborhoods, rehospitalization rates increased from 22% to 27%" while the "30-day rehospitalization rate did not vary significantly across the least disadvantaged 85% of neighborhoods, which had an average rehospitalization rate of 21%" (Kind et al., 2014, para. 7).

The more disadvantaged the neighborhood—as rated by the area deprivation index (ADI)—the more likely the patients will return to the hospital (Kind et al., 2014). Consider the patient with diabetes who is an amputee and cannot walk and, thus, is unable to get to the grocery store and the closest grocery store, defined as one with vegetables and fruits (not a convenience store), is many miles away. The United States Department of Agriculture (USDA) lists the following criteria as contributing to *food deserts:* "accessibility to sources of healthy food, as measured by distance to a store or by the number of stores in an area, individual-level resources that may affect accessibility, such as family income or vehicle availability, neighborhood-level indicators of resources, such as the average income of the neighborhood, and the availability of public transportation" (2013, para. 3–5).

Other examples include a young adult on enteral nutrition due to a malabsorption disorder needing specialized formulas or baby formula for a premature baby. Patients may also need help with housing, have insurance questions, or have food or nutrition questions; these and numerous other needs are essential to and greatly impact health. A knowledgeable home care or hospice nurse in the community knows many people, resources, and access sites to help patients and families. Some of these resources may be churches, WIC (the Women, Infants, and Children program), food banks, local charitable foundations, the local Veterans Affairs medical center, and more. As discussed later in this chapter, the organization's medical social worker can be a great asset in these sometimes complex and Byzantine processes.

Now that the five previsit activities are addressed, it is time for the work to begin: visiting patients in their sacred space—their homes! This is the best part of home care! This is where team members can make all the difference—and, at the end of every call and visit, they should ask themselves, "What was the value that I brought today to improve/move positively Mr. Hinckley's (or any other patients') health status?"

Patients and families usually appreciate the visiting nurses, therapists, and other team members. You and your visit will often be the highlight of their day! The bond and connection is unlike any other healthcare setting or site for healthcare—enjoy this difference.

The Visit!—Performing the Initial Assessment

There is much data gathering, formulating of the plan, and critical thinking that begins the care planning or nursing process. The assessment visit sets the stage for the assessment of all the data, the formulation of the problems, and the creation of a workable and realistic plan—this, in essence, is the nursing or care planning process.

This initial assessment visit can take up to two hours—and sometimes more. It all depends on the patients and their needs. Examples of why the visit might be longer include if there is more data still left to collect or if the patient is unable to participate in one very long visit without breaks. Pain medications, exhaustion from getting back home after hospitalization, disease processes, and other needs unique to each patient can all impact the length of that initial assessment visit. Sometimes it takes more than one visit to complete all the data collection for these reasons as well. Because of the complexity and detail associated with the comprehensive assessment, organizations sometimes have designated "admission" nurses who are trained specifically to perform this task.

HOME CARE NURSING
PATIENT EXEMPLAR CONTINUES: INITIAL
VISIT TO MR. HINCKLEY'S HOME

Mr. Hinckley's discharge date is known and a referral was made for Mr. William Hinckley to be evaluated for home care. On the referral information, it was noted that Mr. Hinckley is 86 and lives alone. He is very frail, and the hospital discharge planner was concerned about his safety, especially since he is living alone and given the condition that brought him in to the emergency department. He was very thin, needed a shave, was unkempt, and in dirty clothes. It was also noted that he had a very poor short-term memory. It was reported that his neighbor had called 911 and had sent him to the emergency department with a plastic bag full of pills. It was also noted that on admission to the hospital he had an open bleeding wound on his lower left leg. The neighbor reported to the emergency medical services team that she thought he had fallen at home and hit his leg on something.

When walking up to the house, the nurse noted the poor maintenance of the home. There were four brick steps to the front door and no rail. The nurse could hear the TV from outside the door. After knocking (the doorbell was noted to be not working and had tape over it), the nurse heard Mr. Hinckley say that he was coming to the door. After waiting for what seems a few minutes, the door very slowly opened. The nurse introduced herself as the home care nurse who had called and showed Mr. Hinckley her nametag from the organization.

Mr. Hinckley welcomed the nurse inside and she followed him into the small vestibule of the house. It was 10:00 a.m. and a clear day, but it was quite dark inside. All the nurse could see were stacks of paper. There was a skinny pathway from the front door all the way to the kitchen, which was at the back of the house. The nurse followed Mr. Hinckley on what seemed a long way back to the kitchen. In addition to the stacks of old newspapers and magazines, there were many unopened boxes from shopping networks that also lined the pathway. The nurse observed that Mr. Hinckley walked painfully slowly with a walker that barely fit along the path in the home. Even with the walker, she noted he was very unsteady in his walking. He frequently leaned on the papers and boxes as he walked since these stacks reached up to his hip level. In the kitchen, the nurse found a very small round table and two chairs. The table was centered on a glass "back door" that was not functional from coats of paint that joined the doorframe with the wallpaper that covered the kitchen. The nurse brought out her visit bag, asked if she could sit down there, and began her assessment.

NOTE: Though the home care nurse is there primarily to meet the medical needs of patients, there is no question that the patient's home conditions and other factors greatly impact care and healthcare. The skills of observation and assessment are perhaps two of the most valued because they help paint the picture of the patient from a holistic perspective. Only in home care is the patient viewed in their unique home environment—be it ever so humble or grand.

Mr. Hinckley's vital signs showed a temperature of 98.4, a pulse of 74, and a blood pressure of 176/90. He was tall, thin, and very frail. The nurse noted that he was very unsteady when going from standing to sitting in the small kitchen chair. Because the nurse had called that morning to confirm their appointment, he had his medications "ready." Mr. Hinckley pulled out his plastic bag full of medications. He also had a shoebox full of old medications, many expired and many with his deceased wife's name on the bottles. On many questions Mr. Hinckley responded that he "had a poor memory and did not know." He reported that since his wife's death 8 months before, he just wanted to sit and watch TV or read. He said he was hungry when the nurse asked what he had had for breakfast. After the nurse respectfully asked if she could look in his refrigerator and was granted permission, she noted some old lettuce and out-of-date milk as well as some very spoiled strawberries. Mr. Hinckley reported he had three children, but they all lived out of state. He only heard from two of them, and those two rarely.

The nurse obtained Mr. Hinckley's consent for care and services, and Mr. Hinckley signed forms and answered many questions. He also walked and showed the nurse what he could do (and could not do) safely. The nurse completed the assessment and other admission forms, performed the physical assessment, provided the specific ordered wound care, provided instructions about elevating his leg and not taking the dressing off the leg wound site, and advised him that she would recheck it when she came back in 2 days. She also helped fill his medication box, which was marked with days of the week. A medication review was done, and it reconciled with the doctor's discharge list that was sent home from hospital. There were two over-the-counter medications, a stool softener, and an herbal sleep aid that the nurse noted she would need to talk to the doctor about to get orders for them to be added to the POC.

Besides the consent, there are numerous forms to be either completed in writing or entered on a tablet or other device while in the home. While the nurse was there, the neighbor came over and told the nurse that she would be bringing Mr. Hinckley meals now that he was back home. In fact, she had come over with a grocery bag and made him coffee and an English muffin with peanut butter while the nurse finished her work and entered data on her device. The neighbor explained that she bought his groceries along with hers when she went to the store. During this time, the nurse continued to observe, ask questions, reflect on answers, and collect more data to develop the individualized POC for Mr. Hinckley. He also told the nurse it was okay to exchange phone numbers with the neighbor as she was "like family." The neighbor and the nurse exchanged phone numbers and information so that they could be in touch as needed. The nurse noted that Mr. Hinckley was very pleased to see his neighbor, who he mentioned was his wife's best friend for over 50 years.

While at Mr. Hinckley's home, the nurse called the doctor's office with the findings and asked for orders so that physical therapy, occupational therapy, a social worker, and a home health aide for personal care and ADL assistance could also come out. She also asked about the PRN medications and verified other information to be able to complete the POC and ensure its accuracy for the initial certification. The face-to-face had already occurred. The nurse at the doctor's office spoke with the physician who approved this plan and these services. The home care nurse also relayed that she would be revisiting Mr. Hinckley in 2 days for his wound care and follow-up. The nurse went on to describe the condition of the inside of the home and her concern about his living alone and his frailty, as well as the stacks of papers and boxes except for the one path through the home. She considered that Mr. Hinckley could be a hoarder given the state of the house. Also while on the phone, the nurse verified the principal diagnoses and the date and time of Mr. Hinckley's next physician office appointment. The nurse made a note to figure out how he was getting there and placed that on her to-do list for the next visit. Mr. Hinckley was known to his local medical doctor because this practice had also cared for Mr. Hinckley's wife through her death.

The nurse created what is called a "home care" or a "soft" chart that is to be left at Mr. Hinckley's home. This soft chart might include:

- Information about the care to be provided, including copies of the forms that Mr. Hinckley's signed

- Organizational forms such as the patient's "Bill of Rights and Responsibilities"

- Hotlines and phone numbers for complaints related to neglect or abuse

- How to access on-call after hours

- The name of his nurse and how to reach his primary nurse should he need to between visits

- A calendar that shows when the nurse will next visit and the projected home visit schedule

- The aide's schedule (and name when scheduled)

- A medication list

- Educational information about his leg care and infection control

- Copies of the visit notes as well as the aide POC and the aide visit notes left in the home or soft chart

- A form/tool completed that addressed emergency management or what would happen with Mr. Hinckley should there be an emergency

As addressed in Chapter 5, emergency preparedness and management is a very important consideration in home. The sample form entitled "Emergency Phone Numbers and Instructions" shown in Figure 7.2 is a good example.

EMERGENCY PHONE NUMBERS AND INSTRUCTIONS

(If different from office phone no.)
ON-CALL PHONE NO. (_____) _____ – _____

EMERGENCY PHONE NUMBERS		
Description	**Name**	**Phone**
Hospital of choice		
Physician to call		
Physician, back-up		
Next of kin		
Alternate contact (e.g., neighbor)		
Local emergency response no.		
Fire		
Police		
Ambulance		
Other _____		
Primary Nurse		
Equipment company rep.		
Pharmacy		
Spiritual counselor (if applicable)		

EMERGENCY GUIDELINES/INSTRUCTIONS

Symptoms to report with call to:
   911 or other (specify) _____
   Physician _____
   On call _____
Personal emergency response system? ❑ No ❑ Yes, specify _____
_____

Preplanned funeral arrangements? ❑ No ❑ Yes, specify_____
_____

Emergency preparedness kit (dependent upon geographical needs) ❑ Not applicable
   ❑ Water   ❑ 3-day food supply   ❑ Flashlight and dry battery
   ❑ Battery-operated radio (emergency broadcast)   ❑ Other, specify _____
_____

Receipt of Home Environment Safety Evaluation ❑ No ❑ Yes, date ____/____/____

ADDITIONAL EMERGENCY GUIDELINES/INSTRUCTIONS

PART 1 – Clinical Record	PART 2 – On-Call Book	PART 3 – Patient

PATIENT NAME – Last, First, Middle Initial | ID#

Form 3536/3P Rev. 6/03 © 1994 BRIGGS, Des Moines, IA (800) 247-2343
Unauthorized copying or use violates copyright law. www.BriggsCorp.com PRINTED IN U.S.A.   **BRiGGS** Healthcare°   EMERGENCY PHONE NUMBERS AND INSTRUCTIONS

Figure 7.2   Emergency Phone Numbers and Instructions Form
Copyright © 1994 Briggs Healthcare. Reprinted with permission.

All these efforts are to help with care coordination and communications so that Mr. Hinckley knows what to do should a change arise or he needs to communicate with a member of the home care team. This also supports Mr. Hinckley being an active participant in his care and care planning! After asking if he had any questions or if she could do anything else for Mr. Hinckley before leaving, the nurse packed up her supplies and equipment, disposed of all biohazardous waste per the agency's policy, and prepared to leave. The nurse again told Mr. Hinckley that he would receive phone calls every morning this week and that she, the nurse, would be back in 2 days. She also wrote this on the calendar that was left in home. She encouraged him to call for any changes or concerns.

This exemplar about Mr. Hinckley shows the importance of the home environment and that home environment's role in maintaining, improving, or otherwise impacting health. See the "Home Assessment Tool" sample form shown in Figure 7.3, which may be useful to determine aspects of safety as well as list who else lives in the home with the patient and other information.

HOME ASSESSMENT TOOL

Home Address: _____ Phone: _____

Who will be living in home with resident: _____

Type of Home:

❑ Mobile Home ❑ Apartment ❑ Single Story Home ❑ Multiple Story Home Will resident use all levels: ❑ Yes ❑ No

---

Approach to Home:

❑ Dirt ❑ Asphalt ❑ Cement ❑ Gravel ❑ Grass ❑ Sidewalk leading to entrance

---

Location of Entrance to be used by Resident:

❑ Front ❑ Back ❑ Side

_____ Number of steps   _____ Width of steps

_____ Depth of steps (if vary in depth, indicate shallowest step)

_____ Height of steps (if vary in height, indicate greatest height)

_____ Total overall height of steps   _____ Measurement of platform if present at top of steps

Railing available? ❑ Yes ❑ No If yes, indicate: ❑ R ❑ L ❑ Both   Ramp available? ❑ Yes ❑ No

---

Entrance Door:

Ramp available: ❑ Yes ❑ No   _____ Width of door   _____ Height of step up into home including door sill

---

Living Room:

Can furniture be re-organized to allow for safer mobility by resident: ❑ Yes ❑ No

_____ Door width _____ Floor type _____ Height of sofa _____ Height of chair resident will use

Are cushions sturdy? ❑ Yes ❑ No

Dining Room:

_____ Door width _____ Floor type _____ Height of table

Kitchen:

_____ Door width _____ Height of counters

Appliances resident will most likely use (Check all that apply):

❑ Refrigerator ❑ Cook range/stove ❑ Oven ❑ Microwave ❑ Small appliances: List _____

Door handles on refrigerator? ❑ L ❑ R

_____ Stove/Range height   _____ Height of oven/stove handle   Stove type: ❑ Gas ❑ Electric

Can utensils/food be re-organized to allow for safer use by resident? ❑ Yes ❑ No

---

NAME–Last	First	Middle	Attending Physician	Record No.	Room/Bed

Form 3748HH 8/02 © BRIGGS, Des Moines, IA (800) 247-2343
Unauthorized copying or use violates copyright law. www.BriggsCorp.com PRINTED IN U.S.A.   **BRIGGS**Healthcare®   **HOME ASSESSMENT TOOL**

Figure 7.3 Home Assessment Tool

Copyright © 2002 Briggs Healthcare. Reprinted with permission.

The OASIS-C, Quality, and Value: Prospective Payment System (PPS) Considerations

Success depends on the clinician's skills and understanding, and accurate, detailed completion of the comprehensive assessment, which determines the needed care and care plan, regardless of the kind of insurer or payer. That assessment is the driver that creates the care plan and related interventions, goals, and desired outcomes. The OASIS, the mandated set of data elements, must be understood as a significant part of the patient's assessment, which it is, and also the structure that underlies the determination of the Prospective Payment System (PPS) case-mix payment. This tool helps to identify the patient's unique care needs and services. One analogy is that the scoring of these OASIS data elements provides the fuel that determines the trajectory of the PPS rocket.

It is very important that all team members are educated on OASIS and OASIS data collection. The regulations about OASIS are located in the Conditions of Participation (CoPs) 484.55 "Comprehensive Assessment of Patients." It is also very important that clinicians learn how to apply these conventions into daily practice, and that clinicians recognize that OASIS is a statistical data collection instrument. There are specific conventions or "rules" that govern data collection, and each individual item has its own set of instructions for data collection that must be followed to assure reliability of the data. Appropriate data collection relies on both interview and observational skills to determine the appropriate responses. It is also important to remember the clinician is to assess the patient's safe ability to perform certain functional tasks and not their actual performance. The ability of the caregiver, although important, is not reported. When in doubt, have an OASIS-specific educator for your team.

The OASIS is administered at specified time intervals: admission, discharge, transfer, death, resumption of care, recertification, and when there is a significant change in the patient's condition that was not anticipated. The OASIS is then used to monitor three major outcomes for specific patient status attributes—improvement, stabilization, and deterioration. The OASIS data are the basis for the Outcome-Based Quality Monitoring (OBQM), Outcome-Based Quality Improvement (OBQI), Process-Based Quality Improvement (PBQI), Home Health Star Ratings, and Home Health Compare reports. These reports are benchmarking tools that identify the organization's status as determined by specified clinical, functional, and service utilization indicators. These reports must be reviewed by agencies and are used for quality improvement purposes. The data analysis and findings can also inform and suggest future adjustments and refinement of the OASIS and PPS to CMS. OASIS reports will be used to determine adjustment to payment under the Home Health Value-Based Purchasing (HHVBP) model that starts in 2016 in select states.

OASIS was developed in order to capture patient-specific data to measure outcomes of care and determine payment. It does not capture all of the information that should be included in a comprehensive assessment. Because of this, clinicians must understand and be competent in the comprehensive patient assessment, including the OASIS data elements. All patients must be assessed accurately on each data element, and each piece of the assessment needs to correlate and be consistent with all other parts of the assessment. This is best accomplished by a thorough orientation to OASIS, training followed by testing, and verification of OASIS skills, consistency, and similar assessment findings (e.g., interrater reliability). OASIS not a "one and done" process; it needs continual refreshers and ongoing training.

The Home Care Team: Who Else Is on It?

Home care and hospice at home is truly a team effort. This is important to note as the assessment or evaluation visit often identifies what other team members, or "who else," should be providing specialized services in a patient's care. Of course, this need is determined by specific findings and other data collected and observed on visit. The following information lists the team members in home care. Sometimes there may be overlapping skillsets, and this may depend on state and other regulations, such as state practice acts and others. Examples include nursing and physical therapy, such as for providing wound care and/or medication management. Similarly, this may be true sometimes for occupational therapy (OT) and/or physical therapy (PT), and it depends on many factors.

Home Health Aide Services

Though Medicare calls aides "home health aides," they may also be called certified nursing assistants depending on their education and the state and policies at specific organizations. The following six services are mentioned specifically in the "Medicare Benefit Policy Manual." They are Nursing, PT, OT, MSW, SLP, and Aides. Not all services will be used in most cases. There are very specific medical-necessity and other rules that govern the use of the services. When in doubt, refer to the Medicare Manual.

Because of the oversight, supervisory, and delegation responsibilities when working with aides, the aide role is highlighted and explained the most. The five others are addressed later in this section.

Aides in all kinds of care at home are very important team members. Aides bring special value to the interdisciplinary team as well as to the patients and families they serve and provide care to. They truly are the "eyes and ears" of the clinical team, and patients confide sometimes more in the aides because the aides may be in the homes more than other team members. Aides provide primarily personal care and ADL assistance and support. Personal care is just that, extremely personal. In what other situation would we meet someone and get a bath from them that same day? Or have them preparing and cooking and serving a meal? Home health aides provide personal care and activities of daily living support and assistance. This is truly the role that helps many older adults remain at home and with dignity.

Aides have a wide scope of activities, all usually related to personal care and ADLs. Some important ones include bathing, grooming, exercising, dressing, meal preparation, meal set-up, light housekeeping related to the patient's area, and numerous other activities. Not surprisingly, when organizations sometimes call a patient to get feedback about the care and services and the agency asks about the nursing, social worker, or therapy services, it is not uncommon that the aide's name is the one that the patient or family remembers most.

It is important to note that the home health and hospice aide plan of care cannot use the term or have "PRN" written on the POC. This is because CMS believes this is outside the scope of practice for the aide—to make such determinations that "PRN" implies, such as what tasks need to be done and when. The nurse must develop the aide plan and identify what tasks and activities the patient needs and the specific frequency of such duties. This is important to note, as the use of PRN in a patient record (or "per patient request") could be cited as a deficiency during a Medicare or accreditation survey. Refer to your supervisor for any clarification or for further information. The aide must adhere to the plan of care exactly or contact the supervisor prior to deviating from the aide care plan.

See the sample "Aide Care Plan" shown in Figure 7.4 and the corresponding "Aide Visit Record" shown in Figure 7.5 for examples of documenting the aide care plan.

AIDE CARE PLAN

Patient Address:_____ Telephone No._____

Directions to Home:_____

Case Manager:_____ Phone No._____

Frequency/Duration:_____

Supervisory visits: ❑ every 2 weeks ❑ every 30 ❑ every 60 ❑ Other_____

Patient problem:_____

PARAMETERS TO NOTIFY CARE MANAGER

Temp_____ BP _____

P _____ R _____

Urine _____

Other (pain)_____

DNR: ❑ Yes ❑ No

PRECAUTIONARY AND OTHER PERTINENT INFORMATION – Check all that apply. Circle the appropriate item if separated by slash.

❑ Lives alone
❑ Lives with other
❑ Alone during the day
❑ Bed bound
❑ Bed rest/BRPs
  ❑ Up as tolerated
❑ Amputee (specify):_____
❑ Partial weight bearing: ❑ R ❑ L

❑ Non weight bearing: ❑ R ❑ L
❑ Fall precautions
❑ Special equipment:_____
❑ Speech/Communication deficit
❑ Vision deficit: ❑ Glasses
  ❑ Contacts
  ❑ Other:_____
❑ Hearing deficit: ❑ Hearing aid

❑ Dentures: ❑ Upper ❑ Lower
  ❑ Partial
❑ Oriented x 3 ❑ Alert
❑ Forgetful/Confused
❑ Urinary catheter
❑ Prosthesis (specify): _____
❑ Allergies (specify):_____

❑ Diabetic ❑ Do not cut nails
  ❑ Diet:_____
❑ Seizure precaution
❑ Watch for hyper/hypoglycemia
❑ Bleeding precautions
❑ Prone to fractures
❑ Other (specify):_____
❑ _____
❑ _____

Check all applicable tasks. Specify by circling the applicable activity for those items separated by slashes. Write additional precautions, instructions, etc. as needed beside the appropriate item.

ASSIGNMENT	Every Visit	Weekly	Other – Comments/Instructions	ASSIGNMENT	Every Visit	Weekly	Other – Comments/Instructions
VITALS Temperature	❑	❑		**ACTIVITY** Assist with Ambulation W/C / Walker / Cane	❑	❑	
Pulse	❑	❑					
Respirations	❑	❑		Mobility Assist Chair / Bed Dangle / Commode Shower / Tub	❑	❑	
Blood Pressure	❑	❑					
Weight	❑	❑					
Pain Rating	❑	❑					
BATH Tub/Shower	❑	❑		ROM Active / Passive Arm R / L Leg R / L	❑	❑	
Bed Bath - Partial/Complete	❑	❑					
Assist Bath - Chair	❑	❑		Positioning - Encourage Assist every ____ hrs	❑	❑	
HYGIENE/GROOMING Personal Care	❑	❑					
Assist with Dressing	❑	❑		Exercise - Per PT / OT / SLP Care Plan	❑	❑	
Hair Care	❑	❑					
Shampoo	❑	❑		Other (specify):	❑	❑	
Skin Care	❑	❑					
Foot Care	❑	❑					
Check Pressure Areas	❑	❑		**NUTRITION** Meal Preparation	❑	❑	
Nail Care	❑	❑		Assist with Feeding	❑	❑	
Oral Care	❑	❑		Limit/Encourage Fluids	❑	❑	
Clean Dentures	❑	❑		Grocery Shopping	❑	❑	
Other (specify):	❑	❑		Other (specify):	❑	❑	
PROCEDURES Assist with Elimination	❑	❑					
Catheter Care	❑	❑		Wash Clothes	❑	❑	
Ostomy Care	❑	❑		**OTHER** Light Housekeeping Bedroom / Bathroom / Kitchen / Change Bed Linen	❑	❑	
Record Intake/Output	❑	❑					
Inspect/Reinforce Dressing (see specifics in comment section)	❑	❑					
Medication Reminder	❑	❑		Equipment Care	❑	❑	
Other (specify):	❑	❑		Other (specify):	❑	❑	

Signature/Title:_____ Date:_____ Review and/or revise at least every 60 days

SIGNATURE/TITLE	DATE	SIGNATURE/TITLE	DATE

PART 1 - Clinical Record   PART 2 - Patient   PART 3 - Care Manager

PATIENT NAME – Last, First, Middle Initial	ID#

Form 3574/3P Rev. 10/12 © 1994 BRIGGS, Des Moines, IA (800) 247-2343
Unauthorized copying or use violates copyright law. www.BriggsCorp.com PRINTED IN U.S.A.

BRIGGS Healthcare°

AIDE CARE PLAN

Figure 7.4 Aide Care Plan

Copyright © 1994 Briggs Healthcare. Reprinted with permission.

AIDE VISIT RECORD

Date_____ Time In_____ Time Out_____

☐ Q5001: Hospice or Home Health Care provided in patient's home/residence   ☐ Q5009: Hospice or Home Health Care provided in place not otherwise specified
☐ Q5002: Hospice or Home Health Care provided in Assisted Living Facility

Check each activity completed during visit, refer to Aide Care Plan.

	ACTIVITIES	REFUSED	COMMENTS		ACTIVITIES	REFUSED	COMMENTS
VITALS/ RESULTS	T_____ P_____			ACTIVITY	Assist with Ambulation W/C / Walker / Cane		
	R_____ B/P_____				Assist with Mobility Chair / Bed / Dangle / Commode Shower / Tub		
	Weight_____ Pain rating_____						
BATH	Tub/Shower						
	Bed Bath - Partial/Complete				ROM Active / Passive Arm R / L Leg R / L		
	Assist Bath - Chair						
	Other (specify):				Positioning - Encourage Assist every _____ hrs		
HYGIENE / GROOMING	Personal Care				Exercise - Per PT / OT / SLP Care Plan		
	Assist with Dressing						
	Hair Care				Other (specify):		
	Shampoo						
	Skin Care			NUTRITION	Meal Preparation		
	Foot Care				Assist with Feeding		
	Check Pressure Areas				Limit / Encourage Fluids		
	Nail Care				Grocery Shopping		
	Oral Care				Other (specify):		
	Clean Dentures						
	Other (specify):			OTHER	Wash Clothes		
PROCEDURES	Assist with Elimination				Light Housekeeping Bedroom / Bathroom / Kitchen Change Bed Linen		
	Catheter Care						
	Ostomy Care				Equipment Care		
	Record Intake/Output				Other (specify):		
	Inspect/Reinforce Dressing						
	Medication Reminder						
	Other (specify):						

Comments/Notes:

_____
_____
_____
_____
_____

Coordination of Care With: ☐ SN ☐ Therapy ☐ PT ☐ OT ☐ SLP ☐ Family & Patient

SIGNATURE/DATE

Employee_____ ___/___/___ Patient_____ ___/___/___
                                              Date   Date

PATIENT NAME - Last, First, Middle Initial	ID#

BRIGGSHealthcare®   AIDE VISIT RECORD

Figure 7.5 Aide Visit Record
Copyright © 2002 Briggs Healthcare. Reprinted with permission.

The RN indicates the specific activities that the home health aide is to perform or complete for a patient on the aide plan of care. Of course, the RN obtained specific physician orders for the aide services prior to the aide visiting or providing any care. The aide can only provide the care checked off and approved by the RN (or in some instances related to therapy, by the therapist). Similarly, the aide should perform only the tasks/activities that are indicated on the aide's POC. These forms list some of the usual activities, duties, and tasks performed by aides for patients.

Readers are referred to the "Medicare Benefit Policy Manual" for the specific services and coverage explanations and examples under the Medicare home care benefit: https://www.cms.gov/Regulations-and-Guidance/Guidance/Manuals/downloads/bp102c07.pdf.

 The RN supervisory visit is a very important time for the nurse, the patient, and the aide. Try to view these with "new eyes" and review what the aide is doing tasks-wise and then what the patient needs. These needs may change across time—such as the patient "graduating" from a bed bath to a shower-assisted one. The aide POC should reflect what the patient needs and what duties the aide is performing.

HOME CARE NURSING
THE AIDE SUPERVISORY VISIT—A CHECKLIST

Approach the supervisory visit as a time for education for the aide and validation of a job well done. The following are some of the fundamental activities for an aide supervisory visit.

✓ Incorporate some kind of education for the aide into every supervisory visit.

✓ Recognize that the number of aides needed in the coming years is staggeringly huge and value them for their contribution to the team—they need to be valued and retained.

✓ Review the aide plan of care with the aide. Is it accurate, up-to-date, and reflective of exactly what the aide does?

✓ Review the aide's visit notes against the aide's plan of care. Are they congruent? If not, is this updated to reflect care?

✓ Does the aide need more PPE or other supplies, such as gloves, paper towels, alcohol-based hand cleanser, or other items to provide safe care?

✓ Observe and validate the aide's hand hygiene and other activities related to infection control and care.

✓ Validate that the aide is staying within the scope of the position description and per state regulations.

✓ What other activities are done during the aide supervisory visit per your organization's policy?

✓ Is there an up-to-date and legible aide care plan in the home?

✓ Is the binder that houses the aide POC and the visit notes professional and organized (i.e., if you had to make that supervisory visit because the regular nurse was sick, could you easily find/know the current/latest aide POC and the corresponding aide documentation? Is documentation on the POC and in the aide visit notes legible and neat if handwritten? Do they "adhere" to the POC?)?

✓ Are there physician orders for the aide services and are they up-to-date?

✓ Is the aide's POC updated as the patient's condition changes?

✓ If a state or accreditation surveyor accompanied you to a home visit, would the aide's notes and POC meet the organization's policies and standards?

✓ Document the aide supervisory visit.

✓ Identify what other activities are a part of an aide supervisory visit at your organization.

Medicare Disciplines and Services—Five More

Readers are referred to the *Medicare Benefit Policy Manual* for the specific discipline's services and coverage explanations and examples under the Medicare home care benefit. See https://www.cms.gov/Regulations-and-Guidance/Guidance/Manuals/downloads/bp102c07.pdf.

1. Skilled Nursing Care

2. Occupational Therapy Services

3. Physical Therapy Services

4. Speech-Language Pathology Services

5. Medical Social Services

It is important to note that these are the Medicare-specific services. Other home care service providers and programs, such as hospice, that make many home visits may have other team members. Whatever they are called, for example the interprofessional or interdisciplinary team, the care coordination and communication that happens between the whole care team, including the patient and caregiver, is key to helping patients achieve desired goals and outcomes.

Other Interdisciplinary Team Members

Other team members might include:

- Physicians

- The patient and family/caregiver and/or patient representative

- Specialty nurses (such as for wound care, psychiatric care, etc.)

- Registered nurses (RN) and licensed practical (LPN) or vocational (LVN) nurses

- Dietitians/nutritional counselors

- Bereavement counselors

- Chaplains/other spiritual counselors

- Homemakers

- Pharmacists

- Respiratory therapists

- Specialty services supporting specific missions of programs such as musical therapy, aromatherapy, massage, pet therapy, and others

- Volunteers for any of these programs (such as hospice, meals-on-wheels, friendly visitors, and others)

- Others based on the organization's mission and policies

The Intersection of Visits and Case Management

In many instances, the nurse is the case manager or primary nurse for a certain patient population or group of patients. In these capacities, the nurse may identify other services that may be appropriate to help the patient achieve predetermined and individualized goals. With this in mind, the nurse may identify members of the interdisciplinary or interprofessional team to also assess the patient and contribute to the POC. Readers are referred to the sample of an "Interdisciplinary Referral" tool form shown in Figure 7.6.

INTERDISCIPLINARY REFERRAL

CARE MANAGER _____

DATE OF REFERRAL _____/_____/_____

USE THE COMMENTS AREA TO FURTHER EXPLAIN CHECKED ITEMS AND/OR TO PROVIDE ADDITIONAL PERTINENT INFORMATION

PHYSICAL THERAPY

REASON FOR REFERRAL: ❏ PT Evaluation ❏ ADL or ambulation ❏ Teach caregiver/spouse ❏ Fall prevention/safety
❏ Adaptive equipment/home medication ❏ Other (specify) _____
COMMENTS:_____

SHOULD BE SEEN WITHIN _____ DAYS/WEEKS   ORDERED/RECOMMENDED (circle) FREQUENCY_____
DATE FAXED/CALLED (circle)_____

OCCUPATIONAL THERAPY

REASON FOR REFERRAL: ❏ OT evaluation ❏ Adaptive equipment home modification ❏ Home management and functional mobility
❏ UE sensorimotor program ❏ Home safety ❏ Energy conservation ❏ Other (specify)_____
COMMENTS:_____

SHOULD BE SEEN WITHIN _____ DAYS/WEEKS   ORDERED/RECOMMENDED (circle) FREQUENCY_____
DATE FAXED/CALLED (circle)_____

SPEECH/LANGUAGE PATHOLOGY

REASON FOR REFERRAL: ❏ Swallowing problems ❏ Communication assistance ❏ Slurred speech ❏ Expression
❏ Other (specify) _____
COMMENTS:_____

SHOULD BE SEEN WITHIN _____ DAYS/WEEKS   ORDERED/RECOMMENDED (circle) FREQUENCY_____
DATE FAXED/CALLED (circle)_____

SOCIAL SERVICE

REASON FOR REFERRAL: ❏ Identified social problem that is impeding effective implementation of POC (specify below)
❏ Community resources ❏ Placement ❏ Counseling/Psychosocial problem(s) ❏ Other (specify) _____
COMMENTS:_____

SHOULD BE SEEN WITHIN _____ DAYS/WEEKS   ORDERED/RECOMMENDED (circle) FREQUENCY_____
DATE FAXED/CALLED (circle)_____

SKILLED NURSING

REASON FOR REFERRAL: ❏ Skilled observation and assessment ❏ Teaching ❏ Medication administration ❏ Diabetic care
❏ Medication program ❏ Skin/Wound care ❏ Venipuncture ❏ Management and evaluation care plan ❏ Bladder/Bowel care
❏ Other (specify)_____
COMMENTS:_____

SHOULD BE SEEN WITHIN _____ DAYS/WEEKS   ORDERED/RECOMMENDED (circle) FREQUENCY_____
DATE FAXED/CALLED (circle)_____

HOME HEALTH AIDE

REASON FOR REFERRAL: ❏ Personal care per care plan ❏ Other (specify)_____
COMMENTS:_____

SHOULD BE SEEN WITHIN _____ DAYS/WEEKS   ORDERED/RECOMMENDED (circle) FREQUENCY_____
DATE FAXED/CALLED (circle)_____

DIETARY

REASON FOR REFERRAL: ❏ Consult by phone ❏ Other (specify)_____
COMMENTS:_____

SHOULD BE SEEN WITHIN _____ DAYS/WEEKS   ORDERED/RECOMMENDED (circle) FREQUENCY_____
DATE FAXED/CALLED (circle)_____

PHYSICIAN_____   PHONE_____
VERBAL ORDER OBTAINED FROM MD FOR REFERRAL TO: ❏ SN ❏ PT ❏ OT ❏ ST ❏ MSW ❏ Aide ❏ Dietary
❏ Other (specify) _____
OTHER DISCIPLINES INVOLVED IN CARE: ❏ SN ❏ PT ❏ OT ❏ ST ❏ MSW ❏ Aide ❏ Dietary
❏ Other (specify) _____

PERSON COMPLETING FORM
SIGNATURE/TITLE_____   DATE_____/_____/_____

PART 1 – Clinical Record	PART 2 – Discipline Referred To
PATIENT NAME – Last, First, Middle Initial	ID #

Form 3582/2P Rev. 12/04 © 1994 BRIGGS, Des Moines, IA. (800) 247-2343
Unauthorized copying or use violates copyright law. www.BriggsCorp.com PRINTED IN U.S.A.

BRIGGS Healthcare®

INTERDISCIPLINARY REFERRAL

Figure 7.6 Interdisciplinary Referral Form
Copyright © 2004 Briggs Healthcare. Reprinted with permission.

Mr. Hinckley and the Team

Varying team members bring their expertise and unique skills to help patients. In the example of Mr. Hinckley, the nurse considered a medical social worker, a physical therapist, an occupational therapist, and the home health aide to help meet his unique care needs. The medical social worker would be involved for assessing and evaluating the possible hoarding, and would work to address depression and safety issues seen in the home as well as the socioeconomic factors that would impact his not being able to meet goals, such as not having food in the home and/ or not being able to afford physician-ordered medications.

Impediments to the POC being implemented should trigger consideration about the need for the expertise of the medical social worker. The physical therapist would assess Mr. Hinckley for his unsteady walking, poor strength, and poor balance, efforts to support function, as well as other safety factors. The aide was called in to assist with Mr. Hinckley's personal care and his activities of daily living, such as grooming, assistance with hygiene, meal preparation, and other duties that the RN identifies on the aide POC.

 Medical social workers are valued members of the care team and bring unique skills to help patients and families. In any instance of suspected neglect or abuse, contact your supervisor and the medical social worker. In addition, individual states have specific laws about reporting of such incidents.

Readers are referred to the "Medicare Benefit Policy Manual" for the specific services and coverage explanations and examples under the Medicare home care benefit: https://www.cms.gov/Regulations-and-Guidance/Guidance/Manuals/downloads/bp102c07.pdf.

HOME CARE NURSING
MR. HINCKLEY: AN UPDATE

As illustrated in the exemplar story, Mr. Hinckley was appropriate for home care. It is important to note that he is an example only. He also met the organization's policies for admission. He was homebound and needed a walker to walk and, even with that, it was noted that he had to hold onto boxes occasionally while walking through the home. In addition, he could not walk without assistance and needed to keep his leg elevated per orders. The nurse later decided to also ask the doctor for a physical therapy evaluation after she saw his walking by following him back to the front door on her way out. She was critically thinking and gathering data to help improve the care plan; experienced home care nurses do this so that the plan of care is active and can be improved, integrating the best of care planning with quality improvement.

Refer to the section "Homebound: A Major Qualifying Criterion" in Chapter 6 (see p. 146) for the definition and examples of *homebound.* The nursing skill that Mr. Hinckley's care necessitated was wound care. Wound care may involve three skills: 1) observation and assessment of the wound, such as observing for infection and healing at the site; 2) teaching and training, such as about elevating the leg, protecting it, and pain medications related to the leg site; and 3) the actual hands-on wound care, such as changing the dressing.

The assessment took a long time—2 hours—because of Mr. Hinckley's frailty and tiredness, which necessitated a lot of breaks. Care coordination and communication occurred when the nurse called the office about an aide to help with personal care and ADL assistance; a physical therapist to assess him with safety related to his walking and balance, strengthening, and a home exercise program; and a medical social worker to visit and assess for possible hoarding, depression, and related safety concerns.

Components of an Effective Visit

Consider the following components of an effective visit:

- At the beginning and end of every visit, ask yourself what was the value (that I) brought to this patient's home that helped improve care and perhaps process measures (e.g., improvement in ambulation, bed transferring, bathing, pain or other distress, wound healing, self-management, and others)?

- Clarify patient expectations and goals. What are the patient's goals for care? This entails having the patient state specifically what his or her unique goals are. Identify how the team can also help the nurse and patient achieve these goals.

- Have a plan for that specific visit, such as the nurse's goals of what to teach. While there is a need, in many situations, for repeated efforts to evaluate a patient/family on an important or complex issue, over time, the education program should address varying aspects of the issues where such education could be of direct benefit to the patient/family to keep the education meaningful.

- Wash your hands and be aware that you are a role model for hand hygiene and infection control and other prevention activities.

- Identify the "skills" needed and to be performed in care and use/reflect/know the Medicare coverage terms when appropriate such as observation and assessment, teaching and training, and others.

- Know and adhere to organizational policies and clinical procedural policies, such as nurse bag techniques, infection control and prevention, and others.

- Complete the assessment and any ordered care (such as wound care, observation and assessment, teaching and training, etc.).

- Ask open-ended questions whenever possible.

- Allow "quiet" time for the patients' family to formulate questions—this is especially true when trying to perform a drug regimen review or a medication reconciliation.

- Drill down further when assessing and noting a problem area. This may include pain, depression, distress, nutritional risks, bleeding and bleeding precautions (such as for patients taking anticoagulants), falls and fall assessments, safety concerns, and any other areas of concern to the patient. Use the organization's assessment tools. See the sample form "Pain Evaluation" shown in Figure 7.7 for an example of documenting pain symptoms.

Patients on pain medications usually need a bowel program to prevent constipation. Think of these two issues as going together so that when the physician orders the pain medication the nurse automatically asks for a bowel regimen. Think of them like peanut butter and jelly—they go together.

People should not have to suffer in pain. There are expert nurses and others whom you can consult. One great nurse reminded me of the acronym "OLD CART," which stands for "Onset, Location, Duration, Characteristics, Aggravating factors, Relieving factors, and Treatment response."

- Identify other team members who should be involved in care.

- Explain and support homebound clearly on admission and then in every visit note or per organizational policy.

- When in doubt about orders or care or any part of the POC, contact the physician to clarify and to verify the next appointment(s).

- Write in any appointments, including physician appointments, on the patient's home calendar if they allow you to, or ensure that they do. Also, consider how the patient is going to get there when the patient cannot drive.

- Identify and write down next visits on the home chart calendar (for patients who may have memory problems, have someone at the office call them to remind them as well).

- Document while in the home when safe and possible.

- For nursing supervisory or recertification visits, look with "new eyes"—pretend the patient is new and create a totally new assessment and plan that reflects the current needs of the patient; update their goals and other data as needed based on this assessment.

- For discharge visits, recognize that this is a very important visit for a number of reasons. Ask questions about the patient and their readiness for discharge. This might include:

  - Is this patient stable enough to remain out of the hospital?

  - Does the patient have self-care and management skills that have been working for them? For example, how is their response to teaching and teach-back?

- The discharge visit is also the last visit encounter from a safety, quality, customer-service, and patient-experience perspective. Make this visit a great one—critically think about the patient and this patient's unique needs.

PAIN EVALUATION

GENERAL INFORMATION

Does the resident have any diagnosis(es) which would give reason to believe he/she would be in pain?   ❑ Yes   ❑ No

If yes, describe cause, origin of pain, radiation of pain, and prior treatment: _____
_____

Ask resident: *"Have you had pain or hurting at any time in the last 5 days?"*   ❑ Yes   ❑ No

If yes, date of pain onset:_____/_____/_____

As the patient describes it, what does the pain feel like? (check all that apply.)

❑ Aching ❑ Heavy ❑ Tender ❑ Splitting ❑ Tiring ❑ Exhausting ❑ Throbbing ❑ Shooting ❑ Stabbing
❑ Sharp ❑ Cramping ❑ Hot/Burning ❑ Tingling ❑ Other:_____

Additional symptoms associated with pain (e.g., nausea, anxiety):_____
_____

Pain is increased by (describe circumstances or activities):_____

Any language and/or cultural barriers: ❑ Yes   ❑ No   If yes, explain:_____

Times when pain is worse: ❑ Early morning (pre-dawn) ❑ Morning ❑ Afternoon ❑ Evening ❑ Night

PAIN LOCATION/TYPE/FREQUENCY/INTENSITY/DURATION

If the resident is able, identify pain type(s) and locations and record below. Label sites as A, B, C, D. Code pain type, frequency and intensity/duration as applicable. If resident is able to interview, use Wong-Baker, if not, use PAINAD.

TYPE	SITE A	SITE B	SITE C	SITE D	FREQUENCY	SITE A	SITE B	SITE C	SITE D
Code: I = Internal; **A** = Acute; **E** = External; **C** = Chronic					Ask resident: *"How much of the time have you experienced pain or hurting over the last 5 days?"* 1. Almost constantly 2. Frequently 3. Occasionally 4. Rarely 9. Unable to answer				

WONG-BAKER

Ask resident: *"Please rate the intensity of your worst pain over the last 5 days, with 0 being no pain and 10 as the worst pain you can imagine."*

Wong-Baker FACES Pain Rating Scale

NO HURT	HURTS LITTLE BIT	HURTS LITTLE MORE	HURTS EVEN MORE	HURTS WHOLE LOT	HURTS WORSE
0 No Pain	2	4 Moderate Pain	6	8	10 Worst Possible Pain

From Wong D.L., Hockenberry, Eaton M., Wilson D., Winkelstein M.L. Schwartz P.: Wong's Essentials of Pediatric Nursing, ed. 6, St. Louis, 2001, p. 1301. Copyrighted by Mosby, Inc. Reprinted by permission.

	SITE A	SITE B	SITE C	SITE D
At Present				
1 Hour After Medication				
3 Hours After Medication				
Worst It Gets				
Best It Gets				

PAINAD: Score each row and total

	0	1	2	SCORE
Breathing Independent of Vocalization	Normal	Occasional labored breathing. Short period of hyperventilation.	Noisy labored breathing. Long period of hyperventilation. Cheyne-Stokes respirations	
Negative Vocalization	None	Occasional moan or groan. Low level speech with a negative or disapproving quality.	Repeated troubled calling out. Loud moaning or groaning. Crying.	
Facial Expression	Smiling, or inexpressive	Sad, Frightened, Frowning	Facial grimacing	
Body Language	Relaxed	Tense, Distressed pacing, Fidgeting	Rigid. Fists clenched, Knees pulled up. Pulling or pushing away. Striking out.	
Consolability	No need to console	Distracted or reassured by voice or touch	Unable to console, distract or reassure.	

Development and Psychometric Evaluation of the Pain Assessment in Advanced Dementia (PAINAD) Scale: Victoria Warden, RN, Ann C. Hurley, RN, DNSc, FAAN, and Ladislav Volicer, MD, PhD, FANN.

TOTAL

NAME–Last	First	Middle	Attending Physician	Record No.	Room/Bed

Form 3690HH-10 9/10 © 1997 BRIGGS, Des Moines, IA (800) 247-2343
Unauthorized copying or use violates copyright law. www.BriggsCorp.com PRINTED IN U.S.A.

BRiGGSHealthcare®

PAIN EVALUATION
❑ Continued on Reverse

Figure 7.7   Pain Evaluation Form

Copyright © 1997 Briggs Healthcare. Reprinted with permission.

Postvisit Activities

The following list includes postvisit activities as care planning and related processes continue:

- Critically think and consider all the data—whether by interview, observation, etc.

- Support medical necessity in your documentation.

- Start to develop plan/goal(s) for next visit(s).

- Develop the plan of care to go to the physician in a timely manner and follow up about the orders.

- Coordinate care and communicate with the patient/family and all involved team members.

- Provide careful and detailed case management.

- Call the physician and follow up to obtain the signed orders per regulatory requirements and state licensure laws.

- When in doubt or if you have questions, contact your manager.

Continue to critically think and develop the plan of care that will assist in meeting goals and outcomes. Some of the best ideas come after leaving the home and you have "quiet" thinking time. Such questions in Mr. Hinckley's example could be:

- How can his ambulation be improved?

- How can his home be made safer?

- How can we support the wound healing?

- How can his nutritional status be improved?

- How can his knowledge of medications and adherence to the medication regimen be improved?

- How does the nurse decrease the need for a (re)hospitalization given his frailty and trajectory while in the hospital?

- How can the nurse and aide work to improve his bathing and hygiene?

- Overall, how can we keep him safe and comfortable at home?

Some of these are measures that are rated and publicly reported with the agency's star ratings. Home care is truly a team effort, and all team members involved with a specific patient must work to together to achieve patient-specific goals.

Document the care! Documentation is initiated with the referral and continues across time and certification(s) through to discharge and includes the discharge summary. In this way, the documentation tells the patient's unique story.

Summary

The visit in home care is the value proposition for practice, quality, and operations. The team, the services, and other aspects of home care all support the patient and exist to provide needed care to patients. There is no question that the assessment visit; the OASIS, which is a part of the comprehensive assessment; and myriad other details all contribute to help create the data from which begins the care planning process and a realistic plan with individualized care and goals developed for that one, new patient.

The integration of best practices, including effective hand hygiene, adherence to organizational policies, and the dual role of admission expert and clinical leader, are just some of the multifaceted components of home care and visits. Though there are different "kinds" of visits, they all have three components. They are the previsit, the visit, and the postvisit activities.

Through an exemplar of Mr. Hinckley, a patient is followed from hospital discharge and through to the admission into home care. Mr. Hinckley is not discharged from home care in this example, but discharge visits are important for a number of reasons. Discharge visits have the added responsibility of trying to discern and predict (another great example of critical thinking in home care) that the patient will be safe and able to self-manage his or her care. In addition, this discharge visit may be the last encounter with a patient and family. From a patient experience perspective the last encounter may impact, in either a good or bad way, the feedback about the patient experience at the home care organization. All of this care, care planning, coordination, and communications naturally leads to the documentation of this patient data.

The next chapter addresses documentation and the important roles it plays in home care practice, quality, and operations. For this reason, and because the assessment is the driver for care and related processes, this will be illustrated in the next chapter. Mr. Hinckley's OASIS-C and POC are shown as examples along with the systems-based care and care planning processes that are a hallmark of effective care, care planning, and documentation.

Questions for Further Consideration and Discussion

1. What are the five steps in the "previsit activities"? Could there be more? What are they?

2. Explain why Mr. Hinckley met the admission criteria for Medicare.

3. Explain two reasons that a home care organization might not admit a patient to their service.

4. What is the nursing or scientific process and how does it integrate with the patient POC?

5. List the six covered services in Medicare and describe the scope of these disciplines/roles.

For Further Reading

- *Handbook of Home Health Standards: Quality, Documentation, and Reimbursement, 5th Edition,* by Tina Marrelli

- *Home Health Aide: Guidelines for Care Handbook, 2nd Edition,* 2008, and the *Home Health Aide: Guidelines for Care: Instructor Manual,* by Tina Marrelli

- "Bag Technique: Preventing and Controlling Infections in Home Care and Hospice" by Mary McGoldrick in *Home Healthcare Nurse,* January 2014, Vol. 32(1): pp. 39–45

- "SHOW ME: Enhancing OASIS Functional Assessment" by Mary Narayan, Joise Salgado, and Ann VanVoorhis in *Home Health-care Nurse*

- The Academy of Nutrition and Dietetics: www.eatright.org

- Certified Diabetes Educator: http://www.ncbde.org/

- Chaplains: www.professionalchaplains.org

- Hospice Nurses: www.hpna.org

- International Home Care Nurses Organization: www.IHCNO.org

- The Visiting Nurses Associations of America: www.VNAA.org

- Occupational therapy: www.aota.org

- Physical therapy: www.apta.org

- Speech language pathology, language and hearing: www.asha.org

- Social workers: www.socialworkers.org

- Visiting Nurse Associations of America Clinical Procedure Manual: http://www.vnaa.org/cpm

- Women, Infants, and Children (WIC) food and nutrition service: www.fns.usda.gov/wic/women-infants-and-children-wic

References

Centers for Medicare & Medicaid Services (CMS). (2015). *Medicare benefit policy manual*, Chapter 7 - Home health services. Retrieved from https://www.cms.gov/Regulations-and-Guidance/Guidance/Manuals/downloads/bp102c07.pdf

Kind, A. J. H., Jencks, S., Brock, J., Yu, M., Bartels, C., Ehlenbach, W., ... Smith, M. (2014). Neighborhood socioeconomic disadvantage and 30-day rehospitalization: A retrospective cohort study. *Annals of Internal Medicine*, 161(11), 765–774.

United States Department of Agriculture (USDA). (2013). Food access research atlas. Retrieved from http://www.ers.usda.gov/data-products/food-access-research-atlas/about-the-atlas.aspx

8

Documentation of Care and Related Processes

There are many kinds of documentation methods and systems in home care and hospice at home. Some are primarily a blend of paper and data entered on a device, such as a tablet. Many organizations have chosen one vendor only to later find a better one—and sometimes it is the clinical documentation system that makes the biggest difference for success. It is intuitive that documentation of the nursing and/or the care planning process be integrated in the system's processes.

The information in this chapter is about documentation, in whatever format your organization uses. Documentation needs to meet a number of objectives to be effective and show value. Documentation describes clinician practice to state or accreditation surveyors, peers, payers, managers, patients, families, and others who may review patient records. Keep in mind that this may also include lawyers and juries. Be aware, too, that there is now more access for patients and families to review and keep their clinical records—which makes sense from a self-management perspective. This is not said to cause you worry, but you should be aware that many people, with permission of course, have access to and read clinical records. This is another reason to clearly and objectively document.

 Value and getting paid or reimbursed "for value" begins and ends with clinical documentation. The question to ask, then, when reviewing documentation—such as a comprehensive assessment, a visit note, or care coordination and/or communication notes to other team members and/or a discharge summary—is this: "Is the value of the care reflected in clear, understandable documentation that paints a picture of that patient's status, healthcare problems, case management, care coordination, care, and interventions directed toward improvement and/or comfort toward the end of life?"

This is how clinical documentation needs to be viewed, through the lens of value and quality. Documentation impacts many areas of practice and care in the healthcare environment generally, and perhaps even more so in the home care and hospice at home environments.

Documentation and the Prevention of Hospitalizations and Rehospitalizations

Now that the patient exemplar (from Chapter 7, "The Home Visit: The Important Unit of Care"), Mr. Hinckley, is back at home, one of the main goals of the home care organization and team is to keep him out of the hospital, thus working to prevent a rehospitalization. How this is best accomplished will continue to be studied, but we do know what works best for some patients. The body of literature and science is growing on this important aspect of care. And efforts toward this goal should be documented.

According to the U.S. Department of Health & Human Services, "the all-cause 30-day hospital readmission rate among Medicare fee-for-service beneficiaries held constant from 2007 to 2011, generally between 19-19.5 percent of beneficiaries readmitted to the hospital within 30 days. This rate fell to 18.5 percent in 2012" (2014, p. 2).

In an important article, "Risk Factors for Hospitalization in a National Sample of Medicare Home Health Care Patients," the authors "determined risk factors at HHC [home health care] admission associated with subsequent acute care hospitalization in a nationally representative Medicare patient sample (N = 374,123). Hospitalization was measured using Medicare claims data; risk factors were measured using Outcome Assessment and Information Set data. Seventeen percent of sample members were hospitalized" (Fortinsky, Madigan, Sheehan, Tullai-McGuiness, & Kleppinger, 2014, para. 1).

From this data, it was postulated that "HHC initiatives that minimize chronic condition exacerbations and actively treat depressive symptoms might help reduce Medicare patient hospitalizations" (Fortinsky et al., 2014, para. 1). "Another important finding was that patients judged by HHC clinicians on the first home visit as having expected minimal improvement in functional status were nearly 50% more likely to be subsequently hospitalized than patients judged to have expected marked improvement in functional status" (Fortinsky et al., 2014, para. 29).

In the patient exemplar of Mr. Hinckley, his nurse also thought he would have minimal improvement; home care nurses are often astute at projecting progress and trajectory. Readers can access this interesting article with its practical implications at http://www.ncbi.nlm.nih.gov/pmc/articles/PMC4008711/.

Numerous tools and indicators suggest that some people may be at higher risk for hospitalizations. Many home care patients have complex and chronic conditions. Some of these include frailty, needing assistance with activities of daily living (ADLs), loneliness, depression, anxiety, use of oxygen or other technology, limited life expectancy, and other factors. For an example, see "Hospitalization Risk Assessment" shown in Figure 8.1. It shows some of the more common areas and provides a format for trying to intervene early and throughout care based on the patient's unique condition and findings.

Consider this checklist of the roles of effective documentation, including:

- Supports Medicare certification and coverage through a knowledge of the "rules" and "requirements," such as a knowledge of "homebound" and "skilled care"

- Supports Medicare, Medicaid, and other programs by showing the "medical necessity" of the care or otherwise supporting tenets of the payer

- Supports the tenet that the care is "reasonable and necessary" for the specific patient

- Demonstrates compliance with specific conditions of participation (such as home health aide supervisory visits) and integrates the knowledge of regulatory information with patient-specific care

- Assists in showing quality care and may be used in quality assurance performance improvement (QAPI) initiatives

- Documents the care provided to a specific patient

- Reflects the current standard of care and shows that it has been maintained

- Is the sole source document of the patient's care

- Is the basis for communication and coordination among the team

- Becomes the foundation of the evaluation of care provided

- May act as the best defense against malpractice or allegations of negligence

- Becomes the source of information about that patient for all team members upon which they make subsequent care decisions

- Helps organizations when they perform audits since it may show that the organization and clinicians "know" the rules and/or provides opportunities for performance improvement

- Shows, factually, the patient's status and responses to interventions and care

- Is presented in an organized, standardized manner

- Supports the tenet that the care is "reasonable and necessary" for the specific patient

- Tells the patient's specific story across time

HOSPITALIZATION RISK ASSESSMENT

INSTRUCTIONS: Fill out this form in accordance with organizational policies and procedures. These are suggestions/recommendations for identifying high risk patients. Check all that apply.

RISK FACTORS

❑ 2 or more ER visits or hospitalizations in the past 12 months

❑ History of falls (obtain Physical Therapy referral if indicated)

Diagnosis of: ❑ CHF ❑ COPD ❑ Neoplasm ❑ Diabetes
              ❑ Chronic Skin Ulcers (E.T. consult if indicated)

Add Comments if Applicable

❑ Socioeconomic/Financial concerns (M0150) _____

❑ Discharge from SNF or hospital (M1000) _____

• ❑ Lives alone (M1100) _____

■ ❑ ADL assistance needed (M1800-M1870, M2100) _____

❑ Poor perception of physical ability _____

❑ Decreased ambulation (M1860) _____

❑ History of non-compliance _____

❑ Urinary catheter _____

❑ Incontinence (M1610) _____

❑ IV therapy or central line care _____

❑ Pressure ulcers (M1306, M1308) _____

❑ Stasis ulcers (M1330, M1332, M1334) _____

❑ Surgical wounds (M1340, M1342) _____

• ❑ Difficulty with comprehension _____

■ ❑ Dyspnea (M1400) _____

❑ Confusion (M1710) _____

❑ Cognitive disorders (M1740) _____

❑ Assistance w/medications (M2020, M2030, M2100) _____

❑ Poor vision (M1200) _____

❑ Multiple medications (M2020, M2030) _____

❑ Medications with high potential of side effects (M2000) _____

Add Details if Applicable

Consider Hospice referral ❑ Yes _____

■ Consider HHA's referral ❑ Yes _____

• Consider MSW referral ❑ Yes _____

The results of this assessment may indicate patients at risk for hospitalization. Consider increasing up front visits for more teaching, follow-up for the first 2 weeks. Additional suggestions are outlined on the back of this form.

PATIENT NAME – Last, First, Middle Initial | ID#

Form 3508P Rev. 12/09 © BRIGGS, Des Moines, IA (800) 247-2343
Unauthorized copying or use violates copyright law. www.BriggsCorp.com PRINTED IN U.S.A. **BRiGGS** Healthcare· **HOSPITALIZATION RISK ASSESSMENT**

Figure 8.1 Hospitalization Risk Assessment Form
Copyright © 2009 Briggs Healthcare. Reprinted with permission.

There may also be other roles of documentation specific to the organization, based on their policies, procedures, and software requirements.

HOME CARE NURSING

MR. HINCKLEY'S COMPREHENSIVE ASSESSMENT AND OASIS-C

The comprehensive assessment and the embedded OASIS items and the Home Health Certification and Plan of Care (what used to be called the Form 485) data elements together are important parts of the patient's admitting, beginning documentation. This documentation begins to "tell the patient's story." Figures 8.2 and 8.3 show sample documentation of an integrated home health plan of care and a start of care comprehensive assessment (OASIS) for the patient exemplar of Mr. Hinckley. The sample form 485/POC is shown in its entirety (22 pages) in Figure 8.3. It is important to note that this is just an example.

As shown in this example documentation, the specifics completed in these forms help to "paint the picture" of the patient, the care environment, his problems, his care plan, and the desired goals. The information housed in the forms and presented together shows that Mr. Hinckley is very frail, homebound, and has care needs meeting skilled care criteria as per Medicare (for example, wound care, observation and assessment, teaching and training, hands-on care related to the wound, and more).

Looking further, the information supports medical necessity and a need for a physical therapy evaluation given his history of falls, his frailty, and the walking problems observed and identified by the nurse. In addition, the medical social worker visit would assess and address his possible depression and hoarding. Both of these factors can impact the medically directed plan of care (POC) from being effectively implemented.

Department of Health and Human Services Centers for Medicare & Medicaid Services			Form Approved OMB No. 0938-0357	
HOME HEALTH CERTIFICATION AND PLAN OF CARE				
1. Patient's HI Claim No. 123456789A	2. Start Of Care Date 02/09/17	3. Certification Period From:02/09/2017 To:04/16/2017	4. Medical Record No. 102345	5. Provider No. 123456

6. Patient's Name and Address
William J. Hinckley
340 Center St
Anywhere, USA 10987

7. Provider's Name, Address and Telephone Number
ST. Elsewhere Home Care
2468 B Street
Anywhere, USA 10987

8. Date of Birth 12/03/1930	9. Sex	M X ☐ F

10. Medications: Dose/Frequency/Route (N)ew (C)hanged

11. ICD S81.802D	Principal Diagnosis Open wound left leg	Date 01/19/17 (O)

Metoprolol Tartate 100mg/tablet; take 1 tablet every day by mouth (C)

12. ICD	Surgical Procedure	Date

Celexa 20 mg/tablet; take 1 tablet every day by mouth (N)

Multiple Vitamin capsule: take 1 capsule every day by mouth

13. ICD	Other Pertinent Diagnoses	Date
I10	Essential Hypertension	01/19/17 (E)
F32.9	Major Depressive Disorder single ep, unspec	01/19/17 (O)
R53.1	Generalized Weakness	01/19/17 (O)
R26.81	Unsteady Gait	01/19/17 (O)
N39.3	Stress Incontinence	01/20/10 (O)
Z91.81	History of falls	
Z87.44	History of UTI	
Z87.01	History of Pneumonia	

Acetaminophen 325 mg/tablet; take 2 tablets by mouth every 4-6 hours as needed for leg pain

14. DME and Supplies
Wound cleanser, 4X4, rolled gauze, hydrogel gauze, elastic bandage, measuring tape, gloves, thermometer probe covers, alcohol swabs, walker

15. Safety Measures
Fall precautions, clear pathways, infection control measures, walker safety

16. Nutritional Req. No added salt

17. Allergies Penicillin

18.A. Functional Limitations

1	☐ Amputation	5	☐ Paralysis	9	☐ Legally Blind
2	X Bowel/Bladder (Incontinence)	6	X Endurance	A	☐ Dyspnea With Minimal Exertion
3	☐ Contracture	7	X Ambulation	B	☐ Other (Specify)
4	X Hearing	8	☐ Speech		

18.B. Activities Permitted

1	☐ Complete Bedrest	6	☐ Partial Weight Bearing	A	☐ Wheelchair
2	☐ Bedrest BRP	7	X Independent At Home	B	X Walker
3	X Up As Tolerated	8	☐ Crutches	C	☐ No Restrictions
4	☐ Transfer Bed/Chair	9	☐ Cane	D	☐ Other (Specify)
5	☐ Exercises Prescribed				

19. Mental Status

1	X Oriented	3	X Forgetful	5	☐ Disoriented	7	☐ Agitated
2	☐ Comatose	4	X Depressed	6	☐ Lethargic	8	☐ Other

20. Prognosis

1	☐ Poor	2	☐ Guarded	3	X Fair	4	☐ Good	5	☐ Excellent

21. Orders for Discipline and Treatments (Specify Amount/Frequency/Duration)
SN 3W1, 2W3, 1W5, with 2 PRN visits/month for wound complications.
SN to observe/assess/evaluate all body systems with emphasis on cardiopulmonary, integument, neuro/emotional/behavioral, nutritional, and genitorurinary systems.
SN to monitor vital signs and report to physician BP< 90/50 or >150/90, P < 60 or >100, R <12 or >26, T <96 or >100.5.
SN to assess wound every visit, monitor closely for signs and symptoms of infection and wound complications. Teach patient/perform wound care to left lower leg 2 times a week using aseptic technique, cleanse with wound cleanser, apply hydrogel impregnated gauze to wound bed, cover with dry 4X4 dressing and secure with rolled gauze and elastic bandage. Measure wound weekly and report negative changes to the physician. Teach patient to elevate legs when sitting.
SN to assess for pain control and evaluate effectiveness of pain medication/ pain relief measures.
SN to evaluate patient's ability to manage medications and teach strategies for compliance. Evaluate patient knowledge of medications and provide medication education as needed. Evaluate for effectiveness of medication and notify physician of ineffectiveness or untoward effects.
SN to teach disease process: HTN, Wound management, depression symptoms and interventions, fall prevention strategies and general home safety.
SN to evaluate incontinence and teach signs and symptoms of UTI and timed voiding strategies.
PT to evaluate and treat for home safety modification, strengthening exercises, and gait training.
OT to evaluate and treat for adaptive equipment and teach energy conservation techniques.
MSW to evaluate and treat for need for community resources and long term care planning and resources for further depression evaluation.
HHA 3W2, 2W7, for personal care for ADL assistance, light meal prep, and light housekeeping.

22. Goals/Rehabilitation Potential/Discharge Plans
Nursing Goals: The Patient wound will decrease in size to 4 cm X 3cm X .5cm and show no signs/symptoms of infection by 03/01/17.
The wound will heal completely without complications by 04/10/17.
The patient will verbalize understanding of disease management for HTN, wound management, depression, fall prevention and home safety by 04/10/17.
The patient will demonstrate compliance with medication regimen as evidence by no missed dosages by 02/28/17.
The patient BP will be within normal range for the patient by 02/28/17.
The patient will verbalize decreased depressive symptoms by 03/08/17.
HHA Goals: The patient personal hygiene needs will be met. Rehabilitation Potential: Good for stated goals. Discharge Plan: Discharge to self with physician follow-up, meals on wheels, and homemaker services.

23. Nurse's Signature and Date of Verbal SOC Where Applicable: *Betty Able* 2/8/17	25. Date of HHA Received Signed POT 2/28/17

24. Physician's Name and Address Charles De La Torrens, D. O. 2525 Division St. Anywhere, USA 10987	26. I certify/recertify that this patient is confined to his/her home and needs intermittent skilled nursing care, physical therapy and/or speech therapy or continues to need occupational therapy. The patient is under my care, and I have authorized services on this plan of care and will periodically review the plan.

27. Attending Physician's Signature and Date Signed *Charles De La Torrens, D. O* 2/27/17	28. Anyone who misrepresents, falsifies, or conceals essential information required for payment of Federal funds may be subject to fine, imprisonment, or civil penalty under applicable Federal laws.

Form CMS-485 (C-3) (12-14) (Formerly HCFA-485) (Print Aligned)

Figure 8.2   Plan of Care Documentation for Mr. Hinckley

Save To Web

COMPREHENSIVE ADULT NURSING ASSESSMENT
INCLUDING SOC/ROC OASIS
ELEMENTS WITH PLAN OF CARE/485 INFORMATION
DATE 02/09/2017

PERFORMANCE INDICATORS:
- R = Risk Adjustment
- ◊ = Outcome Measure
- HH = Home Health Compare
- P = Process Measure
- PA = Potentially Avoidable Event
- S = Reimbursement Potential
- ★ = 5 Star

TIME IN 2pm   TIME OUT 4pm

Follow M numbers in sequence unless otherwise directed.
REASON FOR ASSESSMENT: ☑ Start of Care
☐ Resumption of Care

This Patient Tracking Information must be filled out at start of care and per organizational policy. It is to be maintained as part of the clinical record.

(M0010) CMS Certification Number: (Locator #5) 1 2 3 4 5 6

Branch Identification (M0014) Branch State: __ __

(M0016) Branch ID Number: __ __ __ __ __ __ __ __

(M0018) National Provider Identifier (NPI) for the attending physician who has signed the plan of care:

0 9 8 7 6 5 4 3 2 ☐ UK - Unknown or Not Available

Phone: (Locator #24) 0 0 0 _ 0 0 0 _ 0 0 0 0

Name: (Locator #24) c h a r l e s
(First)   (MI)

D e L a T o r r e s _____ D o
(Last)   (Suffix)

Address: (Street/Apt. No.) (Locator #24)
2 5 2 5   D i v i s i o n   S T

City: (Locator #24)
A n y w h e r e

State: (Locator #24)   ZIP Code: (Locator #24)
U S   1 0 9 8 7

Secondary Referring Physician I.D.#: __ __ __ __ __ __ __ __

Phone: __ __ __ - __ __ __ - __ __ __ __

Name: _____
(First)   (MI)

_____
(Last)   (Suffix)

(M0020) Patient ID Number: (Locator #4)

Medical Record Number if different from M0020

(M0030) Start of Care Date: (Locator #2) 0 2 / 0 9 / 2 0 1 7
                                          month / day / year
P HH PA ★

(M0032) Resumption of Care Date:
☑ NA - Not Applicable P R HH PA ★ __ __ / __ __ / __ __ __ __ month / day / year

(M0040) Patient Name: (Locator #6)

w i l l i a m _____ J
(First)   (MI)

H i n c k l e y
(Last)

_____
(Suffix)

Patient Phone: 0 0 0 _ 0 0 0 _ 0 0 0 0

Patient Address: (Locator #6)
0 0 0   2 3 r d   S T
(Street/Apt. No.)

_____
(City)

(M0050) Patient State of Residence: (Locator #6) F L

(M0060) Patient ZIP Code: (Locator #6) 0 0 0 0 0 _ 0 0 0 0

(M0063) Medicare Number: ☐ NA - No Medicare
0 0 0 0 0 0 0 0 0 A (including suffix)

(M0064) Social Security Number: ☐ UK - Unknown or Not Available
0 0 0 _ 0 0 _ 0 0 0 0

(M0065) Medicaid Number: ☑ NA - No Medicaid

(M0066) Birth Date: (Locator #8) 1 2 / 0 3 / 1 9 3 0 R
                                  month / day / year

Patient's HI Claim No.: (Locator #1)
☑ 1 - Same as M0063   ☐ 2 - Same as M0065

☐ 3 - Other __ __ __ __ __ __ __ __ __ __ __ __

(M0069) Gender: (Locator #9) ☑ 1-Male ☐ 2-Female R

Emergency Preparedness/Acuity Level: level 3
Does the patient have an Advance Directives order? ☐ No ☑ Yes

(M0140) Race/Ethnicity: (Mark all that apply.)
☐ 1 - American Indian or Alaska Native
☐ 2 - Asian
☐ 3 - Black or African-American
☐ 4 - Hispanic or Latino
☐ 5 - Native Hawaiian or Pacific Islander
☑ 6 - White

(M0150) Current Payment Sources for Home Care: (Mark all that apply.) R
☐ 0 - None; no charge for current services
☑ 1 - Medicare (traditional fee-for-service)
☐ 2 - Medicare (HMO/managed care/Advantage plan)
☐ 3 - Medicaid (traditional fee-for-service)
☐ 4 - Medicaid (HMO/managed care)
☐ 5 - Workers' compensation
☐ 6 - Title programs (for example, Title III, V, or XX)
☐ 7 - Other government (for example, TriCare, VA)
☐ 8 - Private insurance
☐ 9 - Private HMO/managed care
☐ 10 - Self-pay
☐ 11 - Other (specify)_____
☐ UK - Unknown

Certification Period: (Locator #3)
From 02/09/2017   To 04/10/2017

PATIENT NAME–Last, First, Middle Initial   ID#

COMPREHENSIVE ADULT NURSING ASSESSMENT
with OASIS ELEMENTS
Page 1 of 22

Figure 8.3   Mr. Hinckley's Comprehensive Assessment
Copyright © 2009 Briggs Healthcare. Reprinted with permission.

Patient Name_____ ID #_____

CLINICAL RECORD ITEMS

(M0080) Discipline of Person Completing Assessment:
☒ 1-RN ☐ 2-PT ☐ 3-SLP/ST ☐ 4-OT

(M0090) Date Assessment Completed: <u>0 2</u> / <u>0 9</u> / <u>2 0 1 7</u>
                    month / day / year

(M0100) This Assessment is Currently Being Completed for the Following Reason: Start/Resumption of Care ⓠ Ⓟ Ⓡ **HH** **PA**
☒ 1 - Start of care—further visits planned
☐ 3 - Resumption of care (after inpatient stay)
   When ROC, review patient tracking information and complete M0032.

(M0102) Date of Physician-ordered Start of Care (Resumption of Care): If the physician indicated a specific start of care (resumption of care) date when the patient was referred for home health services, record the date specified. Ⓟ **HH**

___ / ___ / ___ ___ ___ ___ **[Go to M0110, if date entered]**
month / day / year
☒ NA - No specific SOC date ordered by physician

(M0104) Date of Referral: Indicate the date that the written or verbal referral for initiation or resumption of care was received by the HHA.
<u>0 2</u> / <u>0 7</u> / <u>2 0 1 7</u>
  month / day / year   Ⓟ **HH**

(M0110) Episode Timing: Is the Medicare home health payment episode for which this assessment will define a case mix group an "early" episode or a "later" episode in the patient's current sequence of adjacent Medicare home health payment episodes? ⬙ Ⓡ
☒ 1 - Early
☐ 2 - Later
☐ UK - Unknown
☐ NA - Not Applicable: No Medicare case mix group to be defined by this assessment.

*Early Episode is first or second episode in a sequence of adjacent episodes. **Later** is the third episode and beyond in sequence of adjacent episodes. Adjacent episodes are separated by 60 days or fewer between episodes.

PATIENT HISTORY AND DIAGNOSES

(M1000) From which of the following Inpatient Facilities was the patient discharged within the past 14 days? (Mark all that apply.)
☐ 1 - Long-term nursing facility (NF)   Ⓟ Ⓡ **HH**
☐ 2 - Skilled nursing facility (SNF / TCU)
☒ 3 - Short-stay acute hospital (IPPS)
☐ 4 - Long-term care hospital (LTCH)
☐ 5 - Inpatient rehabilitation hospital or unit (IRF)
☐ 6 - Psychiatric hospital or unit
☐ 7 - Other (specify) _____
☐ NA - Patient was not discharged from an inpatient facility
   [Go to M1017]

(M1005) Inpatient Discharge Date (most recent):
<u>0 2</u> / <u>0 8</u> / <u>2 0 1 7</u> ☐ UK - Unknown Ⓟ **HH**
month / day / year

(M1011) List each Inpatient Diagnosis and ICD-10-C M code at the level of highest specificity for only those conditions actively treated during an inpatient stay having a discharge date within the last 14 days (no V, W, X, Y, or Z codes or surgical codes): Ⓡ

Inpatient Facility Diagnosis	ICD-10-C M Code
a. open wound left leg	S 8 1 . 8 0 2 D
b. UTI	N 3 9 . 0
c. Bacterial pneumonia	J 1 5 . 9
d. Depression	F 3 2 . 9
e. Hypertension	I 1 0 .
f.	.

(M1017) Diagnoses Requiring Medical or Treatment Regimen Change Within Past 14 Days: List the patient's Medical Diagnoses and ICD-10-C M codes at the level of highest specificity for those conditions requiring changed medical or treatment regimen within the past 14 days (no V, W, X, Y, or Z codes or surgical codes): Ⓡ

Changed Medical Regimen Diagnosis	ICD-10-C M Code
a. Open wound left leg	S 8 1 . 8 0 2 D
b. UTI	N 3 9 . 0
c. Bacterial pneumonia	J 1 5 . 9
d. Depression	F 3 2 . 9
e. Hypertension	I 1 0 .
f.	.

☐ NA - Not applicable (no medical or treatment regimen changes within the past 14 days)

(M1018) Conditions Prior to Medical or Treatment Regimen Change or Inpatient Stay Within Past 14 Days: If this patient experienced an inpatient facility discharge or change in medical or treatment regimen within the past 14 days, indicate any conditions that existed <u>prior to</u> the inpatient stay or change in medical or treatment regimen. **(Mark all that apply.)** Ⓡ
☒ 1 - Urinary incontinence
☐ 2 - Indwelling/suprapubic catheter
☐ 3 - Intractable pain
☐ 4 - Impaired decision-making
☐ 5 - Disruptive or socially inappropriate behavior
☐ 6 - Memory loss to the extent that supervision required
☐ 7 - None of the above
☐ NA - No inpatient facility discharge <u>and</u> no change in medical or treatment regimen in past 14 days
☐ UK - Unknown

Form 3491P-15R © 2015 BRIGGS (800) 247-2343 www.BriggsCorp.com. The Outcome and ASsessment Information Set (OASIS) is the intellectual property of the Center for Health Services and Policy Research, Denver, Colorado. It is used with permission.

BRiGGS Healthcare·

**COMPREHENSIVE ADULT
NURSING ASSESSMENT
with OASIS ELEMENTS**
Page 2 of 22

Figure 8.3   Continued

Patient Name_____ ID #_____

PATIENT HISTORY AND DIAGNOSES (Cont'd.)

(M1021/1023/1025) Diagnoses, Symptom Control, and Optional Diagnoses: List each diagnosis for which the patient is receiving home care in Column 1, and enter its ICD-10-C M code at the level of highest specificity in Column 2 (diagnosis codes only - no surgical or procedure codes allowed). Diagnoses are listed in the order that best reflects the seriousness of each condition and supports the disciplines and services provided. Rate the degree of symptom control for each condition in Column 2. ICD-10-C M sequencing requirements must be followed if multiple coding is indicated for any diagnoses. If a Z-code is reported in Column 2 in place of a diagnosis that is no longer active (a resolved condition), then optional item M1025 (Optional Diagnoses - Columns 3 and 4) may be completed. Diagnoses reported in M1025 will not impact payment.

Code each row according to the following directions for each column:

Column 1: Enter the description of the diagnosis. Sequencing of diagnoses should reflect the seriousness of each condition and support the disciplines and services provided.

Column 2: Enter the ICD-10-C M code for the condition described in Column 1 - no surgical or procedure codes allowed. Codes must be entered at the level of highest specificity and ICD-10-C M coding rules and sequencing requirements must be followed. Note that external cause codes (ICD-10-C M codes beginning with V, W, X, or Y) may not be reported in M1021 (Primary Diagnosis) but may be reported in M1023 (Secondary Diagnoses). Also note that when a Z-code is reported in Column 2, the code for the underlying condition can often be entered in Column 2, as long as it is an active on-going condition impacting home health care.

Rate the degree of symptom control for the condition listed in Column 1. Do not assign a symptom control rating if the diagnosis codes is a V, W, X, Y or Z-code. Choose one value that represents the degree of symptom control appropriate for each diagnosis using the following scale:

    0 - Asymptomatic, no treatment needed at this time
    1 - Symptoms well controlled with current therapy
    2 - Symptoms controlled with difficulty, affecting daily functioning; patient needs ongoing monitoring
    3 - Symptoms poorly controlled; patient needs frequent adjustment in treatment and dose monitoring
    4 - Symptoms poorly controlled; history of re-hospitalizations

Note that the rating for symptom control in Column 2 should not be used to determine the sequencing of the diagnoses listed in Column 1. These are separate items and sequencing may not coincide.

Column 3: (OPTIONAL) There is no requirement that HHAs enter a diagnosis code in M1025 (Columns 3 and 4). Diagnoses reported in M1025 will not impact payment.

Agencies may choose to report an underlying condition in M1025 (Columns 3 and 4) when:
- a Z-code is reported in Column 2 AND
- the underlying condition for the Z-code in Column 2 is a resolved condition. An example of a resolved condition is uterine cancer that is no longer being treated following a hysterectomy.

Column 4: (OPTIONAL) If a Z-code is reported in M1021/M1023 (Column 2) and the agency chooses to report a resolved underlying condition that requires multiple diagnosis codes under ICD-10-C M coding guidelines, enter the diagnosis descriptions and the ICD-10-C M codes in the same row in Columns 3 and 4. For example, if the resolved condition is a manifestation code, record the diagnosis description and ICD-10-C M code for the underlying condition in Column 3 of that row and the diagnosis description and ICD-10-C M code for the manifestation in Column 4 of that row. Otherwise, leave Column 4 blank in that row.   M1021, M1023, M1025 = ◈ Ⓡ

(M1021) Primary Diagnosis & (M1023) Other Diagnoses		(M1025) Optional Diagnoses (OPTIONAL) (not used for payment)	
Column 1	Column 2	Column 3	Column 4
Diagnoses (Sequencing of diagnoses should reflect the seriousness of each condition and support the disciplines and services provided)	ICD-10-C M and symptom control rating for each condition. Note that the sequencing of these ratings may not match the sequencing of the diagnoses	May be completed if a Z-code is assigned to Column 2 and the underlying diagnosis is resolved	Complete only if the Optional Diagnosis is a multiple coding situation (for example: a manifestation code)
Description	ICD-10-C M / Symptom Control Rating	Description / ICD-10-C M	Description / ICD-10-C M
(M1021) Primary Diagnosis (Locator #11)	V, W, X, Y codes NOT allowed	V, W, X, Y, Z codes NOT allowed	V, W, X, Y, Z codes NOT allowed
a. Open wound left leg Date 1/19/2017 ☑ O ☐ E	a. S 8 1 . 8 0 2 D ☐0 ☐1 ☐2 ☑3 ☐4	a. _____ (_ _ _ . _ _ _ _)	a. _____ (_ _ _ . _ _ _ _)
(M1023) Other Diagnoses (Locator #13)	All ICD-10-C M codes allowed	V, W, X, Z codes NOT allowed	V, W, X, Y, Z codes NOT allowed
b. Hypertension Date 1/19/2017 ☐ O ☑ E	b. I 1 0 . ☐0 ☐1 ☑2 ☐3 ☐4	b. _____ (_ _ _ . _ _ _ _)	b. _____ (_ _ _ . _ _ _ _)
c. Depression Date 1/19/2017 ☑ O ☐ E	c. F 3 2 . 9 ☐0 ☐1 ☑2 ☐3 ☐4	c. _____ (_ _ _ . _ _ _ _)	c. _____ (_ _ _ . _ _ _ _)
d. Weakness Date 1/19/2017 ☐ O ☑ E	d. R 5 3 . 1 ☐0 ☐1 ☑2 ☐3 ☐4	d. _____ (_ _ _ . _ _ _ _)	d. _____ (_ _ _ . _ _ _ _)
e. Unsteady Gait Date 1/19/2017 ☐ O ☑ E	e. R 2 6 . 8 1 ☐0 ☐1 ☑2 ☐3 ☐4	e. _____ (_ _ _ . _ _ _ _)	e. _____ (_ _ _ . _ _ _ _)
f. Stress Incontinence Date 1/20/2010 ☑ O ☐ E	f. N 3 9 . 3 ☐0 ☐1 ☑2 ☐3 ☐4	f. _____ (_ _ _ . _ _ _ _)	f. _____ (_ _ _ . _ _ _ _)

☐ Check here if a coder or Business Associate was consulted with to complete ICD coding.

Surgical Procedure   **ICD** (Locator #12)

_____ (_____) Date_____

_____ (_____) Date_____

Form 3491P-15R © 2015 BRIGGS (800) 247-2343 www.BriggsCorp.com. The Outcome and ASsessment Information Set (OASIS) is the intellectual property of the Center for Health Services and Policy Research, Denver, Colorado. It is used with permission.

BRiGGS Healthcare

COMPREHENSIVE ADULT
NURSING ASSESSMENT
with OASIS ELEMENTS
Page 3 of 22

Figure 8.3 Continued

Patient Name_____ ID #_____

PATIENT HISTORY AND DIAGNOSES (Cont'd.)

PHYSICIAN: Date last contacted <u>02/09/2017</u>   Date last visited <u>02/08/2017</u>

PRIMARY REASON FOR HOME HEALTH:

Home care required following a 3 week stay in the hospital. The patient's neighbor found him at home following a fall. He had an open wound to his left leg, was disheveled and dirty in appearance and exhibited poor short term memory. EMS was called and the patient was taken to the ED and admitted to the hospital. While in the hospital he was diagnosed with a UTI and bacterial pneumonia, both were treated with antibiotics and resolved prior to discharge. He also reported feeling depressed and was evaluated in the hospital and placed on Celexa. He was also noted to have an increase in his blood pressure requiring a change to his antihypertensive medication regimen. SN is required for wound care to left lower leg, home safety evaluation, effectiveness of new medication changes- metoprolol and celexa, disease management education for wound management, hypertension, and depression. PT/OT for home safety, adaptive equipment, strengthening and gait training. MSW for community resources and HHA for personal care assistance.

HOMEBOUND REASON: (review/consider Face-to-Face documentation)   ☒ Needs assistance for all activities   ☒ Residual weakness
☒ Requires assistance to ambulate   ☐ Confusion, unable to go out of home alone   ☒ Unable to safely leave home unassisted
☐ Severe SOB   ☐ SOB upon exertion   ☒ Dependent upon adaptive device(s)   ☐ Medical restrictions
☒ Other (specify) <u>unsteady even with the use of walker</u>

PERTINENT HISTORY AND/OR PREVIOUS OUTCOMES: (note dates of onset, exacerbation when known)
(Reference M1000, M1005, and M1011)
☒ Hypertension ☐ Cardiac ☐ Diabetes ☐ Respiratory ☐ Osteoporosis ☐ Fractures ☐ Cancer (site:_____)
☐ Infection ☐ Immunosuppressed ☒ Open Wound ☐ Surgeries _____
☒ Other (specify) <u>depression</u>

IMMUNIZATIONS: Within the past 12 months: ☒ Influenza (specifically this year's flu season October 1 to March 31)
According to immunization guidelines: ☒ Pneumonia ☐ Tetanus ☐ Shingles ☐ Other _____
Needs: _____

PRIOR HOSPITALIZATIONS: ☐ No ☒ Yes   Number of times <u>2</u>   Reason(s)/Date(s):

1/19/2017-2/8/2017 for fall weakness, open wound, UTI, pneumonia, depression
10/1/2016-10/6/2016 for gastroenteritis and dehydration

(M1030) Therapies the patient receives at home: **(Mark all that apply.)**
☐ 1 - Intravenous or infusion therapy (excludes TPN)   ⊗ ®
☐ 2 - Parenteral nutrition (TPN or lipids)
☐ 3 - Enteral nutrition (nasogastric, gastrostomy, jejunostomy, or any other artificial entry into the alimentary canal)
☒ 4 - None of the above

(M1033) Risk for Hospitalization: Which of the following signs or symptoms characterize this patient as at risk for hospitalization? **(Mark all that apply.)** ®
☒ 1 - History of falls (2 or more falls - or any fall with an injury - in the past 12 months)
☒ 2 - Unintentional weight loss of a total of 10 pounds or more in the past 12 months
☒ 3 - Multiple hospitalizations (2 or more) in the past 6 months
☒ 4 - Multiple emergency department visits (2 or more) in the past 6 months
☐ 5 - Decline in mental, emotional, or behavioral status in the past 3 months
☐ 6 - Reported or observed history of difficulty complying with any medical instructions (for example, medications, diet, exercise) in the past 3 months
☒ 7 - Currently taking 5 or more medications
☒ 8 - Currently reports exhaustion
☐ 9 - Other risk(s) not listed in 1 - 8
☐ 10 - None of the above

(M1034) Overall Status: Which description best fits the patient's overall status? **(Check one)** ®
☐ 0 - The patient is stable with no heightened risk(s) for serious complications and death (beyond those typical of the patient's age).
☐ 1 - The patient is temporarily facing high health risk(s) but is likely to return to being stable with heightened risk(s) for serious complications and death (beyond those typical of the patient's age).
☒ 2 - The patient is likely to remain in fragile health and have ongoing high risk(s) of serious complications and death.
☐ 3 - The patient has serious progressive conditions that could lead to death within a year.
☐ UK - The patient's situation is unknown or unclear.

ADVANCE DIRECTIVES
☒ Living will   ☐ Education needed
☐ Do not resuscitate   ☒ Copies on file
☐ Organ donor   ☐ Funeral arrangements made
☒ POA   ☐ Healthcare representative
☐ State specific form(s)_____
Comments:

Patient's son James Hinckley is POA
101-202-3030

PROGNOSIS (Locator #20)
☐ 1-Poor ☐ 2-Guarded ☐ 3-Fair ☒ 4-Good ☐ 5-Excellent

(M1036) Risk Factors, either present or past, likely to affect current health status and/or outcome: **(Mark all that apply.)** ®
☐ 1 - Smoking
☐ 2 - Obesity
☐ 3 - Alcohol dependency
☐ 4 - Drug dependency
☒ 5 - None of the above
☐ UK - Unknown

Comments:

Mr. Hinckley lives alone in a single story home, he has 3 children who live out of state and are not involved in care. A neighbor assisting with groceries and meals is the only support the patient receives. Due his recent hospitalization, residual weakness, unsteady gait, wound, changes in medications and reports of depression he is at greater risk for exacerbation and readmission to the hospital.

Form 3491P-15R © 2015 BRIGGS (800) 247-2343 www.BriggsCorp.com. The Outcome and ASsessment Information Set (OASIS) is the intellectual property of the Center for Health Services and Policy Research, Denver, Colorado. It is used with permission.

BRIGGS Healthcare®

COMPREHENSIVE ADULT
NURSING ASSESSMENT
with OASIS ELEMENTS
Page 4 of 22

Figure 8.3   Continued

Patient Name_____ ID #_____

LIVING ARRANGEMENTS/SUPPORTIVE ASSISTANCE

(M1100) Patient Living Situation: Which of the following best describes the patient's residential circumstance and availability of assistance? **(Check one box only.)** [R]

Living Arrangement	Availability of Assistance				
	Around the clock	Regular daytime	Regular nighttime	Occasional/short-term assistance	No assistance available
a. Patient lives alone	☐ 01	☐ 02	☐ 03	▣ 04	☐ 05
b. Patient lives with other person(s) in the home	☐ 06	☐ 07	☐ 08	☐ 09	☐ 10
c. Patient lives in congregate situation (for example, assisted living, residential care home)	☐ 11	☐ 12	☐ 13	☐ 14	☐ 15

Name of facility_____ Phone_____

Primary Caregiver: ▣ Patient ☐ Family
☐ Caregiver (name)_____
Phone Number (if different from patient)_____
Relationship_____
List name/relationship of other caregiver(s) (other than home health staff) and the specific assistance they give with medical cares, ADLs, and/or IADLs:
Mrs. Johnson-Neighbor provides assistance with groceries and meals

Able to safely care for patient? ▣ Yes ☐ No
Comments:

Community resources (for example; Meals on Wheels; adult daycare):
Mr. Hinckley has not accessed any community resources currently or in the past.

EYES

(M1200) Vision (with corrective lenses if the patient usually wears them): [R]
☐ 0 - Normal vision: sees adequately in most situations; can see medication labels, newsprint.
▣ 1 - Partially impaired: cannot see medication labels or newsprint, but can see obstacles in path, and the surrounding layout; can count fingers at arm's length.
☐ 2 - Severely impaired: cannot locate objects without hearing or touching them, or patient nonresponsive.

☐ No Problem ▣ PERRLA
☐ Pupils unequal ▣ Glasses ☐ Glaucoma:☐ R ☐ L ☐ Cataract(s):▣ R ☐ L
☐ Scleral icterus/yellowing ☐ Contacts:☐ R ☐ L ☐ Blurred vision: ▣ R ▣ L
☐ Ptosis:☐ R ☐ L ☐ Prosthesis:☐ R ☐ L ☐ Blind:☐ R ☐ L
☐ Other_____
☐ Infections_____
☐ Cataract surgery: (Right) Date_____
(Left) Date_____
How does the impaired vision interfere/impact their function/safety?
(explain) *Patient reports he has an appointment with the eye doctor next week to get new glasses. He states he is going to discuss cataract removal at this appointment.*

NOSE

▣ No Problem
☐ Congestion ☐ Epistaxis ☐ Loss of smell ☐ Sinus problem
☐ Other (specify)

THROAT

▣ No Problem
☐ Dysphagia ☐ Hoarseness ☐ Lesion(s) ☐ Sore throat
☐ Other (specify)

MOUTH

▣ No Problem
☐ Dentures: ☐ Upper ☐ Lower ☐ Partial ☐ Mass(es) ☐ Tumor(s)
☐ Gingivitis ☐ Ulceration(s) ☐ Toothache ☐ Lesion(s)
☐ Other (specify)

EARS

(M1210) Ability to Hear (with hearing aid or hearing appliance if normally used): [R]
☐ 0 - Adequate: hears normal conversation without difficulty.
▣ 1 - Mildly to Moderately Impaired: difficulty hearing in some environments or speaker may need to increase volume or speak distinctly.
☐ 2 - Severely Impaired: absence of useful hearing.
☐ UK - Unable to assess hearing.

☐ No Problem
☐ HOH: ▣ R ▣ L ☐ Deaf: ☐ R ☐ L ☐ Hearing aid: ☐ R ☐ L
☐ Vertigo ☐ Tinnitus: ☐ R ☐ L
☐ Other (specify) *Patient denies HOH although upon arrival TV on very loud so patient could hear. Must speak loudly*

SPEECH/ORAL (VERBAL) EXPRESSION

(M1220) Understanding of Verbal Content in patient's own language (with hearing aid or device if used): [R]
☐ 0 - Understands: clear comprehension without cues or repetitions.
▣ 1 - Usually Understands: understands most conversations, but misses some part/intent of message. Requires cues at times to understand.
☐ 2 - Sometimes Understands: understands only basic conversations or simple, direct phrases. Frequently requires cues to understand.
☐ 3 - Rarely/Never Understands.
☐ UK - Unable to assess understanding.

(M1230) Speech and Oral (Verbal) Expression of Language (in patient's own language): ◇ [R]
☐ 0 - Expresses complex ideas, feelings, and needs clearly, completely, and easily in all situations with no observable impairment.
▣ 1 - Minimal difficulty in expressing ideas and needs (may take extra time; makes occasional errors in word choice, grammar or speech intelligibility; needs minimal prompting or assistance).
☐ 2 - Expresses simple ideas or needs with moderate difficulty (needs prompting or assistance, errors in word choice, organization or speech intelligibility). Speaks in phrases or short sentences.
☐ 3 - Has severe difficulty expressing basic ideas or needs and requires maximal assistance or guessing by listener. Speech limited to single words or short phrases.
☐ 4 - Unable to express basic needs even with maximal prompting or assistance but is not comatose or unresponsive (for example, speech is nonsensical or unintelligible).
☐ 5 - Patient nonresponsive or unable to speak.

Form 3491P-15R © 2015 BRIGGS (800) 247-2343 www.BriggsCorp.com. The Outcome and ASsessment Information Set (OASIS) is the intellectual property of the Center for Health Services and Policy Research, Denver, Colorado. It is used with permission.

BRiGGS Healthcare

COMPREHENSIVE ADULT NURSING ASSESSMENT with OASIS ELEMENTS
Page 5 of 22

Figure 8.3   Continued

PAIN

Patient Name _____ **ID #** _____

Check box to indicate which pain assessment was used.
- ☑ Wong-Baker
- ☐ PAINAD

Intensity: (using scales below)

Wong-Baker FACES Pain Rating Scale

NO HURT	HURTS LITTLE BIT	HURTS LITTLE MORE	HURTS EVEN MORE	HURTS WHOLE LOT	HURTS WORSE
0 No Pain	2	4 Moderate Pain	6	8	10 Worst Possible Pain

~From Wong D.L., Hockenberry-Eaton M., Wilson D., Winkelstein M.L., Schwartz P.: Wong's Essentials of Pediatric Nursing, ed. 6, St. Louis, 2001, p. 1301. Copyrighted by Mosby, Inc. Reprinted by permission.

Collected using: ☑ FACES Scale ☐ 0-10 Scale (subjective reporting)

☐ No Problem

Is patient experiencing pain? ☑ Yes ☐ No
☐ Unable to communicate

Non-verbals demonstrated: ☐ Diaphoresis ☐ Grimacing
☐ Moaning ☐ Crying ☐ Guarding ☐ Irritability ☐ Anger
☐ Tense ☑ Restlessness ☐ Change in vital signs
☐ Other:

Non-verbals demonstrated: (Cont'd.)
☑ Self-assessment ☐ Implications:

Patient reports when leg hurts he has a hard time walking and getting out of the chair

How does the pain interfere/impact the patient's safety? ☐ N/A
(explain)

the pain can cause the patient to shuffle when walking impacting safe ambulation.

Pain Assessment	Site 1	Site 2	Site 3
Location	left lower leg		
Onset	with movement		
Present level (0-10)	2		
Worst pain gets (0-10)	4		
Best pain gets (0-10)	1		
Pain description (aching, radiating, throbbing, etc.)	aching at wound site		

Pain Assessment IN Advanced Dementia - PAINAD*

ITEMS	0	1	2	SCORE
Breathing Independent of Vocalization	Normal	Occasional labored breathing. Short period of hyperventilation.	Noisy labored breathing. Long period of hyperventilation. Cheyne-Stokes respirations.	
Negative Vocalization	None	Occasional moan or groan. Low level speech with a negative or disapproving quality.	Repeated troubled calling out. Loud moaning or groaning. Crying.	
Facial Expression	Smiling, or inexpressive	Sad, Frightened, Frowning.	Facial grimacing	
Body Language	Relaxed	Tense, Distressed pacing, Fidgeting.	Rigid. Fists clenched, Knees pulled up. Pulling or pushing away. Striking out.	
Consolability	No need to console	Distracted or reassured by voice or touch.	Unable to console, distract or reassure.	

Total scores range from 0 to 10 (based on a scale of 0 to 2 for five items), with a higher score indicating more severe pain 0 = "no pain" to 10 = "severe pain"). **TOTAL****

Instructions: Observe the older person both at rest and during activity/with movement. For each of the items included in the PAINAD, select the score (0, 1, or 2) that reflects the current state of the person's behavior. Add the score for each item to achieve a total score. Monitor changes in the total score over time and in response to treatment to determine changes in pain. Higher scores suggest greater pain severity.

Note: Behavior observation scores should be considered in conjunction with knowledge of existing painful conditions and report from an individual knowledgeable of the person and their pain behaviors. Remember that some individuals may not demonstrate obvious pain behaviors or cues.

*Reference: Warden, V, Hurley AC, Volicer, V. (2003). Development and psychometric evaluation of the Pain Assessment In Advanced Dementia (PAINAD) Scale. *J Am Med Dir Assoc*, 4:9-15. Developed at the New England Document updated 1.10.2013.

(M1240) Has this patient had a formal **Pain Assessment** using a standardized, validated pain assessment tool (appropriate to the patient's ability to communicate the severity of pain)? Ⓟ HH
- ☐ 0 - No standardized, validated assessment conducted
- ☑ 1 - Yes, and it does not indicate severe pain
- ☐ 2 - Yes, and it indicates severe pain

(M1242) Frequency of Pain Interfering with patient's activity or movement: ◇ ◆ Ⓡ HH ★
- ☐ 0 - Patient has no pain
- ☐ 1 - Patient has pain that does not interfere with activity or movement
- ☐ 2 - Less often than daily
- ☑ 3 - Daily, but not constantly
- ☐ 4 - All of the time

Form 3491P-15R © 2015 BRIGGS (800) 247-2343 www.BriggsCorp.com. The Outcome and ASsessment Information Set (OASIS) is the intellectual property of the Center for Health Services and Policy Research, Denver, Colorado. It is used with permission.

BRIGGS Healthcare®

COMPREHENSIVE ADULT NURSING ASSESSMENT with OASIS ELEMENTS
Page 6 of 22

Figure 8.3   Continued

Patient Name_____ ID #_____

PAIN (Cont'd.)	INTEGUMENTARY STATUS

PAIN (Cont'd.)

What makes pain worse? ☒ Movement ☒ Ambulation ☐ Immobility
☐ Other:_____
Is there a pattern to the pain? (explain)

no

What makes pain better? ☐ Heat ☐ Ice ☐ Massage ☐ Repositioning
☒ Rest ☐ Relaxation ☒ Medication ☐ Diversion
☐ Other:_____
How often is breakthrough medication needed? ☒ Never
☐ Less than daily ☐ Daily ☐ 2-3 times/day
☐ More than 3 times/day
Does the pain radiate? ☐ Occasionally ☐ Continuously ☐ Intermittent
Current pain control medications adequate: ☒ Yes ☐ No
Comment:

Patient reports pain is manageable when
acetaminophen is taken every 8-10 hours when
he first starts to feel pain

ENDOCRINE/HEMATOLOGY

☒ **No Problem**
Disorder(s) of endocrine system (type)

☐ Fatigue Intolerance to: ☐ heat ☐ cold
Disorder(s) of blood (type)_____
☐ Anemia (specify if known)_____
☐ Secondary bleed: ☐ GI ☐ GU ☐ GYN ☐ Unknown ☐ Hemophilia
☐ Other _____

☐ Diabetes: ☐ Type I Juvenile ☐ Type II Date of onset _____
☐ Diabetic diet ☐ Oral medication ☐ Injectable medication
☐ Medication name, dose / frequency (specify)

On medication since _____
Administered by: ☐ Self ☐ Caregiver ☐ Nurse ☐ Family
                        ☐ Other_____
☐ Hyperglycemia: ☐ Glycosuria ☐ Polyuria ☐ Polydipsia
☐ Hypoglycemia: ☐ Sweats ☐ Polyphagia ☐ Weak ☐ Faint ☐ Stupor
A1C _____% ☐ Patient reported
    ☐ Lab slip Date:_____
BS _____ mg/dL Date/Time:_____ _____
    ☐ FBS ☐ Before meal ☐ Postprandial ☐ Random ☐ HS
☐ Blood sugar ranges_____
    ☐ Patient ☐ Caregiver ☐ Family Report
    Monitored by: ☐ Self ☐ Caregiver ☐ Family ☐ Nurse
                        ☐ Other_____
    Frequency of monitoring _____
    Competency with use of Glucometer _____
☐ **Disease Management Problems (explain)**

INTEGUMENTARY STATUS

☐ **No Problem**
Disorder(s) of skin, hair, nails (details)

Open wound to left leg as a result of hitting a
coffee table during a fall. Several scars noted to
lower legs bilaterally and forearms. Patient
reports are from previous falls.

Check all applicable conditions listed below:
Turgor: ☒ Good ☐ Poor
☐ Itch ☐ Rash ☐ Dry ☐ Scaling ☐ Redness ☐ Bruises
☐ Ecchymosis ☐ Pallor ☐ Jaundice
☐ Other (specify)

Definitions:
- **Unhealed:** The absence of the skin's original integrity.
- **Non-epithelialized:** The absence of the regeneration of the epidermis
  across a wound surface.
- **Pressure Ulcer:** A *pressure ulcer* is localized injury to the skin and/or
  underlying tissue, usually over a bony prominence, as a result of
  pressure or pressure in combination with shear. *A number of
  contributing or confounding factors also are associated with pressure
  ulcers; the significance of these factors is yet to be elucidated.*

(M1300) Pressure Ulcer Assessment: Was this patient assessed for
Risk of Developing Pressure Ulcers? ⓟ Ⓡ ⒽⒽ
☐ 0 - No assessment conducted *[Go to M1306]*
☐ 1 - Yes, based on an evaluation of clinical factors (for example,
    mobility, incontinence, nutrition) without use of standardized tool
☒ 2 - Yes, using a standardized, validated tool (for example, Braden
    Scale, Norton Scale)

(M1302) Does this patient have a **Risk of Developing Pressure Ulcers**?
☒ 0 - No ☐ 1 - Yes   Ⓡ

(M1306) Does this patient have at least one **Unhealed Pressure Ulcer at
Stage II or Higher** or designated as Unstageable? (Excludes Stage I
pressure ulcers and healed Stage II pressure ulcers) Ⓡ ⓅⒶ
☒ 0 - No *[Go to M1322]* ☐ 1 - Yes

**Complete Braden Scale form per organizational guideline (Briggs
#3166). WOCN Staging Guidelines (see page 9 of 22).**

Definitions:
- **Newly epithelialized:**
  - Wound bed completely covered with new epithelium.
  - No exudate.
  - No avascular tissue (eschar and/or slough).
  - No signs or symptoms of infection.
- **Fully granulating:**
  - Wound bed filled with granulation tissue to the level of the
    surrounding skin.
  - No dead space.
  - No avascular tissue (eschar and/or slough).
  - No signs or symptoms of infection.
  - Wound edges are open.

Form 3491P-15R © 2015 BRIGGS (800) 247-2343 www.BriggsCorp.com. The Outcome and ASsessment Information Set (OASIS)
is the intellectual property of the Center for Health Services and Policy Research, Denver, Colorado. It is used with permission.

BRIGGS Healthcare

**COMPREHENSIVE ADULT
NURSING ASSESSMENT
with OASIS ELEMENTS**
Page 7 of 22

Figure 8.3   Continued

Patient Name_____ ID #_____

INTEGUMENTARY STATUS (Cont'd.)

Definitions: (Cont'd.)

- **Early/partial granulation:**
  - ≥25% of the wound bed is covered with granulation tissue.
  - <25% of the wound bed is covered with avascular tissue (eschar and/or slough).
  - No signs or symptoms of infection.
  - Wound edges open.

- **Not healing:**
  - Wound with ≥25% avascular tissue (eschar and/or slough) OR
  - Signs/symptoms of infection OR
  - Clean but non-granulating wound bed OR
  - Closed/hyperkeratotic wound edges OR
  - Persistent failure to improve despite appropriate comprehensive wound management.

(M1308) Current Number of Unhealed Pressure Ulcers at Each Stage or Unstageable: (Enter "0" if none; Excludes Stage I pressure ulcers and healed Stage II pressure ulcers) ⬦ R (PA)

	Stage Descriptions—unhealed pressure ulcers	Number Currently Present
a.	**Stage II:** Partial thickness loss of dermis presenting as a shallow open ulcer with red pink wound bed, without slough. May also present as an intact or open/ruptured serum-filled blister.	_____
b.	**Stage III:** Full thickness tissue loss. Subcutaneous fat may be visible but bone, tendon, or muscles are not exposed. Slough may be present but does not obscure the depth of tissue loss. May include undermining and tunneling.	_____
c.	**Stage IV:** Full thickness tissue loss with visible bone, tendon, or muscle. Slough or eschar may be present on some parts of the wound bed. Often includes undermining and tunneling.	_____
d.1	Unstageable: Known or likely but Unstageable due to non-removable dressing or device	_____
d.2	Unstageable: Known or likely but Unstageable due to coverage of wound bed by slough and/or eschar.	_____
d.3	Unstageable: Suspected deep tissue injury in evolution.	_____

(M1320) Status of Most Problematic Pressure Ulcer that is Observable: (Excludes pressure ulcer that cannot be observed due to a non-removable dressing/device)
- ☐ 0 - Newly epithelialized
- ☐ 1 - Fully granulating
- ☐ 2 - Early/partial granulation
- ☐ 3 - Not healing
- ☐ NA - No observable pressure ulcer

(M1322) Current Number of Stage I Pressure Ulcers: Intact skin with non-blanchable redness of a localized area usually over a bony prominence. The area may be painful, firm, soft, warmer, or cooler as compared to adjacent tissue. ⬦ R
- ■0 ☐1 ☐2 ☐3 ☐4 or more

(M1324) Stage of Most Problematic Unhealed Pressure Ulcer that is Stageable: (Excludes pressure ulcer that cannot be staged due to a non-removable dressing/device, coverage of wound bed by slough and/or eschar, or suspected deep tissue injury.) ⬦ R (PA)
- ☐ 1 - Stage I
- ☐ 2 - Stage II
- ☐ 3 - Stage III
- ☐ 4 - Stage IV
- ■ NA - Patient has no pressure ulcers or no stageable pressure ulcers

(M1330) Does this patient have a Stasis Ulcer? ⬦ R
- ■0 - No **[Go to M1340]**
- ☐1 - Yes, patient has BOTH observable and unobservable stasis ulcers
- ☐2 - Yes, patient has observable stasis ulcers ONLY
- ☐3 - Yes, patient has unobservable stasis ulcers ONLY (known but not observable due to non-removable dressing/device) **[Go to M1340]**

(M1332) Current Number of Stasis Ulcer(s) that are Observable:
- ☐1 - One ⬦ R
- ☐2 - Two
- ☐3 - Three
- ☐4 - Four or more

(M1334) Status of Most Problematic Stasis Ulcer that is Observable:
- ☐1 - Fully granulating ⬦ R (PA)
- ☐2 - Early/partial granulation
- ☐3 - Not healing

(M1340) Does this patient have a **Surgical Wound?** ◇ R HH
- ■0 - No **[Go to M1350]**
- ☐1 - Yes, patient has at least one observable surgical wound
- ☐2 - Surgical wound known but not observable due to non-removable dressing/device **[Go to M1350]**

(M1342) Status of Most Problematic Surgical Wound that is Observable
- ☐0 - Newly epithelialized ◇ ⬦ R HH (PA)
- ☐1 - Fully granulating
- ☐2 - Early/partial granulation
- ☐3 - Not healing

(M1350) Does this patient have a **Skin Lesion** or **Open Wound** (excluding bowel ostomy), other than those described above, <u>that is receiving intervention</u> by the home health agency? R
- ☐0 - No
- ■1 - Yes

Form 3491P-15R © 2015 BRIGGS (800) 247-2343 www.BriggsCorp.com. The Outcome and ASsessment Information Set (OASIS) is the intellectual property of the Center for Health Services and Policy Research, Denver, Colorado. It is used with permission.

BRIGGS Healthcare

COMPREHENSIVE ADULT NURSING ASSESSMENT with OASIS ELEMENTS
Page 8 of 22

Figure 8.3 Continued

Patient Name_____ ID #_____

INTEGUMENTARY STATUS (Cont'd.)

Pressure Ulcer Stages (NPUAP):

Category/Stage I: Non-blanchable erythema. A Stage I pressure ulcer presents as intact skin with non-blanchable redness of a localized area, usually over a bony prominence. Darkly pigmented skin may not have visible blanching; its color may differ from the surrounding area. The area may be painful, firm, soft, and warmer or cooler as compared to adjacent tissue. Stage I ulcers may be difficult to detect in individuals with dark skin tones and may indicate "at risk" persons (a heralding sign of risk).

Category/Stage II: Partial thickness. A Stage II pressure ulcer is characterized by partial-thickness loss of dermis presenting as a shallow open ulcer with a red-pink wound bed without slough. It also may present as an intact or open/ruptured serum-filled blister. A Stage II ulcer also may present as a shiny or dry shallow ulcer without slough or bruising.* This stage should not be used to describe skin tears, tape burns, perineal dermatitis, maceration, or excoriation. *Bruising indicates suspected deep tissue injury.

Category/Stage III: Full thickness skin loss. A Stage III pressure ulcer is characterized by full-thickness tissue loss. Subcutaneous fat may be visible but bone, tendon, or muscle is not exposed. Slough may be present but does not obscure the depth of tissue loss. Stage III ulcers may include undermining and tunneling. The depth of a Stage III pressure ulcer varies by anatomical location. The bridge of the nose, ear, occiput, and malleolus do not have subcutaneous tissue; Stage III ulcers in these locations can be shallow. In contrast, areas of significant adiposity can develop extremely deep Stage III pressure ulcers. Bone/tendon is not visible or directly palpable.

Category/Stage IV: Full thickness tissue loss. A Stage IV pressure ulcer presents with full-thickness tissue loss with exposed bone, tendon, or muscle. Slough or eschar may be present on some parts of the wound bed. These ulcers often include undermining and tunneling. The depth of a Stage IV pressure ulcer varies by anatomical location. The bridge of the nose, ear, occiput, and malleolus do not have subcutaneous tissue; Stage IV ulcers in these locations can be shallow. Stage IV ulcers can extend into muscle and/or supporting structures (e.g., fascia, tendon, or joint capsule); osteomyelitis is possible. Exposed bone/tendon is visible or directly palpable.

Unstageable/Unclassified: Full thickness skin or tissue loss – depth unknown. Full-thickness tissue loss in which the base of the ulcer is covered by slough (yellow, tan, gray, green or brown) and/or eschar (tan, brown or black) in the wound bed may render a wound unstageable. Until enough slough and/or eschar is removed to expose the base of the wound, the true depth (and therefore, the stage) cannot be determined. Stable (dry, adherent, intact without erythema or fluctuance) eschar on the heels serves as "the body's natural (biological) cover" and should not be removed.

Suspected Deep Tissue Injury – depth unknown. Deep tissue injury may be characterized by a purple or maroon localized area of discolored intact skin or a blood-filled blister due to damage of underlying soft tissue from pressure and/or shear. Presentation may be preceded by tissue that is painful, firm, mushy, boggy, and warmer or cooler as compared to adjacent tissue. Deep tissue injury may be difficult to detect in individuals with dark skin tones. Evolution may include a thin blister over a dark wound bed. The wound may further evolve and become covered by thin eschar. Evolution may be rapid, exposing additional layers of tissue even with optimal treatment.

OASIS-C1 Guidance Document – Content Validated - February, 2014
W.O.C.N. • 15000 Commerce Parkway, Suite C, Mount Laurel, NJ 08054

WOUND CARE: (Check all that apply) ☐ N/A

Wound care done during this visit: ☑ Yes ☐ No

  Location(s) wound site: _Open wound to left lower leg_

☑ Soiled dressing removed by:

  ☐ Patient ☐ Caregiver (name)_____ ☐ Family ☑ RN ☐ PT ☐ Other:_____

Technique: ☐ Sterile ☑ Clean

☐ Wound cleaned with (specify): _wound cleanser_

☐ Wound irrigated with (specify): _____

☐ Wound packed with (specify): _____

☑ Wound dressing applied (specify): _hydrogel impregnated dressing, covered with 4 x4, secured with rolled gauze followed by elastic bandage_

Patient tolerated procedure well: ☑ Yes ☐ No

Comments:
        Patient states wound is getting much better, smaller in size and less pain. Patient wanting to learn how to perform wound care.

DIABETIC FOOT EXAM: (Check all that apply) ☑ N/A

Frequency of diabetic foot exam_____

Done by: ☐ Patient ☐ Caregiver (name)_____ ☐ Family ☐ RN ☐ PT ☐ Other:_____

Exam by clinician this visit: ☐ Yes ☐ No

  Integument findings:

Pedal pulses: Present ☐ right ☐ left   Absent ☐ right ☐ left

  Comment:_____

Loss of sense of: Warm ☐ right ☐ left   Cold ☐ right ☐ left

  Comment:_____

Neuropathy ☐ right ☐ left

Tingling ☐ right ☐ left   Burning ☐ right ☐ left   Leg hair: ☐ Present ☐ right ☐ left ☐ Absent ☐ right ☐ left

Complete LEAP Diabetic Foot Screening (Briggs form 3484P) per organizational guideline

Comments:_____

Form 3491P-15R © 2015 BRIGGS (800) 247-2343 www.BriggsCorp.com. The Outcome and ASsessment Information Set (OASIS) is the intellectual property of the Center for Health Services and Policy Research, Denver, Colorado. It is used with permission.

BRiGGS Healthcare®

COMPREHENSIVE ADULT NURSING ASSESSMENT
with OASIS ELEMENTS
Page 9 of 22

Figure 8.3   Continued

Patient Name_____ ID #_____

INTEGUMENTARY STATUS (Cont'd.)

WOUND/LESION (specify)	#1	#2	#3	#4	#5
Location	left anterior lower leg				
Type: Arterial / Diabetic foot ulcer / Malignancy / Mechanical/Trauma / Pressure ulcer / Surgical / Venous stasis ulcer	Mechanical/tra uma				
Size (cm) (LxWxD)	8cm X 3 cm X 1 cm				
Tunneling/Sinus Tract	length _____ cm @ _____ o'clock	length _____ cm @ _____ o'clock	length _____ cm @ _____ o'clock	length _____ cm @ _____ o'clock	length _____ cm @ _____ o'clock
Undermining (cm)	_____ cm, from _____ to _____ o'clock	_____ cm, from _____ to _____ o'clock	_____ cm, from _____ to _____ o'clock	_____ cm, from _____ to _____ o'clock	_____ cm, from _____ to _____ o'clock
Stage (pressure ulcers only)					
Odor	none				
Surrounding Skin	pink/healthy				
Edema	none				
Stoma	none				
Appearance of the Wound Bed	beefy red granulation tissue				
Drainage/Amount	☐ None ☑ Small ☐ Moderate ☐ Large	☐ None ☐ Small ☐ Moderate ☐ Large	☐ None ☐ Small ☐ Moderate ☐ Large	☐ None ☐ Small ☐ Moderate ☐ Large	☐ None ☐ Small ☐ Moderate ☐ Large
Color	☑ Clear ☐ Tan ☐ Serosanguineous ☐ Other	☐ Clear ☐ Tan ☐ Serosanguineous ☐ Other	☐ Clear ☐ Tan ☐ Serosanguineous ☐ Other	☐ Clear ☐ Tan ☐ Serosanguineous ☐ Other	☐ Clear ☐ Tan ☐ Serosanguineous ☐ Other
Consistency	☑ Thin ☐ Thick	☐ Thin ☐ Thick	☐ Thin ☐ Thick	☐ Thin ☐ Thick	☐ Thin ☐ Thick

SYSTEMS REVIEW

Height: 6'3" ☑ reported ☐ actual   Weight: 130 ☑ reported ☐ actual

Reported Wt. Changes: ☐ Gain ☑ Loss 5 lb. X _____ ☐ wk ☐ mo ☑ yr

VITAL SIGNS

Blood Pressure:	Left	Right	Sitting/Lying	Standing
At rest	176/90	168/88		150/80
With activity				
Post activity				

Temperature: 98.4 ☑ Oral ☐ Axillary ☐ Rectal ☐ Tympanic

Pulse: ☑ Apical 74 ☐ Brachial ☑ Regular ☐ Irregular ☐ Radial ☐ Carotid

Respirations: 20 ☑ Regular ☐ Irregular ☐ Cheynes Stokes
☐ Death rattle ☐ Apnea periods _____ sec. (☐ observed ☐ reported)
☐ Accessory muscles used
☑ Non-smoker ☐ Smoker Last smoked: never

CARDIOPULMONARY

Disorder(s) of heart/respiratory system (type)

10 year history of hypertension managed with medication and diet however has been eating an increase in frozen dinners lately. Hx of pneumonia

Breath Sounds:
(Clear, crackles/rales, wheezes/rhonchi, diminished, absent)
Anterior:
Right rhonchi   Left rhonchi

CARDIOPULMONARY (Cont'd.)

Breath Sounds (Cont'd.):
Posterior:
Right Upper diminished   Left Upper _____
Right Lower diminished   Left Lower diminished

O_2 @ _____ LPM via ☐ cannula ☐ mask ☐ trach O_2 saturation _____ %

Trach size/type _____
Who manages? ☐ Self ☐ RN ☐ Caregiver ☐ Family

Intermittent treatments (C&DB, medicated inhalation treatments, etc.)
☑ No
☐ Yes, explain:

Cough: ☐ No
☑ Yes: ☐ Productive ☑ Non-productive
Describe:

Dyspnea: ☐ At rest ☑ During ADLs
Comments: Pneumonia dx in hospital resolved with residual coarse breath sounds and dyspnea with exertion noted to continue.

Positioning necessary for improved breathing:
☑ No ☐ Yes, describe:

Heart Sounds: ☑ Regular ☐ Irregular ☐ Murmur
☐ Pacemaker: Date_____ Last date checked_____
Type_____

Form 3491P-15R © 2015 BRIGGS (800) 247-2343 www.BriggsCorp.com. The Outcome and ASsessment Information Set (OASIS) is the intellectual property of the Center for Health Services and Policy Research, Denver, Colorado. It is used with permission.

BRIGGS Healthcare®

COMPREHENSIVE ADULT
NURSING ASSESSMENT
with OASIS ELEMENTS
Page 10 of 22

Figure 8.3   Continued

Patient Name_____ ID #_____

CARDIOPULMONARY (Cont'd.)

Chest Pain: ☐ Anginal ☐ Postural ☐ Localized ☐ Substernal
☐ Radiating ☐ Dull ☐ Ache ☐ Sharp ☐ Vise-like
Associated with: ☐ Shortness of breath ☐ Activity ☐ Sweats
Frequency/duration:_____
How relieved:

☐ Palpitations ☐ Fatigue
Edema: ☐ Pedal ☐ Right ☐ Left ☐ Sacral
☐ Dependent:
☐ Pitting ☐ +1 ☐ +2 ☐ +3 ☐ +4 ☐ Non-pitting
Site:_____
☐ Cramps ☐ Claudication
Capillary refill: ☐ Less than 3 sec ☐ Greater than 3 sec
☐ **Disease Management Problems (explain)**

Requires education related to hypertension-s/sx, pathophysiology, diet choices, and pacing activities to prevent SOB following bout of pneumonia.

RESPIRATORY STATUS

(M1400) When is the patient dyspneic or noticeably **Short of Breath?**
☐ 0 - Patient is not short of breath ◇ ❖ Ⓡ ⓗⓗ ★
☐ 1 - When walking more than 20 feet, climbing stairs
☑ 2 - With moderate exertion (for example, while dressing, using commode or bedpan, walking distances less than 20 feet)
☐ 3 - With minimal exertion (for example, while eating, talking, or performing other ADLs) or with agitation
☐ 4 - At rest (during day or night)
☑ **Assessed** ☐ **Reported**

(M1410) Respiratory Treatments utilized at home: **(Mark all that apply.)**
☐ 1 - Oxygen (intermittent or continuous) Ⓡ
☐ 2 - Ventilator (continually or at night)
☐ 3 - Continuous / Bi-level positive airway pressure
☑ 4 - None of the above

NUTRITIONAL STATUS

☐ **No Problem**
☑ NAS ☐ NPO ☐ Controlled Carbohydrate ☐ Other_____

Nutritional requirements (diet) (Locator #16)

☐ Increase fluids_____ amt. ☐ Restrict fluids_____ amt.

Appetite: ☐ Good ☑ Fair ☐ Poor ☐ Anorexic
☐ Nausea ☐ Vomiting:
Frequency_____ Amount_____
☐ Heartburn (food intolerance)
☐ Other Patient reports that he, "just doesn't have much of an appetite since he got sick". Neighbor to bring nutritious low sodium meals while patient recovering. He verbalizes knowledge of a low sodium diet but states while sick was easier to eat frozen prepared meals.

Directions: Check each area with "yes" to assessment, then total score to determine additional risk.	YES
Has an illness or condition that changed the kind and/or amount of food eaten.	☑ 2
Eats fewer than 2 meals per day.	☐ 3
Eats few fruits, vegetables or milk products.	☐ 2
Has 3 or more drinks of beer, liquor or wine almost every day.	☐ 2
Has tooth or mouth problems that make it hard to eat.	☐ 2
Does not always have enough money to buy the food needed.	☐ 4
Eats alone most of the time.	☑ 1
Takes 3 or more different prescribed or over-the-counter drugs a day.	☑ 1
Without wanting to, has lost or gained 10 pounds in the last 6 months.	☑ 2
Not always physically able to shop, cook and/or feed self.	☑ 2
TOTAL	9

Reprinted with permission by the Nutrition Screening Initiative, a project of the American Academy of Family Physicians, the American Dietetic Association and the National Council on the Aging, Inc., and funded in part by a grant from Ross Products Division, Abbott Laboratories Inc.

NUTRITIONAL STATUS (Cont'd.)

INTERPRETATION OF ASSESSMENT

0-2 Good. As appropriate reassess and/or provide information based on situation.
3-5 Moderate risk. Educate, refer, monitor and reevaluate based on patient situation and organization policy.
6 or more High risk. Coordinate with physician, dietitian, social service professional or nurse about how to improve nutritional health. Reassess nutritional status and educate based on plan of care.

Describe at risk intervention and plan:

ENTERAL FEEDINGS - ACCESS DEVICE

☑ **N/A** ☐ **No Problem**
☐ Nasogastric ☐ Gastrostomy ☐ Jejunostomy
☐ Other (specify)_____
☐ Pump: (type/specify)_____
☐ Bolus ☐ Continuous
Feedings: Type (amt./rate)_____
Flush Protocol: (amt./specify)_____
Performed by: ☐ Self ☐ RN ☐ Caregiver ☐ Family
☐ Other_____
☐ Dressing ☐ Site care: (specify)_____

Interventions /Instructions / Comments

ELIMINATION STATUS

Urinary Elimination: ☐ No Problem
Disorder(s) of urinary system (type)
incontinence, Hx of UTI while in hospital, treated with antibiotics and resolved.
(Check all applicable items)
☑ Urgency ☐ Frequency ☐ Retention ☐ Burning ☐ Pain
☐ Hesitancy ☐ Nocturia ☐ Hematuria ☐ Oliguria ☐ Anuria
☑ Incontinence (details if applicable)
The patient reports never sure if he will make it to the bathroom and frequently has episodes of incontinence when he laughs, coughs or lifts heavy objects. He now wears a brief "just in case". Does not use time voiding strategies.

Color: ☑ Yellow/straw ☐ Amber ☐ Brown ☐ Gray ☐ Blood-tinged
☐ Other:_____
Clarity: ☑ Clear ☐ Cloudy ☐ Sediment ☐ Mucous
Odor: ☐ Yes ☑ No ☐ Observed ☐ Reported
☐ Diapers / other:_____
Urinary Catheter: Type_____ Date last changed_____
☐ Foley inserted (date)_____ mL with_____ French
Inflated balloon with_____ mL ☐ without difficulty ☐ Suprapubic
Irrigation solution: Type (specify)_____
Amount_____ mL Frequency_____ Returns_____
Patient tolerated procedure well ☐ Yes ☐ No
☐ Urostomy site (details around skin around stoma):

Ostomy care managed by: ☐ Self ☐ Caregiver ☐ Family
☐ **Disease Management Problems (explain)**

patient would benefit from education regarding timed voiding techniques and signs and symptoms of UTI.

(M1600) Has this patient been treated for a **Urinary Tract Infection** in the past 14 days? ◇ ⒫Ⓐ
☐ 0 - No
☑ 1 - Yes
☐ NA - Patient on prophylactic treatment
☐ UK - Unknown

Form 3491P-15R © 2015 BRIGGS (800) 247-2343 www.BriggsCorp.com. The Outcome and ASsessment Information Set (OASIS) is the intellectual property of the Center for Health Services and Policy Research, Denver, Colorado. It is used with permission.

BRIGGS Healthcare®

COMPREHENSIVE ADULT
NURSING ASSESSMENT
with OASIS ELEMENTS
Page 11 of 22

Figure 8.3   Continued

Patient Name_____ ID #_____

ELIMINATION STATUS (Cont'd.)

(M1610) Urinary Incontinence or Urinary Catheter Presence: ◇ ⬦ R

☐ 0 - No incontinence or catheter (includes anuria or ostomy for urinary drainage) **[Go to M1620]**

☑ 1 - Patient is incontinent

☐ 2 - Patient requires a urinary catheter (specifically: external, indwelling, intermittent, or suprapubic) **[Go to M1620]**

(M1615) When does Urinary Incontinence occur? ◇ R

☐ 0 - Timed-voiding defers incontinence

☑ 1 - Occasional stress incontinence

☐ 2 - During the night only

☐ 3 - During the day only

☐ 4 - During the day and night

Bowel Elimination: ☑ No Problem

Disorder(s) of GI system (type)

☐ Flatulence ☐ Constipation ☐ Fecal impaction ☐ Diarrhea

☐ Rectal bleeding ☐ Hemorrhoids ☐ Last BM_____

☑ Bowel sounds: active ˣ⁴_____

absent_____

hypoactive_____

hyperactive_____

RU	LU
RL	LL

☑ Frequency of stools ᵈᵃⁱˡʸ_____

Bowel regimen/program: drinks prune juice daily

☐ Laxative ☐ Enema use: ☐ Daily ☐ Weekly ☐ Monthly ☐ PRN

☐ Other:_____

☐ Involuntary incontinence (details if applicable)

☐ Diapers/other:_____

☐ Ileostomy ☐ Colostomy site (describe skin around stoma):

Ostomy care managed by: ☐ Self ☐ Caregiver ☐ Family

☐ Other

(M1620) Bowel Incontinence Frequency: ◇ ⬦ R

☑ 0 - Very rarely or never has bowel incontinence

☐ 1 - Less than once weekly

☐ 2 - One to three times weekly

☐ 3 - Four to six times weekly

☐ 4 - On a daily basis

☐ 5 - More often than once daily

☐ NA - Patient has ostomy for bowel elimination

☐ UK - Unknown

(M1630) Ostomy for Bowel Elimination: Does this patient have an ostomy for bowel elimination that (within the last 14 days): a) was related to an inpatient facility stay; <u>or</u> b) necessitated a change in medical or treatment regimen? ⬦

☑ 0 - Patient does <u>not</u> have an ostomy for bowel elimination.

☐ 1 - Patient's ostomy was <u>not</u> related to an inpatient stay and did <u>not</u> necessitate change in medical or treatment regimen.

☐ 2 - The ostomy <u>was</u> related to an inpatient stay or <u>did</u> necessitate change in medical or treatment regimen.

ABDOMEN

☑ No Problem

☐ Tenderness ☐ Pain ☐ Distention ☐ Hard ☐ Soft ☐ Ascites

☐ Abdominal girth_____ cm

☐ Other:_____

GENITALIA

☑ No Problem

☐ Discharge/Drainage: (describe)_____

☐ Lesions ☐ Blisters ☐ Masses ☐ Cysts

☐ Inflammation ☐ Surgical alteration

☐ Prostate problem: ☐ BPH ☐ TURP Date_____

☐ Self-testicular exam Freq._____ Date last exam_____

☐ Menopause ☐ Hysterectomy Date_____

Date last PAP_____ Results_____

☐ Breast self-exam Freq._____ Date last exam_____

☐ Nipple discharge: ☐ R Date_____ ☐ L Date_____

☐ Mastectomy: ☐ R Date_____ ☐ L Date_____

☐ Other (specify)_____

NEURO/EMOTIONAL/BEHAVIORAL STATUS

(M1700) Cognitive Functioning: Patient's current (day of assessment) level of alertness, orientation, comprehension, concentration, and immediate memory for simple commands. ◇ Ⓟ R HH

☐ 0 - Alert/oriented, able to focus and shift attention, comprehends and recalls task directions independently.

☑ 1 - Requires prompting (cuing, repetition, reminders) only under stressful or unfamiliar conditions.

☐ 2 - Requires assistance and some direction in specific situations (for example, on all tasks involving shifting of attention) or consistently requires low stimulus environment due to distractibility.

☐ 3 - Requires considerable assistance in routine situations. Is not alert and oriented or is unable to shift attention and recall directions more than half the time.

☐ 4 - Totally dependent due to disturbances such as constant disorientation, coma, persistent vegetative state, or delirium.

☑ No Problem

Disorder(s) of neurological system (type)

☐ History of a traumatic brain injury Date_____

☐ History of headaches Date of last headache_____

(Type)_____

☐ Aphasic: ☐ Receptive ☐ Expressive

☐ Tremors: ☐ At Rest ☐ With voluntary movement ☐ Continuous

☐ Spasms (for example; back, bladder, legs) Location:_____

☐ History of seizures Date of last_____

(Type)_____

☐ Hemiplegia: ☐ Right ☐ Left

☐ Paraplegia ☐ Quadriplegia/Tetraplegia

How does the patient's condition affect functional ability and safety?

Patient reports that he has noticed an increase in his forgetfulness prior to his hospitalization. State it seems a bit better but still has difficulty with short term memory.

(M1710) When Confused (Reported or Observed Within the Last 14 Days): ◇ Ⓟ R HH Ⓟ

☐ 0 - Never

☐ 1 - In new or complex situations only

☐ 2 - On awakening or at night only

☑ 3 - During the day and evening, but not constantly

☐ 4 - Constantly

☐ NA - Patient nonresponsive

(M1720) When Anxious (Reported or Observed Within the Last 14 Days): ◇ Ⓟ R HH

☐ 0 - None of the time

☑ 1 - Less often than daily

☐ 2 - Daily, but not constantly

☐ 3 - All of the time

☐ NA - Patient nonresponsive

Form 3491P-15R © 2015 BRIGGS (800) 247-2343 www.BriggsCorp.com. The Outcome and ASsessment Information Set (OASIS) is the intellectual property of the Center for Health Services and Policy Research, Denver, Colorado. It is used with permission.

BRiGGS Healthcare·

COMPREHENSIVE ADULT NURSING ASSESSMENT with OASIS ELEMENTS
Page 12 of 22

Figure 8.3 Continued

Patient Name_____ ID #_____

NEURO / EMOTIONAL / BEHAVIORAL STATUS (Cont'd.)

(M1730) Depression Screening: Has the patient been screened for depression, using a standardized, validated depression screening tool?
☐0 - No   Ⓟ Ⓡ ⒽⒽ
☑1 - Yes, patient was screened using the PHQ-2© * scale.

Instructions for this two-question tool: Ask patient: "Over the last two weeks, how often have you been bothered by any of the following problems?"

PHQ-2©*	Not at all 0 - 1 day	Several days 2 - 6 days	More than half of the days 7 - 11 days	Nearly every day 12 - 14 days	NA Unable to respond
a) Little interest or pleasure in doing things	☐0	☑1	☐2	☐3	☐NA
b) Feeling down, depressed, or hopeless?	☐0	☑1	☐2	☐3	☐NA

☐2 - Yes, patient was screened with a different standardized, validated assessment and the patient meets criteria for further evaluation for depression.
☐3 - Yes, patient was screened with a different standardized, validated assessment and the patient does not meet criteria for further evaluation for depression.
*Copyright© Pfizer Inc. All rights reserved. Reproduced with permission.

(M1740) Cognitive, behavioral, and psychiatric symptoms that are demonstrated <u>at least once a week</u> **(Reported or Observed): (Mark all that apply.)** Ⓡ (PA)
☐1 - Memory deficit: failure to recognize familiar persons/places, inability to recall events of past 24 hours, significant memory loss so that supervision is required
☐2 - Impaired decision-making: failure to perform usual ADLs or IADLs, inability to appropriately stop activities, jeopardizes safety through actions
☐3 - Verbal disruption: yelling, threatening, excessive profanity, sexual references, etc.
☐4 - Physical aggression: aggressive or combative to self and others (for example, hits self, throws objects, punches, dangerous maneuvers with wheelchair or other objects)
☐5 - Disruptive, infantile, or socially inappropriate behavior **(excludes** verbal actions)
☐6 - Delusional, hallucinatory, or paranoid behavior
☑7 - None of the above behaviors demonstrated

(M1745) Frequency of Disruptive Behavior Symptoms (Reported or Observed): Any physical, verbal, or other disruptive/dangerous symptoms that are injurious to self or others or jeopardize personal safety. ◈ Ⓡ
☑0 - Never
☐1 - Less than once a month
☐2 - Once a month
☐3 - Several times each month
☐4 - Several times a week
☐5 - At least daily

(M1750) Is this patient receiving **Psychiatric Nursing Services** at home provided by a qualified psychiatric nurse?
☑0 - No
☐1 - Yes

MENTAL STATUS

(Locator #19)
☑1 - Oriented   ☐5 - Disoriented   ☐8 - Other
☐2 - Comatose   ☐6 - Lethargic
☐3 - Forgetful   ☐7 - Agitated
☐4 - Depressed

PSYCHOSOCIAL

Primary language English
☐Language barrier ☐Needs interpreter
  ☐Sign language (type)_____
Learning barrier: ☐Mental ☐Psychosocial ☐Physical ☐Functional
Unable to: ☐Read ☐Write   Educational level 10th grade
☑Spiritual☐Cultural implications that impact care.
Explain No spiritual or cultural implications

PSYCHOSOCIAL (Cont'd.)

Spiritual/Cultural implications that impact care (Cont'd.)
  Spiritual resource none_____
  Phone No._____
Sleep: ☐Adequate ☐Inadequate   Rest: ☑Adequate ☐Inadequate
  Frequency of naps: daily
  Number of hours slept per night: 6-8
  Explain_____
Inappropriate responses to☐Caregivers ☐Clinician ☐Family, in past
Inappropriate follow-through in past
  ☐Angry   ☐Flat affect   ☐Discouraged
  ☐Withdrawn   ☐Difficulty coping   ☑Disorganized
Depressed: ☑Recent ☐Long term
  Treatment: recent death of wife (8 mo ago) and 2 hospitalizations in time. dx in hosp and treated with celexa with good results.
Inability to cope with altered health status as evidenced by:
  ☑Lack of motivation   ☑Inability to recognize problems
  ☐Unrealistic expectations   ☐Denial of problems
Evidence of:☐Abuse ☐Neglect ☐Exploitation ☐Potential ☐Actual
  ☐Verbal ☐Emotional ☐Physical ☐Financial
  MSW referral made: ☑Yes ☐No
  Other intervention:_____
Comments:
home cluttered boxes and stacks creating narrow hallways, fire risk.repairs to front of home required. ramp needed

MUSCULOSKELETAL

☐**No Problem**
Disorder(s) of musculoskeletal system (type)
generalized weakness and unsteady, shuffling gait
☐Fracture (location)_____
☐Swollen, painful joints (specify)_____
☐Contracture(s): Location_____
Hand grips: ☑Equal☐Unequal ☐Strong ☑Weak (specify)_____
Dominant side: ☑R ☐L
☐Motor changes: ☐Fine ☐Gross (specify)_____
☑Weakness: ☑UE ☑LE (details) deconditioned following hospitalization
☐Atrophy_____   ☐Poor conditioning
☑Decreased ROM bilat LE   ☐Paresthesia_____
☑Shuffling☐Wide-based gait
☐Amputation: ☐BK ☐AK ☐UE; ☐R☐L (specify)

☐Other (specify)_____
How does the patient's condition affect their functional ability and safety?
(explain) Patient is unsafe ambulating and performing adls independently

BRiGGSHealthcare®

COMPREHENSIVE ADULT
NURSING ASSESSMENT
with OASIS ELEMENTS
Page 13 of 22

Figure 8.3   Continued

Patient Name_____ ID #_____

FUNCTIONAL LIMITATIONS

(Locator #18A)

- ☐ 1 - Amputation
- ☐ 2 - ☐ Bowel ☐ Bladder (Incontinence)
- ☐ 3 - Contracture
- ☐ 4 - Hearing
- ☐ 5 - Paralysis
- ☑ 6 - Endurance
- ☑ 7 - Ambulation
- ☐ 8 - Speech
- ☐ 9 - Legally blind
- ☐ A - Dyspnea with minimal exertion
- ☐ B - Other (specify)

FALL RISK ASSESSMENT
MAHC 10 - FALL RISK ASSESSMENT TOOL

REQUIRED CORE ELEMENTS Assess one point for each core element "yes". *Information may be gathered from medical record, assessment and if applicable, the patient/caregiver. Beyond protocols listed below, scoring should be based on your clinical judgment.*	Points
Age 65+	1
Diagnosis (3 or more co-existing) Includes only documented medical diagnosis.	1
Prior history of falls within 3 months A unintentional change in position resulting in coming to rest on the ground or at a lower level.	1
Incontinence Inability to make it to the bathroom or commode in timely manner. Includes frequency, urgency, and/or nocturia.	1
Visual impairment Includes but not limited to, macular degeneration, diabetic retinopathies, visual field loss, age related changes, decline in visual acuity, accommodation, glare tolerance, depth perception, and night vision or not wearing prescribed glasses or having the correct prescription.	1
Impaired functional mobility May include patients who need help with IADLs or ADLs or have gait or transfer problems, arthritis, pain, fear of falling, foot problems, impaired sensation, impaired coordination or improper use of assistive devices.	1
Environmental hazards May include but not limited to, poor illumination, equipment tubing, inappropriate footwear, pets, hard to reach items, floor surfaces that are uneven or cluttered, or outdoor entry and exits.	1
Poly Pharmacy (4 or more prescriptions – any type) All PRESCRIPTIONS including prescriptions for OTC meds. Drugs highly associated with fall risk include but not limited to, sedatives, anti-depressants, tranquilizers, narcotics, antihypertensives, cardiac meds, corticosteroids, anti-anxiety drugs, anticholinergic drugs, and hypoglycemic drugs.	1
Pain affecting level of function Pain often affects an individual's desire or ability to move or pain can be a factor in depression or compliance with safety recommendations.	1
Cognitive impairment Could include patients with dementia, Alzheimer's or stroke patients or patients who are confused, use poor judgment, have decreased comprehension, impulsivity, memory deficits. Consider patient's ability to adhere to the plan of care.	1
A score of 4 or more is considered at risk for falling **TOTAL**	10

MAHC 10 reprinted with permission from *Missouri Alliance for* HOME CARE

(M1910) Has this patient had a multi-factor **Falls Risk Assessment** using a standardized, validated assessment tool? Ⓟ Ⓡ ⒽⒽ
- ☐ 0 - No.
- ☐ 1 - Yes, and it does not indicate a risk for falls.
- ☑ 2 - Yes, and it does indicate a risk for falls.

Plan/Comments:

PT ordered for home safety evaluation, strengthening, gait training with least restrictive device, home modification. OT ordered for energy conservation techniques, adaptive equipment, shower chair, raised toilet seat, etc.

ADL/IADLs

(M1800) Grooming: Current ability to tend safely to personal hygiene needs (specifically: washing face and hands, hair care, shaving or make up, teeth or denture care, or fingernail care). ◇ Ⓡ ⒫Ⓐ
- ☐ 0 - Able to groom self unaided, with or without the use of assistive devices or adapted methods.
- ☑ 1 - Grooming utensils must be placed within reach before able to complete grooming activities.
- ☐ 2 - Someone must assist the patient to groom self.
- ☐ 3 - Patient depends entirely upon someone else for grooming needs.

(M1810) Current **Ability to Dress Upper Body** safely (with or without dressing aids) including undergarments, pullovers, front-opening shirts and blouses, managing zippers, buttons, and snaps: ◇ ◈ Ⓡ
- ☐ 0 - Able to get clothes out of closets and drawers, put them on and remove them from the upper body without assistance.
- ☑ 1 - Able to dress upper body without assistance if clothing is laid out or handed to the patient.
- ☐ 2 - Someone must help the patient put on upper body clothing.
- ☐ 3 - Patient depends entirely upon another person to dress the upper body.

(M1820) Current **Ability to Dress Lower Body** safely (with or without dressing aids) including undergarments, slacks, socks or nylons, shoes: ◇ ◈ Ⓡ
- ☐ 0 - Able to obtain, put on, and remove clothing and shoes without assistance.
- ☐ 1 - Able to dress lower body without assistance if clothing and shoes are laid out or handed to the patient.
- ☑ 2 - Someone must help the patient put on undergarments, slacks, socks or nylons, and shoes.
- ☐ 3 - Patient depends entirely upon another person to dress lower body.

(M1830) Bathing: Current ability to wash entire body safely. **Excludes grooming (washing face, washing hands, and shampooing hair).** ◇ ◈ Ⓡ ⒽⒽ ⒫Ⓐ ★
- ☐ 0 - Able to bathe self in shower or tub independently, including getting in and out of tub/shower.
- ☐ 1 - With the use of devices, is able to bathe self in shower or tub independently, including getting in and out of the tub/shower.
- ☐ 2 - Able to bathe in shower or tub with the intermittent assistance of another person:
  (a) for intermittent supervision or encouragement or reminders, OR
  (b) to get in and out of the shower or tub, OR
  (c) for washing difficult to reach areas.
- ☑ 3 - Able to participate in bathing self in shower or tub, but requires presence of another person throughout the bath for assistance or supervision.
- ☐ 4 - Unable to use the shower or tub, but able to bathe self independently with or without the use of devices at the sink, in chair, or on commode.
- ☐ 5 - Unable to use the shower or tub, but able to participate in bathing self in bed, at the sink, in bedside chair, or on commode, with the assistance or supervision of another person.
- ☐ 6 - Unable to participate effectively in bathing and is bathed totally by another person.

(M1840) Toilet Transferring: Current ability to get to and from the toilet or bedside commode safely and transfer on and off toilet/commode. ◇ ◈ Ⓡ ⒫Ⓐ
- ☐ 0 - Able to get to and from the toilet and transfer independently with or without a device.
- ☑ 1 - When reminded, assisted, or supervised by another person, able to get to and from the toilet and transfer.
- ☐ 2 - Unable to get to and from the toilet but is able to use a bedside commode (with or without assistance).
- ☐ 3 - Unable to get to and from the toilet or bedside commode but is able to use a bedpan/urinal independently.
- ☐ 4 - Is totally dependent in toileting.

Form 3491P-15R © 2015 BRIGGS (800) 247-2343 www.BriggsCorp.com. The Outcome and ASsessment Information Set (OASIS) is the intellectual property of the Center for Health Services and Policy Research, Denver, Colorado. It is used with permission.

BRiGGS Healthcare·

COMPREHENSIVE ADULT
NURSING ASSESSMENT
with OASIS ELEMENTS
Page 14 of 22

Figure 8.3   Continued

Patient Name_____ ID #_____

ADL/IADLs (Cont'd.)

(M1845) Toileting Hygiene: Current ability to maintain perineal hygiene safely, adjust clothes and/or incontinence pads before and after using toilet, commode, bedpan, urinal. If managing ostomy, includes cleaning area around stoma, but not managing equipment. ⬧ Ⓡ ㉆

- ☐ 0 - Able to manage toileting hygiene and clothing management without assistance.
- ☑ 1 - Able to manage toileting hygiene and clothing management without assistance if supplies/implements are laid out for the patient.
- ☐ 2 - Someone must help the patient to maintain toileting hygiene and/or adjust clothing.
- ☐ 3 - Patient depends entirely upon another person to maintain toileting hygiene.

(M1850) Transferring: Current ability to move safely from bed to chair, or ability to turn and position self in bed if patient is bedfast.

- ☐ 0 - Able to independently transfer. ⬧ ⬧ Ⓡ ⒣⒣ ㉆ ★
- ☐ 1 - Able to transfer with minimal human assistance or with use of an assistive device.
- ☑ 2 - Able to bear weight and pivot during the transfer process but unable to transfer self.
- ☐ 3 - Unable to transfer self and is unable to bear weight or pivot when transferred by another person.
- ☐ 4 - Bedfast, unable to transfer but is able to turn and position self in bed.
- ☐ 5 - Bedfast, unable to transfer and is unable to turn and position self.

(M1860) Ambulation/Locomotion: Current ability to walk safely, once in a standing position, or use a wheelchair, once in a seated position, on a variety of surfaces. ⬧ ⓟ ⬧ Ⓡ ⒣⒣ ㉆ ★

- ☐ 0 - Able to independently walk on even and uneven surfaces and negotiate stairs with or without railings (specifically: needs no human assistance or assistive device).
- ☐ 1 - With the use of a one-handed device (for example, cane, single crutch, hemi-walker), able to independently walk on even and uneven surfaces and negotiate stairs with or without railings.
- ☐ 2 - Requires use of a two-handed device (for example, walker or crutches) to walk alone on a level surface and/or requires human supervision or assistance to negotiate stairs or steps or uneven surfaces.
- ☑ 3 - Able to walk only with the supervision or assistance of another person at all times.
- ☐ 4 - Chairfast, unable to ambulate but is able to wheel self independently.
- ☐ 5 - Chairfast, unable to ambulate and is unable to wheel self.
- ☐ 6 - Bedfast, unable to ambulate or be up in a chair.

(M1870) Feeding or Eating: Current ability to feed self meals and snacks safely. Note: This refers only to the process of eating, chewing, and swallowing, not preparing the food to be eaten. ⬧ Ⓡ ㉆

- ☑ 0 - Able to independently feed self.
- ☐ 1 - Able to feed self independently but requires:
  (a) meal set-up; OR
  (b) intermittent assistance or supervision from another person; OR
  (c) a liquid, pureed or ground meat diet.
- ☐ 2 - Unable to feed self and must be assisted or supervised throughout the meal/snack.
- ☐ 3 - Able to take in nutrients orally and receives supplemental nutrients through a nasogastric tube or gastrostomy.
- ☐ 4 - Unable to take in nutrients orally and is fed nutrients through a nasogastric tube or gastrostomy.
- ☐ 5 - Unable to take in nutrients orally or by tube feeding.

(M1880) Current **Ability to Plan and Prepare Light Meals** (for example, cereal, sandwich) or reheat delivered meals safely: ⬧ Ⓡ

- ☐ 0 - (a) Able to independently plan and prepare all light meals for self or reheat delivered meals; OR
  (b) Is physically, cognitively, and mentally able to prepare light meals on a regular basis but has not routinely performed light meal preparation in the past (specifically: prior to this home care admission).
- ☑ 1 - Unable to prepare light meals on a regular basis due to physical, cognitive, or mental limitations.
- ☐ 2 - Unable to prepare any light meals or reheat any delivered meals.

(M1890) Ability to Use Telephone: Current ability to answer the phone safely, including dialing numbers, and effectively using the telephone to communicate. ⬧ Ⓡ

- ☑ 0 - Able to dial numbers and answer calls appropriately and as desired.
- ☐ 1 - Able to use a specially adapted telephone (for example, large numbers on the dial, teletype phone for the deaf) and call essential numbers.
- ☐ 2 - Able to answer the telephone and carry on a normal conversation but has difficulty with placing calls.
- ☐ 3 - Able to answer the telephone only some of the time or is able to carry on only a limited conversation.
- ☐ 4 - Unable to answer the telephone at all but can listen if assisted with equipment.
- ☐ 5 - Totally unable to use the telephone.
- ☐ NA - Patient does not have a telephone.

Indications for Home Health Aides: ☑ Yes ☐ No ☐ Refused

Order obtained: ☑ Yes ☐ No

Reason for need:

HHA to assist with personal hygiene, light housekeeping, and meal prep until patient stronger and able to safely perform tasks independently or caregiver trained to meet needs.

(M1900) Prior Functioning ADL/IADL: Indicate the patient's usual ability with everyday activities prior to his/her most recent illness, exacerbation, or injury. Check only one box in each row. Ⓡ

Functional Area	Independent	Needed Some Help	Dependent
a. Self-Care (specifically: grooming, dressing, bathing, and toileting hygiene)	☐ 0	☑ 1	☐ 2
b. Ambulation	☐ 0	☑ 1	☐ 2
c. Transfer	☐ 0	☑ 1	☐ 2
d. Household tasks (specifically: light meal preparation, laundry, shopping, and phone use)	☐ 0	☑ 1	☐ 2

M1910 is on page 14 of 20.

ACTIVITIES PERMITTED

(Locator #18B)

- ☐ 1 - Complete bedrest
- ☐ 2 - ☐ Bedrest ☐ BRP
- ☑ 3 - Up as tolerated
- ☐ 4 - Transfer: ☐ Bed ☐ Chair
- ☐ 5 - Exercises prescribed
- ☐ 6 - Partial weight bearing
- ☑ 7 - Independent in home
- ☐ 8 - Crutches
- ☐ 9 - Cane
- ☐ A - Wheelchair
- ☑ B - Walker
- ☐ C - No restrictions
- ☐ D - Other (specify)

Form 3491P-15R © 2015 BRIGGS (800) 247-2343 www.BriggsCorp.com. The Outcome and ASsessment Information Set (OASIS) is the intellectual property of the Center for Health Services and Policy Research, Denver, Colorado. It is used with permission.

BRiGGS Healthcare

COMPREHENSIVE ADULT
NURSING ASSESSMENT
with OASIS ELEMENTS
Page 15 of 22

Figure 8.3 Continued

Patient Name_____ ID #_____

ALLERGIES

Allergies: (Locator #17) ☐ None known ☐ Aspirin
☑ Penicillin ☐ Sulfa ☐ Pollen ☐ Eggs
☐ Milk products ☐ Insect bites
☐ Other

MEDICATIONS

(M2000) Drug Regimen Review: Does a complete drug regimen review indicate potential clinically significant medication issues (for example, adverse drug reactions, ineffective drug therapy, significant side effects, drug interactions, duplicate therapy, omissions, dosage errors, or non-compliance [non-adherence])? ☐R

☐ 0 - Not assessed/reviewed **[Go to M2010]**
☐ 1 - No problems found during review **[Go to M2010]**
☑ 2 - Problems found during review
☐ NA - Patient is not taking any medications **[Go to M2040]**

(M2002) Medication Follow-up: Was a physician or the physician-designee contacted within one calendar day to resolve clinically significant medication issues, including reconciliation? Ⓟ
☐ 0 - No
☑ 1 - Yes

(M2010) Patient/Caregiver High-Risk Drug Education: Has the patient/caregiver received instruction on special precautions for all high-risk medications (such as hypoglycemics, anticoagulants, etc.) and how and when to report problems that may occur? Ⓟ

☐ 0 - No
☐ 1 - Yes
☑ NA - Patient not taking any high-risk drugs OR patient/caregiver fully knowledgeable about special precautions associated with all high-risk medications

(M2020) Management of Oral Medications: Patient's current ability to prepare and take all oral medications reliably and safely, including administration of the correct dosage at the appropriate times/intervals. **Excludes injectable and IV medications. (NOTE: This refers to ability, not compliance or willingness.)** ◇ ☐R ☐HH ☐PA

☐ 0 - Able to independently take the correct oral medication(s) and proper dosage(s) at the correct times.
☐ 1 - Able to take medication(s) at the correct times if:
   (a) individual dosages are prepared in advance by another person; OR
   (b) another person develops a drug diary or chart.
☐ 2 - Able to take medication(s) at the correct times if given reminders by another person at the appropriate times
☑ 3 - Unable to take medication unless administered by another person.
☐ NA - No oral medications prescribed.

(M2030) Management of Injectable Medications: Patient's current ability to prepare and take all prescribed injectable medications reliably and safely, including administration of correct dosage at the appropriate times/intervals. **Excludes IV medications.** ◇ ☐R

☐ 0 - Able to independently take the correct medication(s) and proper dosage(s) at the correct times.
☐ 1 - Able to take injectable medication(s) at the correct times if:
   (a) individual syringes are prepared in advance by another person; OR
   (b) another person develops a drug diary or chart.
☐ 2 - Able to take medication(s) at the correct times if given reminders by another person based on the frequency of the injection
☐ 3 - Unable to take injectable medication unless administered by another person.
☑ NA - No injectable medications prescribed.

MEDICATIONS

(M2040) Prior Medication Management: Indicate the patient's usual ability with managing oral and injectable medications prior to his/her most recent illness, exacerbation or injury. Check only **one** box in each row. ☐R

Functional Area	Independent	Needed Some Help	Dependent	Not Applicable
a. Oral medications	☐0	☑1	☐2	☐NA
b. Injectable medications	☐0	☐1	☐2	☑NA

Psychotropic drug use: ☑No ☐Yes (see med sheet)
Financial ability to pay for medications: ☑Yes ☐No
If no, was MSW referral made? ☐Yes ☐No/comment

Upon arrival found patient was unsure of the medications he was to be taking. Physician notified and meds reconciled.

INFUSION

☑N/A

☐ Peripheral line ☐ Midline catheter ☐ Central line
Type/brand _____
Size/gauge/length _____
☐Groshong® ☐Non-Groshong ☐Tunneled ☐Non-tunneled
Insertion site_____ Insertion date _____
Lumens: ☐Single ☐Double ☐Triple
Flush solution/frequency _____
Patent: ☐Yes ☐No
Injection cap change frequency_____
Dressing change during visit: ☐Yes ☐No
Dressing change frequency _____
   ☐Sterile ☐Clean
Performed by: ☐Self ☐RN ☐Caregiver ☐Family
   ☐Other _____
Site/skin condition _____
External catheter length_____cm
Other

PICC Specific:
   Circumference of arm_____cm
   X-ray verification: ☐Yes ☐No
IVAD Port Specific:
   Reservoir: ☐Single ☐Double
   Huber gauge/length_____
   Accessed: ☐No ☐Yes, date _____
☐Epidural ☐Intrathecal Access:
   Site/skin condition _____
   Infusion solution (type/volume/rate)_____
☐Pump: (type, specify)_____
Administered by: ☐Self ☐Caregiver ☐RN ☐Family
   ☐Other_____
Purpose of Intravenous Access:_____
☐Antibiotic therapy   ☐Pain control   ☐Lab draws
☐Chemotherapy   ☐Maintain venous access
☐Hydration   ☐Parenteral nutrition
☐Other

Form 3491P-15R © 2015 BRIGGS (800) 247-2343 www.BriggsCorp.com. The Outcome and ASsessment Information Set (OASIS) is the intellectual property of the Center for Health Services and Policy Research, Denver, Colorado. It is used with permission.

BRIGGS Healthcare

COMPREHENSIVE ADULT
NURSING ASSESSMENT
with OASIS ELEMENTS
Page 16 of 22

Figure 8.3   Continued

Patient Name_____ ID #_____

INFUSION (Cont'd.)

☐ Medication(s) administered:
(name of drug)_____
Dose_____ Route_____
Frequency_____
Duration of therapy_____
☐ Medication(s) administered:
(name of drug)_____
Dose_____ Route_____
Frequency_____
Duration of therapy_____

☐ Infusion care provided during visit: ☐ Yes ☐ No
Interventions / Instructions / Comments

CARE MANAGEMENT

(M2102) Types and Sources of Assistance: Determine the ability and willingness of non-agency caregivers (such as family members, friends, or privately paid caregivers) to provide assistance for the following activities, if assistance is needed. Excludes all care by your agency staff. (Check only **one** box in each row.) [R] (PA)

Type of Assistance	No assistance needed – patient is independent or does not have needs in this area	Non-agency caregiver(s) currently provide assistance	Non-agency caregiver(s) need training/supportive services to provide assistance	Non-agency caregiver(s) are not likely to provide assistance OR it is unclear if they will provide assistance	Assistance needed, but no non-agency caregiver(s) available
a. **ADL assistance** (for example, transfer/ambulation, bathing, dressing, toileting, eating/feeding)	☐ 0	☐ 1	☐ 2	☑ 3	☐ 4
b. **IADL assistance** (for example, meals, house-keeping, laundry, telephone, shopping, finances)	☐ 0	☑ 1	☐ 2	☐ 3	☐ 4
c. **Medication administration** (for example, oral, inhaled or injectable)	☐ 0	☐ 1	☐ 2	☑ 3	☐ 4
d. **Medical procedures/ treatments** (for example, changing wound dressing, home exercise program)	☐ 0	☐ 1	☐ 2	☑ 3	☐ 4
e. **Management of Equipment** (for example, oxygen, IV/ infusion equipment, enteral/ parenteral nutrition, ventilator therapy equipment or supplies)	☑ 0	☐ 1	☐ 2	☐ 3	☐ 4
f. **Supervision and safety** (for example, due to cognitive impairment)	☐ 0	☐ 1	☐ 2	☑ 3	☐ 4
g. **Advocacy or facilitation** of patient's participation in appropriate medical care (for example, transportation to or from appointments)	☐ 0	☐ 1	☐ 2	☑ 3	☐ 4

(M2110) How Often does the patient receive **ADL or IADL assistance** from any caregiver(s) (other than home health agency staff)? [R]
☑ 1 - At least daily
☐ 2 - Three or more times per week
☐ 3 - One to two times per week
☐ 4 - Received, but less often than weekly
☐ 5 - No assistance received
☐ UK - Unknown

LIVING ARRANGEMENTS / SUPPORTIVE ASSISTANCE

Safety Measures: (Locator #15)
☐ 1 - Bleeding precautions
☐ 2 - O₂ precautionss
☐ 3 - Seizure precautionss
☑ 4 - Fall precautions
☐ 5 - Aspiration precautions
☐ 6 - Siderails up
☐ 7 - Elevate head of bed
☐ 8 - 24 hr. supervision
☑ 9 - Clear pathways
☐ 10 - Lock w/c with transfers
☑ 11 - Infection control measures
☑ 12 - ☐ Walker ☐ Cane
☐ 13 - Other

Form 3491P-15R © 2015 BRIGGS (800) 247-2343 www.BriggsCorp.com. The Outcome and ASsessment Information Set (OASIS) is the intellectual property of the Center for Health Services and Policy Research, Denver, Colorado. It is used with permission.
BRIGGS Healthcare·

COMPREHENSIVE ADULT
NURSING ASSESSMENT
with OASIS ELEMENTS
Page 17 of 22

Figure 8.3 Continued

Patient Name_____ ID #_____

LIVING ARRANGEMENTS/SUPPORTIVE ASSISTANCE (Cont'd.)

HOME ENVIRONMENT SAFETY

Safety hazards in the home:

Unsound structure	☒Y ☐N
Inadequate heating/cooling/electricity	☐Y ☒N
Inadequate sanitation/plumbing	☐Y ☒N
Inadequate refrigeration	☐Y ☒N
Unsafe gas/electrical appliances or outlets	☐Y ☒N
Inadequate running water	☐Y ☒N
Unsafe storage of supplies/equipment	☒Y ☐N
No telephone available and/or unable to use phone	☐Y ☒N
Insects/rodents	☐Y ☒N
Medications stored safely	☐Y ☒N
Grab bar(s) in bathroom/tub/shower	☐Y ☒N

Emergency planning/fire safety:

Fire extinguisher	☐Y ☒N
Smoke detectors on all levels of home	☒Y ☐N
Tested and functioning	☒Y ☐N
More than one exit	☒Y ☐N
Plan for exit	☒Y ☐N
Plan for power failure	☒Y ☐N
CO₂ detector	☐Y ☒N

Oxygen use:

Signs posted	☐Y ☐N
Handles smoking/flammables safely	☐Y ☐N
Oxygen back-up: ☐Available ☐Knows how to use	
Electrical/fire safety	☐Y ☐N
Is there a need for a Fall Risk Plan?	☒Y ☐N

Summary: Safety plan(s) indicated? ☐Y ☐N

(Plan/Comments)

Front of house with bricks missing and no railing on stairs entering the home. Home is very cluttered and dirty with boxes piled high in the hallways creating safety risk significant risks to safety. No safety measures noted in shower/tub. PT/OT and MSW ordered.

Name of Emergency Preparedness Business/Registry (if applicable)

_____

Contact information (e.g., phone #/email)

_____

Instructions/Materials Provided (Check all applicable items)
- ☒ Rights and responsibilities
- ☒ State hotline number
- ☒ Advance directives
- ☒ Do not resuscitate (DNR)
- ☒ HIPAA Notice of Privacy Practices
- ☒ OASIS Privacy Notice
- ☒ Emergency planning in the event service is disrupted
- ☒ Agency phone number ☒ After hours number
- ☒ When to contact: ☒ Physician ☒ Agency
- ☒ Standard precautions ☐Handwashing
- ☒ Basic home safety
- ☒ Disease (specify) HTN, wound management, depression
- ☒ Medication Regimen☐Medication Administration
- ☐ Other

THERAPY NEED AND PLAN OF CARE

(M2200) Therapy Need: In the home health plan of care for the Medicare payment episode for which this assessment will define a case mix group, what is the indicated need for therapy visits (total of reasonable and necessary physical, occupational, and speech-language pathology visits combined)? **(Enter zero ["000"] if no therapy visits indicated.)** ⊘ Ⓡ

(0 1 2) Number of therapy visits indicated (total of physical, occupational and speech-language pathology combined).

☐ NA - Not Applicable: No case mix group defined by this assessment.

(M2250) Plan of Care Synopsis: (Check only **one** box in each row.) Does the physician-ordered plan of care include the following: Ⓟ HH

Plan / Intervention	No	Yes	Not Applicable	
a. Patient-specific parameters for notifying physician of changes in vital signs or other clinical findings	☐0	☒1	☐NA	Physician has chosen not to establish patient-specific parameters for this patient. Agency will use standardized clinical guidelines accessible for all care providers to reference.
b. Diabetic foot care including monitoring for the presence of skin lesions on the lower extremities and patient/caregiver education on proper foot care	☐0	☐1	☒NA	Patient is not diabetic or is missing lower legs due to congenital or acquired condition (bilateral amputee).
c. Falls prevention interventions	☐0	☒1	☐NA	Falls risk assessment indicates patient has no risk for falls.
d. Depression intervention(s) such as medication, referral for other treatment, or a monitoring plan for current treatment and/or physician notified that patient screened positive for depression	☐0	☒1	☐NA	Patient has no diagnosis of depression AND depression screening indicates patients has: 1) no symptoms of depression; or 2) has some symptoms of depression but does not meet criteria for further evaluation of depression based on screening tool used.
e. Intervention(s) to monitor and mitigate pain	☐0	☒1	☐NA	Pain assessment indicates patient has no pain.
f. Intervention(s) to prevent pressure ulcers	☐0	☐1	☒NA	Pressure ulcer risk assessment (clinical or formal) indicates patient is not at risk of developing pressure ulcers.
g. Pressure ulcer treatment based on principles of moist wound healing OR order for treatment based on moist wound healing has been requested from physician	☐0	☐1	☒NA	Patient has no pressure ulcers OR has no pressure ulcers for which moist wound healing is indicated.

Form 3491P-15R © 2015 BRIGGS (800) 247-2343 www.BriggsCorp.com. The Outcome and ASsessment Information Set (OASIS) is the intellectual property of the Center for Health Services and Policy Research, Denver, Colorado. It is used with permission.

BRIGGSHealthcare·

COMPREHENSIVE ADULT
NURSING ASSESSMENT
with OASIS ELEMENTS
Page 18 of 22

Figure 8.3   Continued

Patient Name_____ ID #_____

PATIENT/CAREGIVER/FAMILY EDUCATION

(Check all that applies)

☒Patient ☐Caregiver ☐Family knowledgeable and able to verbalize and/or demonstrate independence with:

Wound care: ☒Yes ☐No ☐N/A	☒Oral ☐Injected ☐Infused ☐Inhaled	Catheter care: ☐Yes ☐No ☒N/A
Diabetic ☐Foot exam ☐Care: ☐Yes ☐No ☒N/A	medication(s) administration: ☒Yes ☐No ☐N/A	Trach care: ☐Yes ☐No ☒N/A
Insulin administration: ☐Yes ☐No ☒N/A	Pain management: ☒Yes ☐No ☐N/A	Ostomy care: ☐Yes ☐No ☒N/A
Glucometer use: ☐Yes ☐No ☒N/A	Oxygen use: ☐Yes ☐No ☒N/A	Other care(s):
Nutritional management: ☐Yes ☒No ☐N/A	Use of medical devices: ☐Yes ☐No ☒N/A	

☒Patient ☐Caregiver ☐Family need further education with:

wound management, Hypertension disease management, depression signs and symptoms, and home safety.

☐Caregiver ☐Family present at time of visit: ☐Yes ☒No   ☒Patient ☐Caregiver ☐Family educated this visit for (specify):

medication reconciliation and proper administration, signs and symptoms of infection, signs and symptoms of elevated B/P. Pt. verbalized understanding and demonstrated proper medication administration

☒Patient ☐Caregiver ☐Family appears to understand all information given: ☒Yes ☐No

Does the ☒Patient ☐Caregiver ☐Family have an action plan when disease symptoms exacerbate (e.g., when to call the homecare nurse vs.

emergency services): ☒Yes ☐No

Comment(s **Patient requires frequent repetition and information in writing due to short term memory issues.**

SUMMARY CHECKLIST

CARE PLAN: ☐Collaboration with ☒Patient ☐Caregiver ☐Family involvement

MEDICATION STATUS: ☒Medication regimen completed/reviewed (Locator #10)   ☐No change ☒Order obtained

Check if any of the following were identified:

☐Potential adverse effects ☐Drug reactions ☐Ineffective drug therapy ☐Significant side effects ☐Significant drug interactions

☐Duplicate drug therapy ☒Non-compliance with drug therapy

CARE COORDINATION: ☒Physician ☒PT ☒OT ☐ST ☒MSW ☒Aide ☐Other (specify)_____

Was a referral made to MSW for assistance with: ☒Community resources ☐Living will ☒Counseling needs (depression/suicidal ideation)

☒Unsafe environment?

Date 2/9/17   ☒Yes ☐No ☐Refused ☐N/A Comment:_____

Verbal Order obtained: ☐No ☒Yes, specify date (Locator #23) 2/9/17

DME/MEDICAL SUPPLIES

DME Company:_____ Phone:_____ Oxygen Company:_____ Phone:_____

Community organizations/services:

Contact:_____ Phone:_____

Comments:_____

(Locator #14) ☐ NONE USED	IV SUPPLIES (Cont'd.):	FOLEY SUPPLIES (Cont'd.):	SUPPLIES/EQUIPMENT:	SUPPLIES/EQUIPMENT (Cont'd.)
WOUND CARE:	☐ IV pole	☐ Irrigation tray	☐ Augmentative and	☐ Oxygen concentrator
☐ 2x2's	☐ IV start kit	☐ Saline	alternative communication	☐ Pressure relieving device
☒ 4x4's	☐ IV tubing	☐ Straight catheter	device(s) (type)	
☐ ABD's	☐ Syringes size_____	☐ Other		☐ Prosthesis: ☐RUE ☐RLE
☐ Cotton tipped applicators	☐ Tape		☐ Bath bench	☐ LUE ☐LLE☐ Other
☐ Drain sponges	☐ Other	**DIABETIC:**	☐ Brace ☐ Orthotics (specify):	
☐ Hydrocolloids		☐ Chemstrips		☐ Raised toilet seat
☒ Kerlix size_____	**URINARY/OSTOMY:**	☐ Syringes		☐ Special mattress overlay
☐ Nu-gauze	☐ External catheters	☐ Other	☐ Cane	
☐ Saline	☐ Ostomy pouch (brand, size)		☐ Commode	☐ Suction machine
☐ Tape	_____	**MISCELLANEOUS:**	☐ Dressing Aid Kit/Hip Kit	☐ TENS unit
☐ Transparent dressings	☐ Ostomy wafer (brand, size)	☐ Enema supplies	(e.g. reacher, long handle	☐ Transfer equipment:
☒ Wound cleanser		☐ Feeding tube: type_____	sponge, long handle shoe	☐ Board ☐Lift
☐ Wound gel		size _____	horn, etc.)	☐ Bedside commode
☒ Other	☐ Skin protectant	☐ Gloves:	☐ Eggcrate	☐ Ventilator
hydrogel impregnated gauze, elastic wrap	☐ Stoma adhesive tape	☐ Sterile ☒ Non-sterile	☐ Enteral feeding pump	☒ Walker
	☐ Underpads	☐ Staple removal kit	☐ Grab bars: Bathroom/Other	☐ Wheelchair
IV SUPPLIES:	☐ Urinary bag ☐Pouch	☐ Steri strips		☐ Other Supplies Needed
☐ Alcohol swabs	☐ Other	☐ Suture removal kit	☐ Hospital bed:	
☐ Angiocatheter size_____		☐ Other	☐ Semi-electric	
☐ Batteries size_____	**FOLEY SUPPLIES:**		☐ Hoyer lift	
☐ Central line dressing	☐ Acetic acid		☐ Knee scooter	
☐ Extension tubings	☐ _____Fr catheter kit		☐ Medical alert	
☐ Infusion pump	(tray, bag, foley)		☐ Nebulizer	
☐ Injection caps				

Form 3491P-15R © 2015 BRIGGS (800) 247-2343 www.BriggsCorp.com. The Outcome and ASsessment Information Set (OASIS) is the intellectual property of the Center for Health Services and Policy Research, Denver, Colorado. It is used with permission.

BRIGGS Healthcare·

COMPREHENSIVE ADULT NURSING ASSESSMENT with OASIS ELEMENTS
Page 19 of 22

Figure 8.3   Continued

HOME CARE NURSING

Patient Name_____ ID #_____

PROFESSIONAL SERVICES		Locator #21

Utilize this section to assist with completion of 485 (optional)

SN - FREQUENCY/DURATION_____
- ☐ Skilled Observation for

- ☐ Evaluate Cardiopulmonary Status
- ☐ Evaluate: ☐ Nutrition ☐ Hydration ☐ Elimination
- ☐ Evaluate for S/S of Infections
- ☐ Teach Disease Process
- ☐ Teach S/S of Infection and Standard Precautions
- ☐ Teach Diet
- ☐ Teach Home Safety ☐ Falls Prevention
- ☐ Other_____
- ☐ PRN Visits for_____
- ☐ Psychiatric Nursing for_____

MEDICATIONS
- ☐ Medication Teaching
- ☐ Evaluate Med Effects ☐ Compliance
- ☐ Set up Meds Every ____ ☐ Days ☐ Weeks
- ☐ Administer Medication(s) (name, dose, route, frequency)

- ☐ Administer Medication(s) (name, dose, route, frequency)

- ☐ Administer Medication(s) (name, dose, route, frequency)

IV
- ☐ Administer IV Medication (name, dose, route, frequency and duration)

- ☐ Teach IV Administration_____

FLUSHING PROTOCOL/ FREQUENCY (specify)
- ☐ Administer Flush(es)_____
  - ___mL normal saline
  - ___mL normal saline
  - ___mL sterile water
  - ___mL heparin ___unit/mL
  - ___mL heparin ___unit/mL

- ☐ Teach S/S of IV Complications
- ☐ Teach IV Site Care
- ☐ Teach Infusion Pump

- ☐ Teach Complete Parenteral Nutrition
- ☐ Site Care (specify)_____
- ☐ Line Protocol (specify)

- ☐ ___PRN Visits for IV Complications
- ☐ Anaphylaxis Protocol (specify orders)

- ☐ Other_____

RESPIRATORY
- ☐ O₂ at _____ liters per minute
- ☐ Pulse Oximetry: Every Visit
- ☐ Pulse Oximetry: PRN Dyspnea
- ☐ Teach Oxygen: ☐ Use ☐ Precautions
- ☐ Teach Trach Care ☐ Administer Trach Care
- ☐ Other_____

INTEGUMENTARY
- ☐ Wound Care (specify each site)

- ☐ Evaluate: ☐ Wound ☐ Pressure Ulcer for Healing
- ☐ Measure Wound(s) Weekly
- ☐ Teach Wound: ☐ Care ☐ Dressing
- ☐ Other_____

ELIMINATION
- ☐ Foley _____ French inflated balloon with _____mL changed every_____
- ☐ Suprapubic Cath Insertion every_____ with size _____Fr. balloon_____
- ☐ Teach Care of Indwelling Catheter
- ☐ Teach Self - Cath ☐ Teach Ostomy Care
- ☐ Teach Bowel Regime
- ☐ Other_____

GASTROINTESTINAL
- ☐ Teach N/G Tube Feeding
- ☐ Teach G-Tube Feeding
- ☐ Other_____

DIABETES
- ☐ Administer Medication
- ☐ Prepare Insulin Syringes
- ☐ Blood Glucose Monitoring PRN or _____
- ☐ Teach Diabetic Care
- ☐ Other_____

LABORATORY
- ☐ Venipuncture for_____ Frequency_____
- ☐ Other

PT - FREQUENCY/DURATION_____
- ☐ Evaluation and Treatment
- ☐ Pulse Oximetry PRN
- ☐ Home Safety ☐ Falls Prevention
- ☐ Therapeutic Exercise
- ☐ Transfer Training
- ☐ Gait Training
- ☐ Establish Home Exercise Program
- ☐ Modality (specify frequency, duration, (amount)

- ☐ Prosthetic Training
- ☐ Muscle Re-Education
- ☐ Other_____

OT - FREQUENCY/DURATION_____
- ☐ Evaluation and Treatment
- ☐ Pulse Oximetry PRN
- ☐ Home Safety ☐ Falls Prevention
- ☐ Adaptive Equipment
- ☐ Therapeutic Exercise
- ☐ Muscle Re-Education
- ☐ Establish Home Exercise Program
- ☐ Homemaker Training
- ☐ Modality (specify frequency, duration, (amount)

- ☐ Other_____

ST - FREQUENCY/DURATION_____
- ☐ Evaluation and Treatment
- ☐ Voice Disorder Treatment
- ☐ Speech Articulation Disorder Treatment
- ☐ Dysphagia Treatment
- ☐ Receptive Skills
- ☐ Expressive Skills
- ☐ Cognitive Skills
- ☐ Other_____

HOME HEALTH AIDE - FREQUENCY/DURATION_____
- ☐ Personal Care for ADL Assistance
- ☐ Other (specific task for HHA)

HOMEMAKER - FREQUENCY/DURATION_____
- ☐ Other

MSW - FREQUENCY/DURATION_____
- ☐ Evaluate and Treat
- ☐ Evaluate Family Situation
- ☐ Evaluate/Refer to Community Resources
- ☐ Evaluate Financial Status
- ☐ Other_____

Form 3491P-15R © 2015 BRIGGS (800) 247-2343 www.BriggsCorp.com. The Outcome and ASsessment Information Set (OASIS) is the intellectual property of the Center for Health Services and Policy Research, Denver, Colorado. It is used with permission.

BRIGGS Healthcare·

COMPREHENSIVE ADULT
NURSING ASSESSMENT
with OASIS ELEMENTS
Page 20 of 22

Figure 8.3   Continued

Patient Name_____ ID #_____

REHABILITATION POTENTIAL / GOALS
Locator #

Check goal(s), circle for specifics and insert information. Check box to indicate short or long term goal(s).

DISCIPLINE GOALS AND DATE WILL BE ACHIEVED

Nursing:

☐ Demonstrates compliance with medication
by _____ (date) ☐ Short ☐ Long

☐ Stabilization of cardiovascular pulmonary condition
by _____ (date) ☐ Short ☐ Long

☐ Demonstrates competence in following medical regimen
by _____ (date) ☐ Short ☐ Long

☐ Verbalizes pain controlled at acceptable level
by _____ (date) ☐ Short ☐ Long

☐ Demonstrates independence in _____
by _____ (date) ☐ Short ☐ Long

☐ Verbalizes ☐ Demonstrates independence with care
by _____ (date) ☐ Short ☐ Long

☐ Wound healing without complications
by _____ (date) ☐ Short ☐ Long

☐ Expect daily SN visits to end
by _____ (date) ☐ Short ☐ Long

☐ Other_____
by _____ (date) ☐ Short ☐ Long

Physical Therapy:

☐ Demonstrates ability to follow home exercise program
by _____ (date) ☐ Short ☐ Long

☐ Other_____
by _____ (date) ☐ Short ☐ Long

Occupational Therapy:

☐ Demonstrates ability to follow home exercise program by
_____ (date) ☐ Short ☐ Long

☐ Other_____
by _____ (date) ☐ Short ☐ Long

Speech Therapy:

☐ Demonstrate swallowing skills in ☐ Formal ☐ Informal dysphagia
evaluation exercise program by _____ (date)
☐ Short ☐ Long

☐ Completes speech therapy program
by _____ (date) ☐ Short ☐ Long

☐ Other_____
by _____ (date) ☐ Short ☐ Long

Aide:

☐ Assumes responsibility for personal care needs
by _____ (date) ☐ Short ☐ Long

☐ Other_____
by _____ (date) ☐ Short ☐ Long

Medical Social Services:

☐ Verbalize information about community resources and how to obt
assistance by _____ (date) ☐ Short ☐ Long

☐ Other_____
by _____ (date) ☐ Short ☐ Long

DISCHARGE PLANS

☐ Return to an independent level of care (self-care)

☐ Able to remain in residence with assistance of ☐ Primary caregiver ☐ Support from community agencies

☐ When ☐ Patient ☐ Caregiver ☐ Family knowledgeable about when to notify physician

☐ Patient ☐ Caregiver ☐ Family able to understand medication regimen and care related to diagnoses

☐ Medical condition stabilizes

☐ When maximum functional potential reached

☐ Discharge at the end of the episode if the patient is hospitalized

☐ Other_____

☐ Other_____

DISCUSSED WITH: ☐ PATIENT ☐ FAMILY ☐ DESIGNATED CAREGIVER: ☐ Yes ☐ No

REHAB POTENTIAL: ☐ Poor ☐ Fair ☐ Good ☐ Excellent

SIGNATURE / DATES

X_____
Patient/Family Member/Caregiver (if applicable)   Date

X_____
Person Completing This Form (signature/title)   Date

OASIS INFORMATION

Date Reviewed 02/11/2017   **Date Entered & Locked** 02/11/2017   **Date Transmitted** 02/11/2017

Form 3491P-15R © 2015 BRIGGS. (800) 247-2343 www.BriggsCorp.com. The Outcome and ASsessment Information Set (OASIS)
is the intellectual property of the Center for Health Services and Policy Research, Denver, Colorado. It is used with permission.

BRIGGS Healthcare·

COMPREHENSIVE AD
NURSING ASSESSM
with OASIS ELEM
Page 21

Figure 8.3   Continued

ASSESSMENT SUMMARY

Patient Name_____ ID #_____

Reason for Admission: Wound care, home safety, HTN, depression   Homebound Reason: weakness, unsteady gait and dyspnea with moderate exertion

86 year old male patient admitted to home care following 3 week hospitalization. Recent history includes: 1/19/2017 the patients neighbor found the patient disheveled with dirty clothes and a bleeding open wound on his left lower leg thought to be the result of a fall. He also exhibited poor short term memory. EMS was called and the patient was taken to the emergency department where he was subsequently admitted. While in the hospital his wound was evaluated as a full thickness tissue loss trauma wound requiring close oversight and wound care. He was diagnosed with a urinary tract infection, and bacterial pneumonia, both treated with antibiotics and resolved prior to discharge home. He also experienced a recent exacerbation of his hypertension requiring a change to his metroprolol dose. He reported while in the hospital an increase feeling of depression resulting from his hospitalization and recent death of his wife and was placed on celexa. He will require skilled nursing for continued wound assessment and dressing changes until patient taught to perform independently, then weekly evaluation of wound healing, evaluation of medication effectiveness for new medication, medication compliance, disease management education for wound management, hypertension, depression and home safety for which the patient has requested information. He will require PT for home modification, strengthening exercises and gait training with least restrictive device, OT for energy conservation and adaptive equipment needs, MSW for community resources for meals and hoarding tendencies, and further depression evaluation, and HHA to support personal hygiene and ADL/IADL's.

PHYSICIAN VERBAL ORDER (Complete if applicable per agency policy)

☑ Physician (name) Dr. De La Torrens _____ called to report comprehensive assessment findings (including medical, nursing, rehabilitative, social and discharge planning needs).

☑ Verbal order received to initiate home health intermittent (reasonable and necessary) skilled services for:

SN 3w/1,2w/4,1w/5, PT Eval and Treat, OT Eval and Treat, MSW Eval and Treat, HHA 3w2, 2w7

(specify amount/frequency/duration for discipline(s) and treatment(s)

X_____ 02/09/2017 4:30pm
Signature/Title of Person Who Received Verbal Order   Date   Time

X_____   Date
Physician Signature for Verbal Order

SIGNATURE/DATES

X_____   Date
Person Completing This Form (signature/title)

Agency Name _____ Phone Number _____

Form 3491P-15R © 2015 BRIGGS (800) 247-2343 www.BriggsCorp.com. The Outcome and ASsessment Information Set (OASIS) is the intellectual property of the Center for Health Services and Policy Research, Denver, Colorado. It is used with permission.

BRIGGS Healthcare

COMPREHENSIVE ADULT NURSING ASSESSMENT with OASIS ELEMENTS Page 22 of 22

Figure 8.3 Concluded

About OASIS

Figure 8.3 illustrated a sample completed OASIS form. Common questions related to OASIS are frequently about "who or which patients need them done and when?" OASIS requirements apply to traditional fee-for-service Medicare as well as Medicare managed care such as a health maintenance organization insurer. They are also usually required by Medicaid, both in traditional fee-for-service and HMO/managed care. When in doubt, ask your state association about your state's rules and programs relating to OASIS. The comprehensive assessment and OASIS data collection must be conducted at the following time points:

- At the start of care
- At the resumption of care
- Re-certification
- Other follow-up
- Upon discharge

OASIS data needs to be collected at transfer and death at home, but no comprehensive assessment is needed. The exceptions to the OASIS collection and transmission are pediatric patients, which are defined as those under age 18; maternity patients; those patients only receiving homemaker or chore services (in other words, when the patient is only receiving unskilled care or are aide-only cases); and patients who are non-Medicare and non-Medicaid.

There are, however, times when OASIS data will be collected in excluded populations and that occurs when the payer reimburses the agency for care using the Medicare PPS model. For more information, see the Centers for Medicare & Medicaid Services (CMS) OASIS-C Guidance Manual at https://www.cms.gov/Medicare/Quality-Initiatives-Patient-Assessment-Instruments/HomeHealthQualityInits/HHQIOASISUserManual.html.

Case Management, Communication, and Coordination Considerations

Effective case or care management and ongoing communications and coordination among those involved in the patient's care are hallmarks of effective care. Be proud of your care and work and get credit for these important and required activities! There is no doubt that they take time, but without communication among and across the team, the physician, the patient, and caregiver(s), there can be "disconnects." It is well documented in the healthcare literature that communications, or the lack thereof, contribute to medical errors and other untoward outcomes and problems.

Being proactive and communicative with others involved is a quality indicator. And, if you are accredited, this is a requirement. In the proposed Medicare Conditions of Participation (CoPs), care coordination and quality are linked together. When reviewing a chart, the care coordination should be readily seen. The following are some examples of effective communication and coordination that should be documented:

- Calling or otherwise communicating with the physician or another team member to update about a change or additional information that is known that may impact the POC.

- Attending interdisciplinary or interprofessional meetings at the organization. This could be documented in the weekly meeting agenda and patient-specific information that can be updated into the patient's record.

- Receiving a call from a family member that the patient was started on a new antibiotic for a urinary tract or other infection. (And then that information is communicated to the infection control coordinator and entered into the infection surveillance tool for the quality assurance and performance improvement process.)

- Calling other team members when notified that the patient went to the hospital or the physician's office for a new problem.

- Visiting together for a joint visit. Purposes for these home visits may be a supervisory visit or a therapist and a nurse overlapping to revise short- and long-term goals with the patient if the patient is improving or otherwise changing.

- Communicating with family caregivers about changes to the POC. Examples might be frequency or new physician orders, such as a medication change.

- Notifying the care team, the physician, and the patient and family when a projected discharge date is determined based on the patient's progress.

- Calling the home health or hospice aide to discuss the patient's personal care needs and any changes to the aide POC.

- Documenting phone calls, meetings, or other communications about patients and their status and the care that is needed— these are all coordination and communication, so give yourself credit.

- Documenting the progress of pediatric patients toward reaching developmental and other goals.

Other communication examples can be as unique as the organization; some examples might include calling in a report or communicating about an emergent care situation, such as a patient fall and/or a patient change in condition with its subsequent notification to the physician. This would also include communicating with the rest of the care team, the identification a sentinel event, noting when a patient is not at home for a scheduled home visit, and others. All these are examples that reflect care coordination and communication and need to be documented in some way.

Ask your supervisor if you have questions about the documentation-related policies at your organization. Documentation is usually a key component of orientation for those new to home care, as well as for those experienced team members joining a new organization. Take advantage of any education related to documentation that your organization offers, or that is offered outside of your organization in your area. Many state associations and national organizations usually offer sessions on this important topic. Appendix A lists state and other organizations related to home care and hospice provided at home.

HOME CARE NURSING
TIPS FOR EFFECTIVE DOCUMENTATION

- Try to look objectively at the documentation—does it support coverage and show the care provided to a specific patient?

- Ensure that each note or shift shows why the skills of a nurse or care by an aide are needed.

- Ensure that the patient's responses to the interventions are noted (for example, after changing/dressing a wound, suctioning, giving a breathing treatment, etc.).

- Make sure all the documentation is clear. Are words spelled out so that others can understand them? Abbreviations can sometimes be problematic from a safety perspective—ask your organization for a list of approved abbreviations. When in doubt, spell it out for clarity/safety since there may be unapproved or confusing abbreviations, especially those related to medications.

- Go over the stated goals. Are there goals related to or corresponding with interventions? Are they realistic? Short- and long-term when needed?

- Infection control and prevention activities should be integrated throughout the documentation.

- The documentation should provide information about movement toward goals and their achievement. If it does not, what steps or intervention are changed in the POC?

- The POC orders should be very specific. This includes such things as the specific wound care orders with the specific type of dressing, the order(s) for the treatment, sterile or aseptic, use of other products, etc.

- The POC is the "road map" for all involved. For example, if the nurse called in sick or could not be there one day for a visit or care, would another nurse know and understand the specific care regimens and "what to do" based on the POC? They should be able to through clear, effective, and up-to-date documentation.

- Allergies should be noted, such as to drugs, medications, shellfish, latex, bee stings, peanuts, and myriad other things that patients can be allergic to. Are these allergies documented somewhere else and communicated (read: care communication and coordination) to other team members, such as to the aide who may prepare/make meals and needs to know of food allergies?

- Depending on the organization and internal operational processes, it may be the nurse or coder who verifies the diagnosis. This should match on the OASIS, POC, and then the claim.

- Ensure that the "principal diagnosis" is defined by the regulations and ICD-10 use conventions. (In addition, these POC codes should align with/match exactly the claim.) This includes the same number and order of the diagnoses. Primary and secondary diagnoses should be reported and sequenced consistently on the comprehensive assessment, POC, and the claim following the ICD-10 official guidelines for coding and reporting.

- When working with clinical experts, such as wound or infection control specialists, be sure their contributions to the care plan and communications with other team members are integrated into care planning to improve care and practice.

- The documentation should tell the patient's story from admission through care and service through their discharge.

- Refrain from using judgmental terms, such as *messy, lazy, angry,* or other terms that are subjective. Instead, describe the circumstances or situation that led to that judgment. Make specific notes about what the situation entailed, how the patient or family spoke, or what the home "looked like." For example, document that "the patient spoke in a very loud voice saying, 'You cannot come in here!'" or note that "the path to the kitchen was approximately 2 feet wide with papers and magazines stacked 3 feet high on either side."

- Corrections or addendums should be done per the organizational policy.

- Adherence to policy and procedural manuals related to care and documentation should be evident.

- The history and physical from the hospital (or physician) to help with care coordination and to help in the transition of care should be included in the record.

- The Form 485/POC data elements and the comprehensive assessment should be congruent. Does it sound like the same patient? For example, if the patient is noted to have high blood pressure (hypertension), is this information reflected in the "cardiovascular system" section of the assessment?

- Because care and documentation are often systems-based from a quality perspective, the correct "systems" should be reviewed for care and interventions. In the exemplar of Mr. Hinckley, this would have included caring for an older, frail adult (which includes safety related to his history of falls, and a fall-assessment tool would need to be completed), the integumentary system because of his lower leg wound, the cardiovascular system with his documented hypertension, etc. Thinking from this systems-based perspective helps 'frame' the POC and is a natural with the emphasis and movement toward population health.

- Ensure that the patient's emergency plan is on the chart, complete, up-to-date, and realistic. (And does that information also go to the "on-call" team or is it somehow housed "offsite" if there is a disaster to the building?)

- The frequency of visits ordered on the POC should match those made in a record review.

- Similarly, the aide's visit notes should match the aide's POC created by the RN supervisor. Does the frequency noted on the 485 for the aide match the documentation of the aide's frequency of visits? Does the aide's documentation match the aide's POC?

- The documented supplies and medical equipment on the POC should also match what is seen in the home.

- The documented medication should also match what is seen in the home and what is used by the patient.

- Document that all prescriptions, OTC, herb, and other products the patient uses are listed on the medication list. Is there documentation about medication teaching and management?

- The documentation of each visit should be independent and standalone from any other visits. It should answer the question, "What is the value of this visit?" and be reflected in the documentation.

Documentation in home care and hospice is multifaceted, complex, and meets numerous requirements while playing important roles in quality. This is a brief overview of some of the important tenets. Readers are referred to the *Handbook of Home Health Standards: Quality, Documentation, and Reimbursement* (Marrelli, 5th Edition, 2012) for in-depth and detailed information about documentation. As emphasized throughout this book, knowledge of rules related to coverage and reimbursement are key to compliance and quality. Medicare Administrative Contractors (MACs) are responsible for medical review and claims processing and related processes in different states and regions. See the map of MACs in Appendix C, beginning on p. 301.

Quality and Documentation Considerations

Consider these quality and documentation issues:

1. What are the signs/symptoms reported/experienced by the patient?

2. Is the patient's pain assessed, addressed, and managed effectively?

3. Is the patient's (and caregiver's) anxiety/depression/mood alteration assessed and managed effectively?

4. Is the patient's functional ability/status (ADLs/instrumental activities of daily living [IADLs]) clearly documented?

5. Are infection control and prevention and safety efforts identified and implemented?

6. Do the patient and caregiver have access to food, supplies, medications, and other items needed to implement the POC? If not, are they referred to appropriate community or other needed resources to assist in meeting the identified goals on the POC?

7. What progress is the patient making toward reaching established goals and discharge? Are they realistic? If not, what is being changed and tried?

8. Is there evidence of case conferencing, care coordination, and communications with the physician and others involved in the care?

9. For patients with known safety risks identified, are they placed on fall, bleeding, hip, or other precautions as needed based on their health problems? Are these risks communicated to and documented in the aide's POC and communicated to other team members?

10. Can the patient and family verbalize their goals for care, and what it would "look like" when they are achieved?

11. Does the documentation paint a picture of the patient's care, including detailed assessments, interventions, and the response to care and interventions in the notes/clinical records?

12. Does the documentation explain reasons for monitoring, observation and assessment, teaching and training, for example, medication management for new, changed, symptomology, side effects, etc.?

13. Does the discharge summary review why the patient was admitted, the care provided, and the status on discharge and across the course of care?

Summary

Home care documentation is complex and detailed. Whether you are working with an automated system or a blend of a system and handwritten documentation, the documentation must be clear, understandable, and, when handwritten, legible. Readers are encouraged to ask their supervisors for specific policies and procedures related to the documentation of patient care and related processes. This may include the correction policy for the handwritten and/or electronic documentation.

The best documentation paints a picture of the patient, the patient's status, the interventions provided, the patient's response to that care, and their movement toward individualized goals. Home care nurses and other clinicians and team members have an important role to play in the lives of home care patients and their families and caregivers—telling their unique story. Embrace this honor!

Questions for Further Consideration and Discussion

1. List eight of the roles of effective documentation.

2. Describe five examples of care coordination that should be documented in the patient's record.

3. There is a statement that the patient plan of care (POC) is the "road map" for care and for all of the clinicians involved in the care. Explain why the POC is the "road map" and why this is so important.

4. Other than clinical team reviewing the patient's clinician record, who else might be viewing/reading the documentation?

5. What are four common reasons for medical review denials?

For Further Reading

- *Handbook of Home Health Standards: Quality, Documentation, and Reimbursement, 5th Edition,* by Tina Marrelli

- *Survivor! Ten Practical Steps to Survey Survival,* by Nancy Allen

- "SHOW ME: Enhancing OASIS Functional Assessment" by Mary Narayan in *Home Healthcare Nurse,* January 2009, Vol. 27(1): pp. 19–23

References

Fortinsky, R. H., Madigan, E. A., Sheehan, T. J., Tullai-McGuinness, S., & Kleppinger, A. (2014). Risk factors for hospitalization in a national sample of Medicare home health care patients. *Journal of Applied Gerontology, 33*(4), 474–93.

U.S. Department of Health & Human Services. (2014, May 7). New HHS data shows major strides made in patient safety, leading to improved care and savings. Retrieved from https://innovation.cms.gov/Files/reports/patient-safety-results.pdf

9

Where to From Here? Or Welcome to the Most Exciting Healthcare Setting There Is!

Those who are immersed in home care in any capacity can get used to how things "are"—but home care, like all healthcare, undoubtedly will continue to shift and change. For instance, the Centers for Medicare & Medicaid Services (CMS) proposed a pre-claim review demonstration project. The states identified for the pre-claim review demonstration are (in order of participation): Illinois, Florida, Texas, Michigan, and Massachusetts.

In another change, the Home Health Consumer Assessment of Health-care Providers and Systems (CAHPs), a program from the U.S. Agency for Healthcare Research and Quality (AHRQ), makes scores available, which can be accessed by the public on the website Home Health Compare: www.medicare.gov/homehealthcompare/.

By 2018, the goal is to have all Medicare providers in alternative pay-ment models. This means value-based care. One example of a bundled model that goes across all involved care settings and providers is the program that is in place for mandatory hip and knee replacement in certain markets. Of interest to home care is that the bundle does not just include the hospital-related care but also all additional care during the 90 days after hospital discharge.

Think about accountable care organizations, bundled payments, and other models that are value-based. The Home Health Value-Based Purchasing (HHVBP) model includes all Medicare-certified agencies in the nine states of Arizona, Florida, Iowa, Maryland, Massachusetts, Nebraska, North Carolina, Tennessee, and Washington (CMS, n.d.-a). This model began in 2016 and runs through the end of calendar year 2022 (CMS, n.d.-a).

The good news, in this time of complexity and change, is that population health provides the vision of common goals across all healthcare settings. Post-acute care (PAC), of which home care is a part, "has been of increased interest to policymakers as a result of a 2013 Institute of Medicine (IOM—now called The Health and Medicine Division—HMD) report that identified the sector as the source of 73 percent of the variation in Medicare spending" (American Hospital Association, 2015, p.1).

Those already working in home care have the expertise to offer to others who are seeking partners and who need to better understand home care. This is especially true as care becomes more similar across care settings, including the development of cross-setting measures, and as the harmonization of healthcare continues. Nowhere is this more apparent than in the CARE Tool, which is the acronym for the Continuity Assessment Record and Evaluation (CARE) Item Set.

"The CARE Item Set measures the health and functional status of Medicare beneficiaries at acute discharge, and measures changes in severity and other outcomes for Medicare post-acute care patients. The CARE Item Set is designed to standardize assessment of patients' medical, functional, cognitive, and social support status across acute and post-acute settings, including long-term care hospitals (LTCHs), inpatient rehabilitation facilities (IRFs), skilled nursing facilities (SNFs), and home health agencies (HHAs). The goal was to standardize the items used in each of the existing assessment tools" (CMS, n.d.-b, para. 6).

Such a tool makes sense from a continuity of care perspective and supports a movement toward a time when all providers use the same tools and metrics, and perhaps receive the same reimbursement, regardless of care setting. This is another example of the movement toward the standardization of care and process.

The Numbers Increase and Complexity Continues

"In 2011, there were approximately 3.3 million adult 30-day all-cause hospital readmissions in the United States, and they were associated with about $41.3 billion in hospital costs" (Hines, Barrett, Jiang, & Steiner, 2014, p. 1). The three conditions that were associated with the largest number of readmissions for Medicare patients were 1) congestive heart failure, 2) septicemia, and 3) pneumonia (Hines et al., 2014).

"These conditions resulted in about $4.3 billion in hospital costs" (Hines et al., 2014, p. 1).

For Medicaid patients, the three conditions were mood disorders, schizophrenia, and diabetes (Hines et al., 2014). These numbers have implications for all working in home care. The exemplar patient, Mr. Hinckley, had pneumonia (as well as other co-morbidities) and, therefore, would clearly be at risk for a readmission within 30 days. In addition, the Medicaid numbers illustrate how mood disorders contribute to hospitalizations. Similarly, our patient, Mr. Hinckley, was thought to be grieving and may have had other factors contributing to his alterations in mood. These are the kinds of problems and comorbidities that can be addressed, when identified.

Home care leaders need to know and act upon data and findings such as these for determining their practical implications. They can be used as a way to improve care through quality improvement processes. For example, consider that patients with the previously mentioned six diagnoses (or others) be more carefully managed and mechanisms initiated to further help such at-risk patients remain at home safely.

Careful Case Management

Careful case management is one way to care for these more complex patient populations. Every visit should be specifically planned and tailored, or "framed," to help achieve a goal for that visit and the care. These visits need to be purposeful, goal-oriented, and bring value. Ask "What did my visit, care, intervention, case management, or other activity contribute to helping the patient reach their predetermined, agreed-upon goals?"

For example, in reviewing a patient's care, think about whether or not the actions contribute to or were attributable to patient(s) having an "improvement in bed transferring." Or, if pain was identified, was a holistic, comprehensive pain assessment performed to effectively manage the patient's pain? Or, if the patient "seemed sad," was a depression assessment conducted so that the information could be analyzed and a plan developed based on that data?

Similarly, for falls and pressure ulcers, is further data gathered and assessed about the patient's situation and then acted upon to improve the plan and care? Home care nurses and managers have the data, power, and responsibility to improve patient care and patients' quality of life.

Compassionate and Comfortable Care

Healthcare models are changing to support improved and more compassionate, "comfortable" care to a large and growing number of Medicare populations. The oldest old, those 85 and older, are the fastest growing segment of older adults and particularly need our care, expertise, and support. We see frailty and other problems that have not been seen before on an increasing basis, and there is, therefore, a dearth of knowledge about the best management practices for this fragile and growing population.

American home care organizations are not alone in trying to address and care for older adults and the oldest old in particular. According to the World Health Organization (WHO), "between 2000 and 2050, the proportion of the world's population over 60 years will double from about 11% to 22%" (WHO, 2014, para. 1). "The absolute number of people aged 60 years and over is expected to increase from 605 million to 2 billion over the same period" (WHO, 2014, para. 1). The main burdens on healthcare providers in the United States and across the globe are from chronic and complex diseases in this population. We have much to learn from other countries, who have much larger populations of aged people to care for.

We need to be advocates for patients and families with the focus truly on "patient- and family-centered care." This is a key component of case management. Perhaps the model should be "slow medicine" with comfort and fun as part of the goals. When I was visiting a pediatric hospital, it dawned on me that we should try to provide that comfort and care (and often with fun integrated into the process) for all patients.

The hospice tenet of making "every day the best it can be" should not just be for those who are dying. Think about this—what was the one most enjoyable or fun thing you and your patient did today? The visiting team members are often the "highlight" of the patient's day. Imagine not being able to leave the house due to illness, complexity, and technology, and being homebound for many days, weeks, and months at a time. Then think of what pediatric units and rooms, and some homes, "look like"—stuffed animals, music (probably from *Frozen*), and lots of color!

Changing models and innovations are helping to fuel the increase in acquisitions, partnerships, consolidation, and other relationships including those directed toward integrating varying components into one system. Some of examples of these changing models might be skilled nursing facilities becoming connected to home care and hospice or organizations seeking to provide more and varied types of care and services through the vision of being able to provide a larger menu of needed services. Now think of all the skillful leadership that entails. From data aggregation, analysis, and other projects, it is easy to see how healthcare has become so complex. It is expected these alignments and consolidations may continue as the move to value-based care and the emphasis of only paying for quality (read: expected improvement and/or planned outcomes) continues, regardless of the care setting.

Professional Growth and Development: More Important Than Ever

This is the time to stay up-to-date. Consider picking one or two meetings that you might not usually attend—step out of your comfort zone and maybe go to one from another part of the health system, such as a hospital or a skilled nursing facility, hospice and palliative care, rehabilitation center, or other meetings. Other conferences could be population health–focused, international, and otherwise different from the norm. When you do this, you will find it easier to see the similarities and differences in use of terms and the glossary of healthcare and perhaps benchmarks that are used across care other healthcare settings. This could also be one way to effectively build a bridge across and with other care settings. Such interfaces and relationship building may also help one get and maintain a "seat at the table."

People skills, likability, and relationship-building attributes have never been as important in the integration and delivery of healthcare. It has been said that our words have a bigger impact than we know and sometimes determine our destiny. Pick a topic that you get energized about and develop a knowledge base around that topic. Think of giving a presentation at your organization about that aspect of improving home care *and* health because I believe the two terms will be more and more linked as home care becomes the primary setting for most healthcare.

What are the retention numbers for registered nurses (RNs), licensed practical nurses (LPNs), and aides where you work? This information needs to be measured, analyzed, and valued. In *The Atlantic* article entitled, "The U.S. is Running Out of Nurses," Grant states that "America's 3 million nurses make up the largest segment of the healthcare workforce in the U.S., and nursing is currently one of the fastest-growing occupations in the country. *Despite that growth, demand is outpacing supply. By 2022, The Bureau of Labor Statistics projects, there will be more than a million job openings for nurses, a considerable shortfall* [emphasis added]." (Grant, 2016, para. 4).

I cringe when I hear the word *handoff* in the discussion of transitions of care. It sounds like (and is!) a football term where one quickly passes something to someone else. Patients are not footballs being passed between people, and I believe they should not be compared that way either. In this context, the word *handoff* is used when moving patients across transitions points, such as from the hospital to the home or from the hospital to the rehabilitation center.

I think this term should be reframed and should become *handovers*—think instead of an infant or someone we wish to protect or ensure their safety until that person is on the "other side," in this case, until settled into the new setting, after the transition occurs. This is just one example of how healthcare needs to "soften," look, be, and act mission-driven (might for right!), and truly care for patients. Home care team members are the experts in this and can be the change that we all seek to see in healthcare.

Home care clinicians and managers are in a great position to show and put the "care" and "caring" back into healthcare and care. Healthcare organizations are trying some innovative ideas and models. This chapter and book have listed some that might help patients stay at home and also get their holistic needs met.

Whatever our role in patient care, it is important to stay up-to-date and apprised of changes and new regulations. As this book goes to press, the new OASIS C-2 tool and related instructions have been released. This information can be located at https://www.cms.gov/Medicare/Quality-Initiatives-Patient-Assessment-Instruments/HomeHealthQualityInits/OASIS-Data-Sets.html. This newest version of OASIS will go into effect January 2017.

Home care, whatever it "looks like," will continue to grow and is expanding all around the globe. Interestingly, when observing home care and home care clinicians and managers in other countries, their humanity and the more caring and personal aspects of home care often shine through. Some years ago, I had an idea for a grassroots and international organization for home care nurses—wherever in the world they live and practice. Starting with a small group of nurse leaders, this became the International Home Care Nurses Organization (IHCNO) (www.IHCNO.org). We invite you to join us! I can be reached about this organization at tina.marrelli@ihcno.org.

Summary

From a long-time perspective in home care, it appears that home care is going back to its roots of community-based care, where home care was a part of that model. In some realms, the vocabulary is already changing to keep up. In 2016, the Institute of Medicine went through a name change to become the Health and Medicine Division to reflect its increased focus on a wider range of health matters. The goal is health! Some of this sounds like "back to the future," but the fundamentals worked in the past. Organizations are employing people who are aides, technicians, navigators, care managers, care coordinators, transition coaches, or any number of other titles. Whatever the title, they have one goal in mind, to help the frail, the vulnerable, the economically disadvantaged, and the otherwise at-risk to get the care and health they need and to help them stay out of hospital.

Some of these activities are so fundamental, but they can make a big difference in people's lives and the healthcare systems they use. Examples include taking people to appointments; getting them to the labs for medically necessary blood tests, or otherwise facilitating some testing process; and coordinating meal delivery services or otherwise making sure nutritious food is in the home. Other activities might include making sure that medications do not "run out" and that patients have their prescriptions and medications when needed and finding them assistance if they cannot afford them.

Such common sense, focused interventions sometimes make the difference between someone being (re)hospitalized or being able to stay at home. Home care nurses must be patient advocates in the full sense of the phrase—they negotiate for and communicate for people who do not have those skillsets due to behavioral health issues, or those who literally do not have a speaking voice, such as those with aphasia after a stroke, or those who cannot speak for themselves for other reasons, such as advanced dementia.

Step back for a moment and think about this—it does not take the skills of a nurse or a therapist or other professional specialty to be a patient advocate. It takes a very caring person who is an effective communicator and one who recognizes the myriad factors that impact health, healthcare, and its success. When you read the quote cited earlier in the chapter about needing a million more nurses in the not too distant future, you can see the need for different and more functional, sustainable care models to go with those nurses. All this change is being reframed to be in alignment with other models, care settings, and processes.

And, as always, we need to ask the question: "Is this the best use of a certain skillset, especially when our resources are limited?" These and other policy and fiscal questions are a part of the quality and cost dilemma. Our part in this big picture includes the important "so what" factor. The question remains, "What interventions, care, data sources, and other attributes and information make a positive impact on care and are translatable and actionable to improve outcomes?"

Providing and enhancing value through objective indicators, outcomes, and metrics is here to stay. Collectively it is up to all of us to "reframe" care and home care and where it should rightfully reside—at the center of healthcare—the patient's home.

We have the responsibility to do the "right things right" through skillful care and while adhering to the rules and structure of home care. Together, and if done right, home care will remain a viable model in the bigger health system. It is up to all of us to be the exemplars of how best this is accomplished—for both care and business models. We need to be seen as the "best care" setting for patients and families, where they live—in their homes. This is truly the heart of healthcare.

Questions for Further Consideration and Discussion

1. What is advocacy and why is it so important to patients meeting desired goals and improving outcomes?

2. The author poses the idea that healthcare is moving back into the community—looking at home care and healthcare, do you agree or disagree and why?

3. What are the most common reasons at your organization that patients come back to the hospital? What would the findings be if a root cause analysis was done on the top five reasons and a sample of the last few patient readmissions? Could this be useful for quality assurance performance improvement processes as one way to decrease rehospitalizations?

4. What are the skills needed for clinicians and managers in home care to work together to improve home care and its value from a holistic, big-picture healthcare perspective?

5. What is the value that home care and home care organizations bring to other care settings? Consider what home care can do and does that others may not.

For Further Reading

- "The U.S. Is Running Out of Nurses" by Rebecca Grant (*The Atlantic*, February 3, 2016)

- *The Future of Nursing: Leading Change, Advancing Health* from the Institute of Medicine (http://www.nationalacademies. org/hmd/Reports/2010/The-Future-of-Nursing-Leading-Change-Advancing-Health.aspx)

- Home Health Value-Based Purchasing Model from CMS: https://innovation.cms.gov/initiatives/home-health-value-based-purchasing-model

- "Population Health Case Reports, From Clinic to Community," from the *Journal of the American Medical Association* (http://jama.jamanetwork.com/article.aspx?articleID=2520367)

References

American Hospital Association (AHA). (2015). The role of post-acute care in new care delivery models. Retrieved from http://www.aha.org/research/reports/tw/15dec-tw-postacute.pdf

Centers for Medicare & Medicaid Services (CMS). (n.d.-a). Home health value-based purchasing model. Retrieved from https://innovation.cms.gov/initiatives/home-health-value-based-purchasing-model

Centers for Medicare & Medicaid Services (CMS). (n.d.-b). CARE Item Set and B-CARE. Retrieved from https://www.cms.gov/Medicare/Quality-Initiatives-Patient-Assessment-Instruments/Post-Acute-Care-Quality-Initiatives/CARE-Item-Set-and-B-CARE.html

Centers for Medicare & Medicaid Services (CMS). (2016). Federal Register Volume 81, Number 24. Retrieved from https://www.gpo.gov/fdsys/pkg/FR-2016-02-05/html/2016-02277.htm

Grant, R. (2016, February 3). The U.S. is running out of nurses. *The Atlantic.* Retrieved from http://www.theatlantic.com/health/archive/2016/02/nursing-shortage/459741/

Hines, A. L., Barrett, M. L., Jiang, J., & Steiner, C. A. (2014). Conditions with the largest number of adult hospital readmissions by payer, 2011. AHRQ Statistical Brief #172. Retrieved from http://www.hcup-us.ahrq.gov/reports/statbriefs/sb172-Conditions-Readmissions-Payer.pdf

National Association for Home Care and Hospice (NAHC). (2016). Medicare prior authorization proposed for home health services. Retrieved from http://www.nahc.org/NAHCReport/nr160208_1/

World Health Organization (WHO). (2014). Facts about ageing. Retrieved from http://www.who.int/ageing/about/facts/en/

A

Home Care and Hospice/ Palliative Care Organizations/ Associations

As explained throughout the book, consolidation and cooperation are the future because all of the varied segments of healthcare must ultimately work together. There are many other kinds of trade organizations such as hospital associations, nursing home associations, case management organizations, geriatric associations, nursing- and other discipline-specific specialty organizations, professional associations, and more that may also be of interest. This listing is not all-inclusive, and some organizations or associations are undergoing name and other changes to better reflect the members they serve.

National and International Organizations

Alliance for Home Care Quality and Innovation (AHHQI)

2121 Crystal Drive, Suite 750
Arlington, VA 22202
(571) 527-1532
www.ahhqi.org

The Council of State Home Care Associations

www.thehomecarecouncil.org

The International Home Care Nurses Organization (IHCNO)

www.IHCNO.org

National Association for Home Care & Hospice (NAHC)

228 7th Street SE
Washington, DC 20003
(202) 547-7424
www.nahc.org

National Hospice and Palliative Care Organization (NHPCO)

1731 King Street
Alexandria, VA 22314
(703) 837-1500
www.nhpco.org

Visiting Nurses Associations of America (VNAA)

2121 Crystal Drive, Suite 750
Arlington, VA 22202
(571) 527-1520
www.vnaa.org

State Associations for Home Care and/or Hospice/Palliative Care

Alabama

Alacare Home Health and Hospice

2400 John Hawkins Parkway
Birmingham, AL 35244
(205) 981-8000
Email: john.beard@alacare.com

Alabama Hospice and Palliative Care Organization

12532 County Road 9
Shorter, AL 36075
(334) 421-8884
www.alhospice.org

Alaska

Alaska Home Care & Hospice Association

Julie Yonkers, President
3701 East Tudor Road, Suite 208
Anchorage, AK 99507
(907) 274-1066
Jyomker@peacehealth.org
www.ahcha.org

Arizona

Arizona Association for Home Care

Marie Fredette, CAE, Executive Director
4015 S. McClintock Drive, Suite 101
Tempe, AZ 85282
(480) 491-0540
Email: info@azhomecare.org
www.azhomecare.org

Arizona Hospice and Palliative Care Organization/Arizona Association for Home Care

3933 S. McClintock Drive
Suite 505
Tempe, AZ 85282
(480) 491-0540
www.ahpco.org
info@ahpco.org

Arkansas

HomeCare Association of Arkansas

Nancy Elphingstone, Executive Director
411 South Victory
Suite 204
Little Rock, AR 72201
(501) 376-2273
Email: hcaaark@sbcglobal.net

Hospice and Palliative Care Association of Arkansas

411 S. Victory Street, Suite 205
Little Rock, AR 72201
(501) 375-1300
www.hpcaa.org

California

California Association for Health Services at Home (CAHSAH)

Dean Chalios, President
3780 Rosin Court
Suite 190
Sacramento, CA 95834
(916) 641-5795
Email:dchalios@cahsah.org
www.cahsah.org

California Hospice and Palliative Care Association (CA & NV)

3841 North Freeway Blvd., Suite 225
Sacramento, CA 95834
(916) 925-3770
www.calhospice.org

Colorado

Home Care Association of Colorado

Don Knox, Executive Director
9200 E Mineral Avenue
Suite 1140
Centennial, CO 80112
(877) 940-7798
Email: admin@civicamanagement.com
www.homecareofcolorado.org

Hospice & Palliative Care Association of the Rockies (CO and WY)

2851 S. Parker Road, Suite 250
Aurora, CO 80014
(303) 848-2522
www.COCHPC.org

Connecticut

Connecticut Association for Home Care, Inc.

Deborah R. Hoyt, President & CEO
110 Barnes Road
PO Box 90
Wallingford, CT 06492-0090
(203) 774-4939
Email: hoyt@cthealthcareathome.org
www.cthealthcareathome.org

Delaware

No listings

Florida

Home Care Association of Florida

Bobby Lolley, Executive Director
1363 East Lafayette Street, Suite A
Tallahassee, FL 32301-2600
(850) 222-8967
Email: blolley@homecareFLA.org
www.homecareFLA.org

Florida Hospice & Palliative Care Association

Paul Ledford, Executive Director
2000 Apalachee Parkway, Suite 200
Tallahassee, FL 32301
(850) 878-2632
Email: info@floridahospices.org
www.floridahospices.org

Georgia

Georgia Association for Home Health Agencies, Inc.

Judy Adams, Executive Director
2146 Roswell Road
Suite 108 - PMB 1107
Marietta, GA 30062
(770) 565-4531

Email: gahomehealth@earthlink.net
www.gahha.org

Georgia Hospice & Palliative Care Organization

3032 Briarcliff Road
Atlanta, GA 30328-5350
(404) 323-9397
www.ghpco.org

Hawaii

Healthcare Association of Hawaii

Andrew Takuya Garrett, MPA, Associate Vice President, Post-Acute Care & Operations
707 Richards Street, PH2
Honolulu, HI 96813
(808) 521-8961
Email: rwong@hah.org
hah.org

Kokua Mau Hawaii Hospice and Palliative Care Organization

P.O. Box 62155
Honolulu, HI 96839
(808) 585-9977
www.kokuamau.org

Idaho

Idaho Association of Home Health Agencies

Katherine M. Jones, Executive Director
c/o 2504 Kootenai
Boise, ID 83705
(208) 866-6360
Email: kjones@cableone.net
idahohomecare.org

Idaho End-of-Life Coalition

P.O. Box 4320
Ketchum, ID 83340-4320
(208) 841-1862
www.idqol.org

Illinois

Illinois HomeCare & Hospice Council

Janet S. Grimes, Executive Director
100 East Washington
Springfield, IL 62701
(217) 753-4422
Email: jangrimes@ilhomecare.org
www.ilhomecare.org

Illinois Hospice & Palliative Care Organization

The PMC Group
902 Ash Street
Winnetka, IL 60093
(847) 441-7200
www.il-hpco.org

Indiana

Indiana Association for Home & Hospice Care, LLC

Evan Reinhardt, Executive Director
6320-G Rucker Road
Indianapolis, IN 46220
(317) 775-6675
Email: evan@iahhc.org
www.iahhc.org

Indiana Hospice & Palliative Care Organization

P.O. Box 68829
Indianapolis, IN 46268-0829
(317) 464-5145
www.ihpco.org

Iowa

Iowa Alliance in Home Care

Greg Boattenhamer, Executive Director
100 East Grand Avenue, Suite 118
Des Moines, IA 50309
(515) 282-3965
Email: BoattenhamerG@ihaonline.org
www.iahc.org

Hospice & Palliative Care Organization of Iowa

100 East Grand Avenue, Suite 120
Des Moines, IA 50309
(515) 243-1046
www.hpcai.org

Kansas

Kansas Home Care Association

Jane Kelly, Executive Director
2738 SW Santa Fe Drive
Topeka, KS 66614
(785) 478-3640
Email: jkelly@kshomecare.org
www.kshomecare.org

Kansas Hospice and Palliative Care Organization

26 Maverick
Wichita, KS 67220
(316) 207-1764
www.khpco.org

Kentucky

Kentucky Home Care Association

Annette Gervais, Executive Director
2331 Fortune Drive
Suite 280
Lexington, KY 40509
(859) 268-2574
Email: annette@khca.net
www.khca.net

Kentucky Association of Hospice & Palliative Care

Brandy Cantor, Executive Director
305 Ann St, Suite 308
Frankfort, KY 40601-2847
(502) 875-1176
www.kah.org

Louisiana

HomeCare Association of Louisiana

Warren Hebert, CHCE, CEO
850 Kaliste Saloom Road
Lafayette, LA 70508
(337) 231-0080
Email: warren@hclanet.org
www.hclanet.org

Louisiana-Mississippi Hospice & Palliative Care Organization

717 Kerlerec Street
New Orleans, LA 70116-2005
(504) 945-2414
www.lmhpco.org

Maine

Home Care & Hospice Alliance of Maine

Vicki Purgavie, Executive Director
30 Association Drive, PO Box 227
Manchester, ME 04351-0227
(207) 213-6125
Email: vicki@homecarealliance.org
www.homecarealliance.org

Maine Hospice Council & Center for the End-of-Life Care

295 Water Street, Suite 303
Augusta, ME 04330
(207) 626-0651
www.mainehospicecouncil.org

Maryland—District of Columbia

Maryland National Capital Homecare Association

Ann Horton, Executive Director
10125 Colesville Road
Suite 294
Silver Spring, MD 20901
(301) 920-2069
Email: ahorton@mncha.org
www.mncha.org

Hospice & Palliative Care Network of Maryland

201 International Drive, Suite 230
Hunt Valley, MD 21030
(410) 891-5741
www.hnmd.org

Massachusetts

Home Care Alliance of MA

Pat Kelleher, Executive Director
31 St. James Avenue, Suite 780
Boston, MA 02116
(617) 482-8830
Email: pkelleher@thinkhomecare.org
www.thinkhomecare.org

Hospice & Palliative Care Federation of Massachusetts

1420 Providence Highway, Suite 277
Norwood, MA 02062
(781) 255-7077
www.hospicefed.org

Visiting Nurse Associations of New England, Inc.

Marlborough, MA
President and CEO, Ed DeVaney
edevaney@vnane.org

Massachusetts Council for Home Care Aide Services

Lisa Gurgone, Executive Director
174 Portland Street
Boston, MA 02114
(617) 224-4141
Email: lgurgone@mahomecareaides.com
www.mahomecareaides.com

Michigan

Michigan HomeCare and Hospice Association

Barry S. Cargill, Executive Director
2140 University Park Dr.
Suite 220
Okemos, MI 48864
(517) 349-8089
Email: barryc@homecaremi.org
www.homecaremi.org

Minnesota

Minnesota HomeCare Association

Kathy Messerli, Executive Director
1711 West County Road B
Suite 211S
St. Paul, MN 55113-4036
(651) 635-0607
Email: kmesserli@mnhomecare.org
www.mnhomecare.org

Minnesota Network of Hospice & Palliative Care

2365 McKnight Rd. North Suite 2
North St. Paul, MN 55109
(651) 917-4616
www.mnhpc.org

Mississippi

Mississippi Association for Home Care

Mary Lea Nations, Executive Director
Mississippi Association for Home Care
134 Fairmont Street, Suite B
Clinton, MS 39056
(601) 924-2275
Email: mnations@mahc.org
http://mahc.org

Louisiana–Mississippi Hospice & Palliative Care Organization

717 Kerlerec Street
New Orleans, LA 70116-2005
(504) 945-2414
www.lmhpco.org

Missouri

Missouri Alliance for Home Care

Mary Schantz, Executive Director
Missouri Alliance for Home Care
2420 Hyde Park Road, Suite A
Jefferson City, MO 65109
(573) 634-7772
Email: mary@homecaremissouri.org
www.homecaremissouri.org

Missouri Hospice & Palliative Care Association

2222 Weathered Rock Road, Suite C
Jefferson City, MO 65101
(573) 634-5514
www.mohospice.org

Montana

Montana Hospital Association, an Association of Montana Healthcare Providers

Casey Blumenthal, Vice President
2625 Winne Avenue
Helena, MT 59601 Phone(406) 442-1911
Email: casey@mtha.org
www.mtha.org

Nebraska

Nebraska Home Care Association

Janet Seelhoff, CAE, Executive Director
1633 Normandy Court, Suite A
Lincoln, NE 68512
(402) 423-0718
Email: jseelhoff@assocoffice.net
www.nebraskahomecare.org

Nebraska Hospice & Palliative Care Association

1200 Libra Drive, St. 100
Lincoln, NE 68512
(402) 477-0204
www.nehospice.org

Nevada

Nevada Homecare Association

David Lampron, Treasurer
10200 W. Flamingo Road
Suite 4, PMB 118
Las Vegas, NV 89145-8394
(800) 559-6580
Email: NVHOMECAREASSOC@aol.com
www.nvhca.com

California Hospice and Palliative Care Association (CA & NV)

3841 North Freeway Blvd., Suite 225
Sacramento, CA 95834
(916) 925-3770
www.calhospice.org

New Hampshire

Home Care Association of New Hampshire

Gina Balkus, CEO
Home Care Association of New Hampshire
8 Green Street, Suite 2
Concord, NH 03301-4012
(603) 225-5597
Email: gbalkus@homecarenh.org
www.homecarenh.org

New Hampshire Hospice and Palliative Care Organization

125 Airport Road
Concord, NH 03301
(603) 415-4298
www.nhhpco.org

New Jersey

Home Care Association of New Jersey

Chrissy Buteas, President & CEO
485D Route 1 South
Suite 210
Iselin, NJ 08830
(732) 877-1100
Email: chrissy@homecarenj.org
www.homecarenj.org

New Jersey Hospital Association

Elizabeth A. Ryan, Esq., President & CEO
760 Alexander Road
PO Box 1
Princeton, NJ 08543-0001
(609) 275-4102
Email: tedelstein@njha.com
www.njha.com

Home Care Council of New Jersey

Ken Wessel, MSW, ACSW, LSW, President
74 Haas Rd.
Basking Ridge, NJ 07920
(862) 812-3677
kenwessel@homecarecouncilnj.org
www.homecarecouncilnj.org

New Jersey Hospice and Palliative Care Organization

1044 Route 22 West Suite 2
Mountainside, NJ 07092
(908) 233-0060
www.njhospice.org

New Mexico

New Mexico Association for Home & Hospice Care

Joie Glenn, RN, MBA, CAE, Executive Director
3200 Carlisle Boulevard, NE
Suite 117
Albuquerque, NM 87110
(505) 889-4556
Email: joieg@nmahc.org
www.nmahc.org

Texas & New Mexico Hospice Organization

1108 Lavaca, Suite 727,
Austin, TX 78701
(512) 454-1247
www.txnmhospice.org

New York

Home Care Association of NY State

Joanne Cunningham, President
Home Care Association of New York State
914 Washington Avenue, Suite 400
Albany, NY 12210
(518) 426-8764 Ext. 214
Email: jcunningham@hcanys.org
www.hcanys.org

New York State Association of Health Care Providers, Inc.

Claudia Hammar, President
20 Corporate Woods Boulevard, 2nd floor
Albany, NY 12211
(518) 463-1118
Email: hammar@nyshcp.org
www.nyshcp.org

Hospice & Palliative Care Association of New York State

Timothy Nichols, President
2 Computer Drive West, Suite 105
Albany, NY 12205-1141
(518) 446-1483
www.hpcanys.org

North Carolina

Association for Home & Hospice Care of North Carolina, Inc.

Timothy Rogers, President & CEO
3101 Industrial Drive, Suite 204
Raleigh, NC 27609
(919) 848-3450
Email: timrogers@homeandhospice-care.org
www.homeandhospicecare.org

The Carolinas Center for Hospice and End of Life Care

Carol Meyer, CEO/President

North Carolina1230 S.E. Maynard Road, Suite 203, Cary, NC 27511; (919) 459-5380

South Carolina1350 Browning Road, Columbia, SC 29210; (803) 509-1021

Email: akiser@cchospice.org

www.cchospice.org

North Dakota

North Dakota Association for Homecare

Erica Cermak, Association Executive (APT, Inc.)
PO Box 2175
Bismarck, ND 58502-2175
701-224-1815
http://www.aptnd.com/ndahc/
Email: erica@exchange.aptnd.com

Ohio

Ohio Council for Home Care & Hospice

Garry Moon, CAE, Executive Director
Ohio Council for Home Care & Hospice
1105 Schrock Road
Suite 120
Columbus, OH 43229
(614) 885-0434
Email: garry@ochch.org
www.ochch.org

LeadingAge Ohio/Midwest Care Alliance

Jeffrey Lycan, RN, BS
President & CEO
2233 North Bank Drive
Columbus, OH 43220
(614) 763-0036

Toll Free(800) 776-9513
Email: jeff.lycan@midwestcarealliance.org
www.midwestcarealliance.org

Oklahoma

Oklahoma Association for Home Care & Hospice

Annette Mays, Executive Director
755 West Covell Road, Suite 100
Edmond OK 73003
(405) 210-7857
Email: abisel@swbell.net
www.OAHC.com

Oklahoma Hospice & Palliative Care Association

P.O. Box 1466
Ardmore, OK 73402
(405)513-8602
http://www.okhospice.org/

Oregon

Oregon Association for Home Care

Fawn Barrie, Executive Director
Oregon Association for Home Care
4676 Commercial Street, SE
Suite 449
Salem, OR 97302
(503) 364-2733
Email: fbarrie@oahc.org
www.oahc.org

Oregon Hospice Association

P.O. Box 10796
812 SW 10th, Suite 204
Portland, OR 97296-0796
(503) 228-2104
www.oregonhospice.org
fbarrie@oahc.org

Pennsylvania

Pennsylvania Homecare Association

Vicki Hoak, Executive Director
600 N. 12th Street
Suite 200
Lemoyne, PA 17043
(717) 975-9448
Email: vhoak@pahomecare.org
www.pahomecare.org

Pennsylvania Hospice Network

475 W. Governor Road, Suite 7
Hershey, PA 17033
(717) 533-4002
www.pahospice.org

VNAs of the Mid-Atlantic

St. Mary's, PA
Executive Director, Denise Kneidel Bish
vna.midatlantic@gmail.com

Puerto Rico

Puerto Rico Hospice and Palliative Care Association Care Association

PO Box 460 Mantín PR 00674
(787) 309-8246
(787) 621-7535
http://www.prhpca.com

Rhode Island

Rhode Island Partnership for Home Care, Inc.

Nicholas A. Oliver, MPA, CAE, Executive Director
260 West Exchange Street, Suite 5
Providence, RI 02903
(401) 351-1010
Email: director@riphc.org
www.riphc.org

South Carolina

South Carolina Home Care & Hospice Association

Tim Rogers, President & CEO
3101 Industrial Drive, Suite 204
Raleigh, NC 27609
(919) 848-3450
Email: timrogers@homeandhospicecare.org
www.schomehealth.org

The Carolinas Center for Hospice and End of Life Care

Carol Meyer, CEO/President
North Carolina1230 S.E. Maynard Road, Suite 203, Cary, NC 27511; (919) 459-5380
South Carolina1350 Browning Road, Columbia, SC 29210; (803) 509-1021
Email: akiser@cchospice.org
www.cchospice.org

South Dakota

South Dakota Association of Healthcare Organizations

Wendy Mead, VP, Communications and Education
3708 Brooks Place
Sioux Falls, SD 57106
(605) 361-2281
Email: wendy.mead@sdaho.org
www.sdaho.org

Tennessee

Tennessee Association for Home Care, Inc.

Gayla Sasser, Executive Director
PO Box 140087
Nashville, TN 37027-7540
(615) 885-3399
Email: gayla.sasser@tahc-net.org
www.tahc-net.org

Tennessee Hospice Organization

500 Interstate Blvd. S
Nashville, TN 37210-4634
(615) 256-8240
www.tnhospice.org

Tennessee Hospital Association Home Care Alliance

Mike Dietrich, Vice President
5201 Virginia Way
Brentwood, TN 37027
(615) 256-8240
Email: mdietrich@tha.com

Texas

Texas Association for Home Care & Hospice, Inc.

Rachel Hammon, Executive Director
3737 Executive Center Drive
Suite 268
Austin, TX 78731
 (512) 338-9293
Toll Free(800) 880-8893
Email: rachel@tahch.org
www.tahch.org

Texas & New Mexico Hospice Organization

1108 Lavaca, Suite 727,
Austin, TX 78701
(512) 454-1247
www.txnmhospice.org

Utah

Utah Association for Home Care

Ed Dieringer, Executive Director
2654 South 1500 East
Salt Lake City, UT 84106
http://www.uthomecare.org/
Email: info@ua4hc.org

Utah Hospice & Palliative Care Organization

1327 South 900 East
Salt Lake City, UT 84105-2301
(801) 582-2245
http://utahhospice.org/
Email: uahchosp@gmail.com

Vermont

VNAs of Vermont

Peter Cobb, Executive Director
173 Elm Street
Montpelier, VT 05602
(802) 229-0579
Email: vnavt@comcast.net
vnavt.com

Hospice and Palliative Care Council of Vermont

137 Elm Street #3, Montpelier
Vermont, 05602
(802) 229-0579
http://www.hpccv.org/

Virginia

Virginia Association for Home Care & Hospice

Marcia Tetterton, MS, CAE, Executive Director
3761 Westerre Parkway
Suite B
Henrico, VA. 23233
(804) 285-8636
Email: mtetterton@vahc.org
www.vahc.org

Virginia Association for Hospices & Palliative Care

PO Box 70025
Richmond, VA 23255
(804) 740-1344
www.virginiahospice.org

Washington

Home Care Association of Washington

Doris Visaya, Executive Director
P.O. Box 65009
Vancouver, WA 98665
(425) 775-8120
Email: dorisv.hcaw@gmail.com
www.hcaw.org

Washington State Hospice & Palliative Care Organization

PO Box 5352
Olympia, WA 98507
(541)490-9073
www.wshpco.org

West Virginia

West Virginia Council of Home Care Agencies, Inc.

Laura Friend, Executive Director
2554 Elk Fork Road
Middlebourne, WV 26149
Phone(800) 210-4663
Fax(304) 758-4354
Email: wvhomecare@hughes.net
www.wvhomecareassociation.com

Hospice Council of West Virginia

1804 Rolling Hills Rd
P.O. Box 4222 or 1063 Maple Drive
Charleston, WV 25314
(304) 206-8929
www.hospicecouncilofwv.org

Wisconsin

Wisconsin Association for Home Care, Inc.

Eric Ostermann, MBA, CAE, Executive Director
563 Carter Court, Suite B
Kimberly, WI 54136
(920) 560-5632
Email: eric@badgerbay.com
www.wiahc.org

The HOPE of Wisconsin

3240 University Avenue, Suite 2
Madison, WI 53705-3570
(608) 233-7166
www.wisconsinhospice.org

Wyoming

Hospice & Palliative Care Association of the Rockies (CO and WY)

2851 S. Parker Road, Suite 250
Aurora, CO 80014
(303) 848-2522
www.COCHPC.org

The compiler wishes to thank Tracey Moorhead, (VNAA), Warren Hebert (LAHC), Jennifer Kennedy (NHPCO), Joie Glenn (NMAHHC), and others who contributed their time on reviews of this project.

Adapted with permission from the Visiting Nurse Associations of America (VNAA).

B

Resources for Clinicians and Patient/Caregiver Education

Alzheimer's Disease

- Caregiver Resources from alzheimers.gov: http://www.alzheimers.gov/caregiver_resources.html

- Caring for Someone from alzheimers.gov: http://www.alzheimers.gov/caring.html

- About Alzheimer's Disease: Symptoms, from the National Institute on Aging: http://www.nia.nih.gov/alzheimers/topics/symptoms

- Alzheimer's Disease, from the Centers for Disease Control and Prevention: http://www.cdc.gov/aging/aginginfo/alzheimers.htm

- Home Safety for People with Alzheimer's Disease, from the National Institute on Aging: http://www.nia.nih.gov/sites/default/files/home_safety_for_people_with_alzheimers_disease.pdf

- Alzheimer's: When to Stop Driving, from the Mayo Clinic: http://www.mayoclinic.org/healthy-living/caregivers/in-depth/alzheimers/art-20044924

- The Alzheimer's Association offers brochures and other resources for professionals and families; includes information on getting the right diagnosis and a 24/7 helpline: www.alz.org; 1-800-272-3900

Amputation

- Lower Extremity Amputation Prevention (LEAP): http://www.hrsa.gov/hansensdisease/leap/

- The U.S. Department of Veterans Affairs offers information on their Rehabilitation and Prosthetic Services page: http://www.prosthetics.va.gov

- The Amputee Coalition offers information for on amputations and support groups: http://www.amputee-coalition.org/

- MedlinePlus offers a foot amputation discharge information page, including self-care guidelines: http://www.nlm.nih.gov/medlineplus/ency/patientinstructions/000013.htm

- The National Amputation Foundation offers information and support: www.nationalamputation.org; 1-516-887-3600

Arthritis

- The American Academy of Orthopaedic Surgeons offers resources and information related to arthritis: www.aaos.org

- The Arthritis Foundation offers information about different types of arthritis as well as tips for eating well and staying active on its website: http://www.arthritis.org/; 1-800-283-7800

- The Arthritis Foundation publishes the *Arthritis Today* magazine: http://www.arthritis.org/arthritis-today-magazine/

- The Arthritis Foundation also offers a resource specifically for caregivers: http://www.arthritistoday.org/what-you-can-do/everyday-solutions/caregiving/

- The National Institute of Arthritis and Musculoskeletal and Skin Diseases offers an information page about rheumatoid arthritis in particular: http://www.niams.nih.gov/health_info/rheumatic_disease/rheumatoid_arthritis_ff.asp; 1-877-226-4267

- The Centers for Disease Control and Prevention (CDC) offers resources including basic information about arthritis: http://www.cdc.gov/arthritis

- MedlinePlus offers information about arthritis, including common types and treatment options: http://www.nlm.nih.gov/medlineplus/ency/article/001243.htm

Cancer

- Caring for the Caregiver from the National Cancer Institute: http://www.cancer.gov/publications/patient-education/caring-for-the-caregiver

- Complementary and Alternative Medicine from the National Cancer Institute: http://www.cancer.gov/cancertopics/cam

- Cancer Treatment from the National Cancer Institute: http://www.cancer.gov/cancertopics/treatment

- Organizations and Resources from the National Cancer Institute for adolescents and young adults: http://www.cancer.gov/cancertopics/aya/resources

- Coping with Cancer from the National Cancer Institute: http://www.cancer.gov/cancertopics/coping

- The American Cancer Society offers support groups such as "I Can Cope" and "Look Good … Feel Better" for women undergoing chemotherapy or radiation. It also offers resources and information on various cancers for patients, families, and professionals: www.cancer.org

- The Oncology Nursing Society offers a "Breast Cancer Patient Resource Area" and links to organizations and journals to help patients: www.ons.org

- Cancer Care offers information for those dealing with cancer—patients, family members, friends, and health professionals providing care: www.cancercare.org; 1-800-813-HOPE (4673)

- The Oral Cancer Foundation: http://oralcancer.org/

Cardiac Care

- The American Heart Association offers professional and patient resources: www.americanheart.org; 1-800-AHA-USA1 (8721)

- The National Heart, Lung, and Blood Institute offers information about heart failure (what it is, the signs and symptoms, treatment options, how it is diagnosed, etc.): www.nhlbi.nih.gov; 1-301-592-8573

- Get Moving: Easy Tips to Get Active!, from the American Heart Association: http://www.heart.org/HEARTORG/HealthyLiving/PhysicalActivity/GettingActive/Get-Moving-Easy-Tips-to-Get-Active_UCM_307978_Article.jsp#.V18uNPkrLIU

Caregivers

- Caregiver Resources, from alzheimers.gov: http://www.alzheimers.gov/caregiver_resources.html

- Caring for Someone, from alzheimers.gov: http://www.alzheimers.gov/caring.html

- Caring for the Caregiver, from the National Cancer Institute: http://www.cancer.gov/publications/patient-education/caring-for-the-caregiver

- Caregiving Resources, from the Centers for Disease Control and Prevention: http://www.cdc.gov/cancer/survivorship/caregivers/resources.htm

- Medicare pays for certain immunizations and information and links to other important immunization websites, such as the Centers for Disease Control and Prevention (CDC): www.cms.hhs.gov/AdultImmunizations

Chronic Obstructive Pulmonary Disease (COPD)

- Overdose on Oxygen? from Patient Safety Network: https://psnet.ahrq.gov/webmm/case/172/overdose-on-oxygen

- The American Academy of Allergy Asthma & Immunology offers an explanation of the differences between asthma and COPD: http://www.aaaai.org/conditions-and-treatments/library/asthma-library/asthma-and-copd--differences-and-similarities.aspx

- MedlinePlus offers a COPD section explaining the disease and common symptoms: http://www.nlm.nih.gov/medlineplus/copd.html

- The Centers for Disease Control and Prevention offers a "What is COPD?" resource: http://www.cdc.gov/copd/

- The National Heart, Lung, and Blood Institute also offers a "What is COPD?" resource, including treatment and living with the disease sections: http://www.nhlbi.nih.gov/health/health-topics/topics/copd

- The National Heart, Lung, and Blood Institute offers a "What Are the Lungs?" page as well for more information on how this organ is affected: http://www.nhlbi.nih.gov/health/health-topics/topics/hlw/

- NIH Senior Health offers information about treating COPD: http://nihseniorhealth.gov/copd/treatingcopd/01.html

- The COPD Foundation offers a frequently asked questions page for caregivers: http://www.copdfoundation.org/Learn-More/For-Patients-Caregivers/FAQ-for-Caregivers.aspx

Diabetes

- Diabetes resources from PublicHealthCorps: http://publichealthcorps.org/diabetes/

- Lower Extremity Amputation Prevention (LEAP): http://www.hrsa.gov/hansensdisease/leap/

- The American Association of Diabetes Educators (AADE) is dedicated to integrating successful self-management as a key outcome in the care of people with diabetes and related health problems: www.diabeteseducator.org

- The American Diabetes Association (ADA) offers resources for patients, families, and professionals: www.diabetes.org; 1-800-DIABETES (342-2383)

- The Joslin Diabetes Center offers educational resources on managing diabetes: www.joslin.org; 1-617-732-2400

- The National Amputation Foundation offers information and support: www.nationalamputation.org; 1-516-887-3600

Education

- "Uniting Academia and Practice in Nursing: Using QSEN to Improve the Quality and Safety of Healthcare" by Patricia Patrician (*American Nurse Today*, 2016)

- Quality and Safety Education for Nurses Project: http://qsen.org/

- Robert Wood Johnson Foundation: http://www.rwjf.org/

- "A Game-Based Strategy for the Staff Development of Home Health Care Nurses" by Inna Popil and Darlene Dillard-Thompson (*Journal of Continuing Education and Nursing*, 2015)

Emergency Preparedness and Management

- Technical Resources from the Healthcare Emergency Preparedness Information Gateway from the U.S. Department of Health and Human Services: https://asprtracie.hhs.gov/technical-resources

- *Five Days at Memorial: Life and Death in a Storm-Ravaged Hospital* by Sheri Fink (American Library Association Notable Books for Adults, 2013)

- Emergency Preparedness and Response from the CDC: http://emergency.cdc.gov/

- NOAA Weather Radio All Hazards (NWR): http://www.nws.noaa.gov/nwr/

- "Preparedness for Natural Disasters Among Older US Adults: A Nationwide Survey" by Tala M. Al-rousan, Linda M. Rubenstein, and Robert B. Wallace (*American Journal of Public Health*)

- Understanding the Proposed Rule on Emergency Preparedness from the Centers for Medicare & Medicaid Services (CMS): https://www.youtube.com/watch?v=8splScqEEQM

- The U.S. Department of Health and Human Services offers the Cultural Competency Curriculum for Disaster Preparedness and Crisis Response: https://cccdpcr.thinkculturalhealth.hhs.gov/

Falls

- Preventing Falls: A Guide to Implementing Effective Community-Based Fall Prevention Programs from the Centers for Disease Control and Prevention (CDC): http://www.cdc.gov/homeandrecreationalsafety/falls/community_preventfalls.html

- Check for Safety: A Home Fall Prevention Checklist for Older Adults from the Centers for Disease Control and Prevention (CDC): http://www.cdc.gov/HomeandRecreationalSafety/pubs/English/booklet_Eng_desktop-a.pdf

- The American Occupational Therapy Association (AOTA): http://www.aota.org

Gastrointestinal and Tube-Related Care

- The Oley Foundation offers support and information options that include a *Lifeline Letter* bi-monthly newsletter for people living with home parenteral and/or enteral nutrition and fact sheets such as Questions New Tube Feeders Should Be Asking. Information also provided in Spanish: www.oley.org; 1-800-776-OLEY

- The Oral Cancer Foundation offers an information page on nutrition and feeding systems include tube feeding systems and more: www.oralcancer.org

- Verifying NG Feeding Tube Placement In Pediatric Patients by Beth Lyman, Jane Anne Yaworksi, Lori Duesing, and Candice Moore: http://www.americannursetoday.com/verifying-ng-feeding-tube-placement-pediatric-patients/

Home and Community Environment

- The website HealthyPeople.gov offers information and tools for learning about and using the Healthy People 2020 objectives to guide health education program planning and evaluation. The site contains links to online lessons for students, professionals, and community health leaders who want to learn more about the nation's health goals and efforts to reach them.

- Social Determinants of Health from HealthyPeople.gov: http://www.healthypeople.gov/2020/topics-objectives/topic/social-determinants-of-health

- American Academy of Home Care Medicine promotes the practice of medicine in the home environment: http://www.aahcm.org/

- The International Home Care Nurses Organization (IHCNO) is a resource for nurses practicing home care for wherever home care patients live in the world: http://ihcno.org/

Hospice, End-of-Life, and Palliative Care

- HospiScript: http://www.hospiscript.com/

- *Dying in America: Improving Quality and Honoring Individual Preferences Near the End of Life* from the National Academies Press: http://iom.nationalacademies.org/Reports/2014/Dying-In-America-Improving-Quality-and-Honoring-Individual-Preferences-Near-the-End-of-Life.aspx

- End-of-Life Nursing Education Consortium (ELNEC): http://www.aacn.nche.edu/elnec

- The American Academy of Hospice and Palliative Medicine provides position statements and other resources regarding important issues in hospice and palliative care: www.aahpm.org

- The Compassionate Friends: www.compassionatefriends.org

- The Hospice and Palliative Nurses Association (HPNA) is the nation's largest and oldest professional nursing organization dedicated to promoting excellence in hospice and palliative nursing: www.hpna.org; 1-412-787-9301

- The National Hospice and Palliative Care Organization: www.nhpco.org

- *Palliative Nursing: Scope and Standards of Practice* from the American Nurses Association (ANA) and the Hospice and Palliative Nurses Association (HPNA): http://www.nursesbooks.org/Main-Menu/Standards/Palliative-Nursing.aspx

Infection Control and Prevention

- *Home Care Infection Prevention and Control Program* by Mary McGoldrick (2016, Home Health Systems)

- Home Health Systems, Inc., provides consultation and education services on infection prevention and control strategies, contracted infection preventionist services, and home care and hospice mock surveys and consultation on The Joint Commission standards: www.homecareandhospice.com

- Infection Prevention and You, from the Association for Professionals in Infection Control and Epidemiology (APIC): http://consumers.site.apic.org/

- AHRQ Safety Program for Reducing CAUTI in Hospitals: http://www.ahrq.gov/sites/default/files/publications/files/implementation-guide_0.pdf

- The Centers for Disease Control and Prevention (CDC) offers handwashing guidelines: http://www.cdc.gov/handwashing/

Medicare

- For more information about Medicare and to check if a "test, item, or service" is covered: https://www.medicare.gov/

- Home Health Agency Center offers links to sites within CMS on home health agencies: www.cms.hhs.gov/center/hha.asp

- Medicare & You 2016: https://www.medicare.gov/Pubs/pdf/10050.pdf

- Medicare Learning Network is the official site for Centers for Medicare & Medicaid Services (CMS) national provider education products to promote national consistency of Medicare provider information developed for CMS initiatives: https://www.cms.gov/outreach-and-education/medicare-learning-network-mln/mlngeninfo/index.html

- The Home Health Quality Improvement (HHQI) National Campaign: www.homehealthquality.org

- Medicare Administrative Contractor (MAC): https://www.cms.gov/Medicare/Medicare-Contracting/Medicare-Administrative-Contractors/What-is-a-MAC.html

- Home Health Compare provides information about home health agencies for consumers: https://www.medicare.gov/homehealthcompare/

- The Office of the Inspector General (OIG) website provides information on reports issues, guidance, and related information on fraud, waste, and abuse issues in healthcare organizations: www.oig.hhs.gov

- *Medicare Benefit Policy Manual* Chapter 7—Home Health Services: https://www.cms.gov/Regulations-and-Guidance/Guidance/Manuals/Downloads/bp102c07.pdf (for the full manual see: https://www.cms.gov/Regulations-and-Guidance/Guidance/Manuals/Internet-Only-Manuals-Ioms-Items/Cms012673.html)

- *Handbook of Home Health Care Administration*, 6th edition, by Marilyn Harris (2015, Jones & Bartlett Learning)

- Center for Medicare Advocacy: http://www.medicareadvocacy.org/

- Centers for Medicare & Medicaid Services State Operations Manual: https://www.cms.gov/Regulations-and-Guidance/Guidance/Manuals/Internet-Only-Manuals-IOMs-Items/CMS1201984.html

- Centers for Medicare & Medicaid Services OASIS User Manual: https://www.cms.gov/Medicare/Quality-Initiatives-Patient-Assessment-Instruments/OASIS/UserManual.html

- Marrelli, T. (2012). Handbook of home health standards: Quality: documentation, and reimbursement (5th edition, revised reprint). St. Louis, MO: Mosby.

Medications and Medication Safety

- Beers Criteria for Potentially Inappropriate Medication Use in Older Adults from the American Geriatrics Society: http://geriatricscareonline.org/ProductAbstract/american-geriatrics-society-updated-beers-criteria-for-potentially-inappropriate-medication-use-in-older-adults/CL001

- PainEDU Improving Pain Treatment Through Education: https://www.painedu.org/

- The American Pharmacists Association (APhA) is the largest association of pharmacists in the United States: www.pharmacist.com

- The Institute for Safe Medication Practices (ISMP) offers information about medication-error prevention and safe medication use and offers numerous resources related to medication safety information, including a fact sheet on oral medications that should not be crushed: www.ismp.org/Tools/DoNotCrush.pdf

- The Institute for Safe Medication Practices (ISMP) offers a List of High-Alert Medications in Community/Ambulatory Healthcare: https://www.ismp.org/communityRx/tools/ambulatoryhighalert.asp

- The National Institute on Drug Abuse offers useful resources related to medication interactions and drug abuse: www.nida.nih.gov

- MedWatch: The FDA Safety Information and Adverse Event Reporting Program: http://www.fda.gov/Safety/MedWatch/

- Guide to Preventing Readmissions Among Racially and Ethnically Diverse Medicare Beneficiaries: https://www.cms.gov/About-CMS/Agency-information/OMH/Downloads/OMH_Readmissions_Guide.pdf

- "Integrating a Pharmacist Into a Home Healthcare Agency Care Model: Impact on Hospitalizations and Emergency Visits" by Shannon Reidt, Tom Larson, Ronald Hadsall, Donald Uden, Mary Ann Blade, and Rachel Branstad (*Home Healthcare Nurse*, 2014)

- HospiScript: http://www.hospiscript.com/

Mental Health and Depression

- National Alliance of Mental Illness: http://www.nami.org/

- The American Psychiatric Nurses Association (APNA) is a resource for mental health nursing: www.apna.org

- The Depression and Bipolar Support Alliance offers information about depression, anxiety, bipolar disorder, and other mood-altering disorders that includes causes, signs, and treatment options: www.dbsalliance.org; 1-800-826-3632

Musculoskeletal

- The American Academy of Orthopaedic Surgeons: http://www.aaos.org

- The Amputee Coalition offers information for on amputations and support groups: http://www.amputee-coalition.org/

- The Myasthenia Gravis Foundation of America offers information and patient support groups: www.myasthenia.org; 1-800-541-5454

- The National Osteoporosis Foundation offers professional and patient information: www.nof.org

Neurologic (See Also Alzheimer's Disease)

- The American Stroke Association: www.strokeassociation.org; 1-888-4-STROKE [478-7653]

- The Amyotrophic Lateral Sclerosis Association (ALSA): www.alsa.org

- The National Institute of Neurological Disorders and Stroke: www.ninds.nih.gov; 1-800-352-9424

Nurse Safety

- NIOSH Hazard Review: Occupational Hazards in Home Healthcare from the National Institute for Occupational Safety and Health (NIOSH) and the Centers for Disease Control and Prevention (CDC): http://www.cdc.gov/niosh/docs/2010-125/pdfs/2010-125.pdf

Nutrition

- The Oral Cancer Foundation nutrition information: http://oralcancer.org/nutrition/

- The Academy of Nutrition and Dietetics promotes optimal nutrition, health, and well-being: www.eatright.org

- The American Diabetes Association (ADA) offers resources for patients, families, and professionals: http://www.diabetes.org; 1-800-DIABETES (342-2383)

- FoodFit provides information on healthy eating, healthy cooking, fitness, healthy weight loss plans, and menu planners, an email newsletter that offers fitness tips, recipes, and nutrition information: www.foodfit.com

- The Food and Nutrition Information Center: http://fnic.nal.usda.gov

- Your Guide to Lowering Your Blood Pressure with DASH: https://www.nhlbi.nih.gov/files/docs/public/heart/new_dash.pdf

- Nutrition.gov offers information on food for consumers: http://www.nutrition.gov/

Older Adults

- The American Geriatrics Society: http://www.americangeriatrics.org/

- Geriatric Pain: www.geriatricpain.org

- The National Council on Aging: www.ncoa.org

- The National Institute on Drug Abuse offers useful resources related to medication interactions and drug abuse in the older adult population: www.nida.nih.gov

- Health in Aging: http://www.healthinaging.org/

- BenefitsCheckUp from the National Council on Aging can help you find out if you qualify for services in your area: https://www.benefitscheckup.org/

- Healthy Living from the Centers for Disease Control and Prevention (CDC): www.cdc.gov/healthyliving and www.cdc.gov/aging

- Eldercare Locator from the U.S. Administration on Aging: www.eldercare.gov; 1-800-677-1116

- The National Academy of Elder Law Attorneys (NAELA): www.naela.org

- The National Center on Elder Abuse (NCEA): http://www.ncea.aoa.gov/

- The National Eye Institute (NEI): www.nei.nih.gov; 1-301-496-5248

- The National Institute on Aging: www.nia.nih.gov; 1-800-222-2225

- NIH Senior Health: www.nihseniorhealth.gov

- Geriatric Examination Tool Kit: http://geriatrictoolkit.missouri.edu/

Pain and Pain Management

- Geriatric Pain: www.geriatricpain.org

- Opioids Dosage Conversion app for iOS: https://itunes.apple.com/us/app/opioids-dosage-conversion/id382383903?mt=8

- PainEDU's "Improving Pain Treatment Through Education": https://www.painedu.org/

- End-of-Life Nursing Education Consortium (ELNEC): http://www.aacn.nche.edu/elnec
- The Agency for Healthcare Research and Quality (AHRQ): www.ahrq.gov; 1-800-358-9295
- The American Pain Society: www.ampainsoc.org
- The Hospice and Palliative Nurses Association: www.hpna.org; 1-412-787-9301
- Management of opioid therapy for chronic pain, from the Department of Veterans Affairs: http://www.va.gov/painmanagement/docs/cpg_opioidtherapy_summary.pdf

Pediatric Care

- The American Cancer Society offers information and support groups for children and adolescents with cancer: www.cancer.org; 1-800-227-2345
- The City of Hope National Medical Center offers information on adult and pediatric cancers of all kinds for patients and care-givers, families, and professionals: www.cityofhope.org; 1-626-256-4673
- The Compassionate Friends is an organization that offers grief support for families after the death of a child: www.compassionatefriends.org; 1-877-969-0010
- The Make-A-Wish Foundation fulfills special wishes for children with a life-threatening illness and their families: www.wish.org; 1-800-722-WISH (9474)
- The Muscular Dystrophy Association offers resources related to muscular dystrophy: www.mda.org; 1-800-752-1717
- The United Cerebral Palsy (UCP) association provides information and resources related to cerebral palsy and advocates for

the rights of persons with any disability: www.ucp.org; 1-800-872-5827

- The American Diabetes Association (ADA) offers resources for patients, families, and professionals: www.diabetes.org; 1-800-DIABETES [342-2383]

- The Juvenile Diabetes Research Foundation International promotes education in diabetes and offers an online support team: www.jdrf.org

- "Verifying NG Feeding Tube Placement in Pediatric Patients" by Beth Lyman, Jane Anne Yaworksi, Lori Duesing, and Candice Moore: http://www.americannursetoday.com/verifying-ng-feeding-tube-placement-pediatric-patients/

Practice Resources

- The Visiting Nurse Associations of America (VNAA) Clinical Procedure Manual: http://www.vnaa.org/cpm

- The Visiting Nurse Associations of America (VNAA) Blueprint for Excellence: http://www.vnaablueprint.org/

- The Joint Commission (TJC) is a not-for-profit organization for standards-setting and accrediting in healthcare that focuses on improving the quality and safety of care: www.jointcommission.org

- The Accreditation Commission for Healthcare provides accreditation services and seeks to improve healthcare quality by accrediting health programs that pass a rigorous, comprehensive review: www.ACHC.org

- *Home Health Nursing: Scope and Standards of Practice*, 2nd edition, from the American Nurses Association (ANA): http://www.nursesbooks.org/Main-Menu/eBooks/eStandards/ebook-Home-Health-Nursing-2nd.aspx

- *Palliative Nursing: Scope and Standards of Practice* from the Hospice and Palliative Nurses Association (HPNA): http://www.nursesbooks.org/Main-Menu/Standards/Palliative-Nursing.aspx

- The Alliance for Home Health Quality and Innovation offers information about the value of home healthcare: http://www.ahhqi.org/

- "How to Succeed as a Home Care Nurse" by Tina Marrelli (*American Nurse Today*, 2015)

- "10 Tips for Transitioning from Home Care Nurse to Nurse Manager" by Tina Marrelli (*American Nurse Today*, 2016)

Professional Boundaries

- A Nurse's Guide to Professional Boundaries from the National Council of State Boards of Nursing: https://www.ncsbn.org/ProfessionalBoundaries_Complete.pdf

- "When Professional Kindness is Misunderstood: Boundaries and Stalking Issues—A Case Study for the Home Health Clinician" by Cheryl Holz (2009, *Home Healthcare Nurse*)

Respiratory

- Help with quitting smoking: www.smokefree.gov

- The American Association for Respiratory Care (AARC) is the professional society for respiratory therapists working in a variety of settings, including homes and nursing homes: www.aarc.org; 1-972-243-2272

- The American Lung Association: www.lung.org

- Tuberculosis information from the Centers for Disease Control and Prevention (CDC): http://www.cdc.gov/tb/

Safety

- The American Burn Association offers the *Fire and Burn Safety for Older Adults: Educator's Guide*: http://www.ameriburn.org/Preven/BurnSafetyOlderAdultsEducator'sGuide.pdf

- The National Fire Protection Association offers helpful resources on their site: http://www.nfpa.org/

- The Consumer Product Safety Commission offers *Safety for Older Consumers—Home Safety Checklist*: http://www.cpsc.gov/PageFiles/122038/701.pdf

- Beers Criteria for Potentially Inappropriate Medication Use in Older Adults from the American Geriatrics Society: http://geriatricscareonline.org/ProductAbstract/american-geriatrics-society-updated-beers-criteria-for-potentially-inappropriate-medication-use-in-older-adults/CL001

- The National Safety Council was established to educate and influence people to prevent accidental injury and death and offers information and resources related to these safety issues: www.nsc.org

- The Occupational Safety & Health Administration: www.osha.gov

- The Joint Commission (TJC) is a not-for-profit organization for standards-setting and accrediting in healthcare that focuses on improving the quality and safety of care: www.jointcommission.org

Social Work

- The National Association of Social Workers (NASW) works to enhance professional growth and development and maintain professional standards in social work: http://www. socialworkers.org

Spirituality

- The Association of Professional Chaplains (APC) is an interfaith professional association serving people's physical, spiritual, or mental needs in diverse settings: http://www. professionalchaplains.org

Telehealth/Telemedicine

- The American Telemedicine Association: www.americantelemed. org

- The National Library of Medicine National Telemedicine Initiative: www.nlm.nih.gov/research/telemedinit.html

Therapy

- The American Occupational Therapy Association (AOTA) supports the professional community of occupational therapists: www.aota.org

- The American Physical Therapy Association (APTA): www.apta. org

- The American Speech-Language-Hearing Association (ASHA) supports speech-language pathologists; audiologists; and speech, language, and hearing professionals: http://www.asha.org; 1-800-498-2071

Urinary and Catheter Care

- The American Urological Association (AUA) offers information for patients and professionals: www.auanet.org

- There are physician-created resources for pediatric and adult conditions on the Urology Care Foundation website: www. urologyhealth.org

- The National Association for Continence (NAFC) offers information on incontinence that includes treatment options, explanations, and how to find help: www.nafc.org; 1-800-BLADDER [252-3337]

- The National Kidney and Urologic Diseases Information Clearinghouse offers information on treatment and booklets: www. kidney.niddk.nih.gov

- The Wound, Ostomy and Continence Nurses Society offers fact sheets and patient guides for incontinence and more: www. wocn.org

- Coalition for Supportive Care of Kidney Patients: http://www. kidneysupportivecare.org/Home.aspx

- "Perceived Value" of a Urinary Catheter Self-Management Program in the Home by Mary Wilde, Feng Zhang, Eileen Fairbanks, Shivani Shah, Margaret McDonald, and Judith Brasch (*Home Healthcare Nurse*, 2013)

Veteran Health

- Veterans Health Library: http://www.veteranshealthlibrary.org/

Wound Care

- The National Pressure Ulcer Advisory Panel (NPUAP): www.npuap.org; 1-202-521-6789

- The Paralyzed Veterans of America (PVA): www.pva.org

- The United Ostomy Associations of America: http://www.ostomy.org/Home.html; 1-800-826-0826

- The Wound, Ostomy and Continence Nurses Society offers fact sheets and patient guides for incontinence and more: www.wocn.org

C
Home Health & Hospice MAC Areas

Home Health & Hospice MAC Areas
as of December 2015

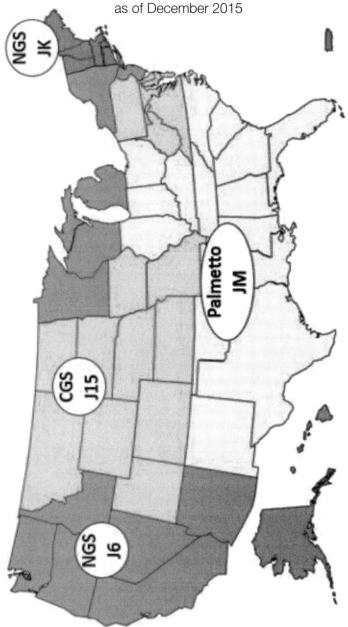

Source: https://www.cms.gov/Medicare/Medicare-Contracting/Medicare-Administrative-
Contractors/Downloads/Home-Health-and-Hospice-Area-Map-Dec-2015.pdf

D

Medicare Benefit Policy Manual:

Chapter 7—Home Health Services

The following text is the complete Chapter 7, Home Health Services, of the *Medicare Benefit Policy Manual.* This version was retrieved on 31 May 2016. Always verify you have the most recent information from https://www.cms.gov/Regulations-and-Guidance/Guidance/Manuals/downloads/bp102c07.pdf.

Medicare Benefit Policy Manual
Chapter 7 - Home Health Services

Table of Contents
(Rev. 208, 05-11-15)

Transmittals for Chapter 7

10 - Home Health Prospective Payment System (*HH* PPS)
(Rev. 208, Issued: 04-22-15, Effective: 01-01-15, Implementation: 05-11-15)

The unit of payment under *the HH* PPS is a national 60-day episode rate with applicable adjustments. The episodes, rate, and adjustments to the rates are detailed in the following sections.

10.1 - National 60-Day Episode Rate
(Rev. 208, Issued: 04-22-15, Effective: 01-01-15, Implementation: 05-11-15)

A. Services Included

The law requires the 60-day episode to include all covered home health services, including medical supplies, paid on a reasonable cost basis. That means the 60-day episode rate includes costs for the six home health disciplines and the costs for routine and nonroutine medical supplies. The six home health disciplines included in the 60-day episode rate are:

1. Skilled nursing services

2. Home health aide services;

3. Physical therapy;

4. Speech-language pathology services;

5. Occupational therapy services; and

6. Medical social services.

The 60-day episode rate also includes amounts for nonroutine medical supplies and therapies that could have been unbundled to Part B prior to *HH* PPS. *(*See §*10.11*.C for those services.)*

B. Excluded Services

The law specifically excludes durable medical equipment *(DME)* from the 60-day episode rate and consolidated billing requirements. DME continues to be paid on the fee schedule outside of the *HH* PPS rate.

The osteoporosis drug (injectable calcitonin), which is covered where a woman is postmenopausal and has a bone fracture. This drug is also excluded from the 60-day episode rate but must be billed by the home health agency (HHA) while a patient is under a home health plan of care since the law requires consolidated billing of osteoporosis drugs. The osteoporosis drug continues to be paid on a reasonable cost basis.

10.2 - Adjustments to the 60-Day Episode Rates

(Rev. 208, Issued: 04-22-15, Effective: 01-01-15, Implementation: 05-11-15)

A. Case-Mix Adjustment

A case-mix methodology adjusts payment rates based on characteristics of the patient and his/her corresponding resource needs (e.g., diagnosis, clinical factors, functional factors, service needs). The 60-day episode rates are adjusted by case-mix methodology based on data elements from the *Outcome and Assessment Information Set (*OASIS*)*. The data elements of the case-mix adjustment methodology are organized into three dimensions to capture clinical severity factors, functional severity factors, and service utilization factors influencing case mix. In the clinical, functional, and service utilization dimensions, each data element is assigned a score value. The scores are summed to determine the patient's case-mix group.

B. Labor Adjustments

The labor portion of the 60-day episode rates is adjusted to reflect the wage index based on the site of service of the beneficiary. The beneficiary's location is the determining factor for the labor adjustment. The *HH* PPS rates are adjusted by the pre-floor and pre-reclassified hospital wage index. The hospital wage index is adjusted to account for the geographic reclassification of hospitals in accordance with §§1886(d)(8)(B) and 1886(d)(10) of the Social Security Act (the Act.) According to the law, geographic reclassification only applies to hospitals. Additionally, the hospital wage index has specific floors that are required by law. Because these reclassifications and floors do not apply to HHAs, the home health rates are adjusted by the pre-floor and pre-reclassified hospital wage index.

NOTE: The pre-floor and pre-reclassified hospital wage index varies slightly from the numbers published in the Medicare inpatient hospital PPS regulation that reflects the floor and reclassification adjustments. The wage indices published in the home health final rule and subsequent annual updates reflect the most recent available pre-floor and pre-reclassified hospital wage index available at the time of publication.

10.3 - Continuous 60-Day Episode Recertification
(Rev. 1, 10-01-03)
HH-201.3

Home health PPS permits continuous episode recertifications for patients who continue to be eligible for the home health benefit. Medicare does not limit the number of continuous episode recertifications for beneficiaries who continue to be eligible for the home health benefit.

10.4 - Counting 60-Day Episodes
(Rev. 208, Issued: 04-22-15, Effective: 01-01-15, Implementation: 05-11-15)

A. Initial Episodes

The "From" date for the initial certification must match the start of care (SOC) date, which is the first billable visit date for the 60-day episode. The "To" date is up to and including the last day of the episode which is not the first day of the subsequent episode. The "To" date can be up to, but never exceed a total of 60 days that includes the SOC date plus 59 days.

B. Subsequent Episodes

If a patient continues to be eligible for the home health benefit, the *HH* PPS permits continuous episode recertifications. At the end of the 60-day episode, a decision must be made whether or not to recertify the patient for a subsequent 60-day episode. An eligible beneficiary who qualifies for a subsequent 60-day episode would start the subsequent 60-day episode on day 61. The "From" date for the first subsequent episode is day 61 up to including day 120. The "To" date for the subsequent episode in this example can be up to, but never exceed a total of 60 days that includes day 61 plus 59 days.

NOTE: The certification or recertification visit can be done during a prior episode. *The Medicare Conditions of Participation, at 42 CFR 484.55(d)(1), require that the recertification assessment be done during the last 5 days of the previous episode (days 56-60).*

10.5 - Split Percentage Payment Approach to the 60-Day Episode
(Rev. 208, Issued: 04-22-15, Effective: 01-01-15, Implementation: 05-11-15)

In order to ensure adequate cash flow to HHAs, the *HH* PPS has set forth a split percentage payment approach to the 60-day episode. The split percentage occurs through the request for anticipated payment (RAP) at the start of the episode and the final claim at the end of the episode. For initial episodes, there will be a 60/40 split percentage payment. An initial percentage payment of 60 percent of the episode will be paid at the beginning of the episode and a final percentage payment of 40 percent will be paid at the end of the episode, unless there is an applicable adjustment. For all subsequent episodes for beneficiaries who receive continuous home health care, the episodes will be paid at a 50/50-percentage payment split.

10.6 - Physician Signature Requirements for the Split Percentage Payments
(Rev. 1, 10-01-03)
HH-201.6
A. Initial Percentage Payment

If a physician-signed plan of care is not available at the beginning of the episode, the HHA may submit a RAP for the initial percentage payment based on physician verbal orders OR a referral prescribing detailed orders for the services to be rendered that is signed and dated by the physician. If the RAP submission is based on a physician's verbal orders, the verbal order must be recorded in the plan of care, include a description of the patient's condition and the services to be provided by the home health agency, and include an attestation (relating to the physician's orders and the date received per Code of

Federal Regulation (CFR) 42 CFR 409.43). The plan of care is copied and immediately submitted to the physician. A billable visit must be rendered prior to the submission of a RAP.

The CMS has the authority to reduce or disapprove requests for anticipated payments in situations when protecting Medicare program integrity warrants this action. Since the request for anticipated payment is based on verbal orders and is not a Medicare claim for purposes of the Act (although it is a claim for purposes of Federal, civil, criminal, and administrative law enforcement authorities, including but not limited to the Civil Monetary Penalties Law, Civil False Claims Act, and the Criminal False Claims Act), the request for anticipated payment will be canceled and recovered unless the claim is submitted within the greater of 60 days from the end of the episode or 60 days from the issuance of the request for anticipated payment.

B. Final Percentage Payment

The plan of care must be signed and dated by a physician who meets the certification and recertification requirements of 42 CFR 424.22 before the claim for each episode for services is submitted for the final percentage payment. Any changes in the plan of care must be signed and dated by a physician.

10.7 - Low Utilization Payment Adjustment (LUPA)
(Rev. 208, Issued: 04-22-15, Effective: 01-01-15, Implementation: 05-11-15)

An episode with four or fewer visits is paid the national per visit amount by discipline adjusted by the appropriate wage index based on the site of service of the beneficiary. Such episodes of four or fewer visits are paid the wage-adjusted per visit amount for each of the visits rendered instead of the full episode amount. The national per visit amounts by discipline (skilled nursing, home health aide, physical therapy, speech-language pathology, occupational therapy, and medical social services) are updated and published annually by the applicable market basket for each visit type.

Beginning in CY 2008, to offset the full cost of longer, initial visits in some LUPA episodes, CMS has modified the LUPA by increasing the payment by an add-on amount for LUPAs that occur as the only episode or the initial episode during a sequence of adjacent episodes.

10.8 - Partial Episode Payment (PEP) Adjustment
(Rev. 208, Issued: 04-22-15, Effective: 01-01-15, Implementation: 05-11-15)

A. PEP Adjustment Criteria

The PEP adjustment accounts for key intervening events in a patient's care defined as:

- A beneficiary elected transfer; or

- A discharge *and return* to *home health* during the 60-day episode.

The intervening event defined as the beneficiary elected transfer or discharge and return to *home health* during the 60-day episode warrants a new 60-day episode for purposes of payment. A start of care OASIS assessment and physician certification of the new plan of care are required. When a new 60-day episode begins due to the intervening event of the *beneficiary elected* transfer or discharge and return to *home health* during the 60-day episode, the original 60-day episode is proportionally adjusted to reflect the length of time the beneficiary remained under the agency's care prior to the intervening event.

Home health agencies have the option to discharge the patient within the scope of their own operating policies. However, an HHA discharging a patient as a result of hospital (*skilled nursing facility (*SNF) or rehab facility) admission with the patient returning to home health services at the same HHA during the 60-day episode will not be recognized by Medicare as a discharge for billing and payment purposes, and thus a Partial Episode Payment (PEP) adjustment would not apply. An intervening hospital (SNF or rehab facility) stay will result in a full 60-day episode spanning the start of care date prior to the hospital (SNF or rehab facility) admission, through and including the days of the hospital admission, and ending 59 days after the original start of care date.

B. Methodology Used to Calculate PEP Adjustment

The PEP adjustment for the original 60-day episode is calculated to reflect the length of time the beneficiary remained under the care of the original HHA based on the first billable visit date through and including the last billable visit date. The PEP adjustment is calculated by determining the actual days served by the original HHA (first billable visit date through and including last billable visit date as a proportion of 60 multiplied by the original 60-day episode payment).

C. Application of Therapy Threshold to PEP Adjusted Episode

The therapy threshold item included in the case-mix methodology used in *the HH* PPS is not combined or prorated across episodes. Each episode whether full or proportionately adjusted is subject to the therapy threshold for purposes of case-mix adjusting the payment for that individual patient's resource needs.

D. Common Ownership Exception to PEP Adjustment

If an HHA has a significant ownership as defined in 42 CFR 424.22, then the PEP adjustment would not apply in those situations of beneficiary elected transfer. Those situations would be considered services provided under arrangement on behalf of the originating HHA by the receiving HHA with the ownership interest until the end of the episode. The common ownership exception to the transfer PEP adjustment does not apply if the beneficiary moved out of their *Metropolitan Statistical Area (*MSA) or non-MSA during the 60-day episode before the transfer to the receiving HHA.

E. Beneficiary Elected Transfer Verification

In order for a receiving HHA to accept a beneficiary elected transfer, the receiving HHA must document that the beneficiary has been informed that the initial HHA will no longer receive Medicare payment on behalf of the patient and will no longer provide Medicare covered services to the patient after the date of the patient's elected transfer in accordance with current patient rights requirements at 42 CFR 484.10(e). The receiving HHA must also document in the record that it accessed the *Medicare contractor's* inquiry system to determine whether or not the patient was under an established home health plan of care and it must contact the initial HHA on the effective date of transfer. In the rare circumstance of a dispute between HHAs, the *Medicare contractor* is responsible for working with both HHAs to resolve the dispute. If the receiving HHA can provide documentation of its notice of patient rights on Medicare payment liability provided to the patient upon transfer and its contact of the initial HHA of the transfer date, then the initial HHA will be ineligible for payment for the period of overlap in addition to the appropriate PEP adjustment. If the receiving HHA cannot provide the appropriate documentation, the receiving HHA's RAP and/or final claim will be cancelled, and full episode payment will be provided to the initial HHA. For the receiving HHA to properly document that it contacted the initial HHA on the effective date of transfer it must maintain similar information as the initial HHA, including the same basic beneficiary information, personnel contacted, dates and times. The initial HHA must also properly document that it was contacted and it accepted the transfer. Where it disputes a transfer, the initial HHA must call its *Medicare contractor* to resolve the dispute. The *Medicare contractor* is responsible for working with both HHAs to resolve the dispute.

10.9 - Outlier Payments
(Rev. 139, Issued: 02-16-11, Effective: 01-01-11, Implementation: 03-10-11)

When cases experience an unusually high level of services in a 60-day period, Medicare systems will provide additional or "outlier" payments to the case-mix and wage-adjusted episode payment. Outlier payments can result from medically necessary high utilization in any or all-home health service disciplines. CMS makes outlier payments when the cost of care exceeds a threshold dollar amount. The outlier threshold for each case-mix group is the episode payment amount for that group or the PEP adjustment amount for the episode, plus a fixed dollar loss amount, which is the same for all case-mix groups. The outlier payment is a proportion of the amount of imputed costs beyond the threshold. CMS calculates the imputed cost for each episode by multiplying the national per visit amount of each discipline by the number of visits in the discipline and computing the total imputed cost for all disciplines. If the imputed cost for the episode is greater than the sum of the case-mix and wage-adjusted episode payment plus the fixed dollar loss amount (the outlier threshold), a set percentage (the loss sharing ratio) of the difference between the imputed amount and outlier threshold will be paid to the HHA as a wage-adjusted outlier payment in addition to the episode payment. The amount of the outlier payment is determined as follows:

1. Calculate the case-mix and wage-adjusted episode payment (including non-routine supplies (NRS));

2. Add the wage-adjusted fixed dollar loss amount. The sum of steps 1 and 2 is the outlier threshold for the episode;

3. Calculate the wage-adjusted imputed cost of the episode by first multiplying the total number of visits for each home health discipline by the national per visit amounts, and wage-adjusting those amounts. Sum the per discipline wage-adjusted imputed amounts to yield the total wage-adjusted imputed cost for the episode;

4. Subtract the total imputed cost for the episode (total from Step 3) from the sum of the case-mix and wage-adjusted episode payment and the wage-adjusted fixed dollar loss amount (sum of Steps 1 and 2 - outlier threshold);

5. Multiply the difference by the loss sharing ratio; and

6. That total amount is the outlier payment for the episode.

Effective January 1, 2010, an outlier cap precludes any HHA from receiving more than 10 percent of their total home health payment in outliers.

10.10 - Discharge Issues
(Rev. 208, Issued: 04-22-15, Effective: 01-01-15, Implementation: 05-11-15)

A. Hospice Election Mid-Episode

If a patient elects hospice before the end of the episode and there was no PEP or LUPA adjustment, the HHA will receive a full episode payment. *The HH* PPS does not change the current rules that permit a hospice patient to receive home health services for a condition unrelated to *the terminal illness and related conditions.* Consistent with all episodes in which a patient receives four or fewer visits, the episode with four or fewer visits in which a patient elects hospice would be paid at the low utilization payment adjusted amount.

B. Patient's Death

The documented event of a patient's death would result in a full episode payment, unless the death occurred in a low utilization payment adjusted episode. Consistent with all episodes in which a patient receives four or fewer visits, if the patient's death occurred during an episode with four or fewer visits, the episode would be paid at the low utilization payment adjusted amount. In the event of a patient's death during an adjusted episode, the total adjusted episode would constitute the full episode payment.

C. Patient is No Longer Eligible for Home Health (e.g., no longer homebound, no skilled need)

If the patient is discharged because he or she is no longer eligible for the Medicare home health benefit and has received more than four visits, then the HHA would receive full episode payment. However, if the patient becomes subsequently eligible for the Medicare home health benefit during the same 60-day episode and transferred to another HHA or returned to the same HHA, then *this* would result in a PEP adjustment.

D. Discharge Due to Patient Refusal of Services or is a Documented Safety Threat, Abuse Threat or is Noncompliant

If the patient is discharged because he or she refuses services or becomes a documented safety, abuse, or noncompliance discharge and has received more than four visits, then the HHA would receive full episode payment unless the patient becomes subsequently eligible for the Medicare home health benefit during the same 60-day episode and transferred to another HHA or returned to the same HHA, then *this* would result in a PEP adjustment.

E. Patient *Enrolls in* Managed Care Mid-Episode

If a patient's enrollment in a Medicare Advantage (MA) plan becomes effective mid episode, the 60-day episode payment will be proportionally adjusted with a PEP adjustment since the patient is receiving coverage under MA. Beginning with the effective date of enrollment, the MA plan will receive a capitation payment for covered services.

F. Submission of Final Claims Prior to the End of the 60-day Episode

The claim may be submitted upon discharge before the end of the 60-day episode. However, subsequent adjustments to any payments based on the claim may be made due to an intervening event resulting in a PEP adjustment or other adjustment.

G. Patient Discharge and Financial Responsibility for Part B Bundled Medical Supplies and Services

As discussed in detail under §10.11, below, the law governing the Medicare *HH* PPS requires the HHA to provide all bundled home health services (except DME) either directly or under arrangement while a patient is under a home health plan of care during an open episode. Once the patient is discharged, the HHA is no longer responsible for providing home health services including the bundled Part B medical supplies and therapy services.

H. Discharge Issues Associated With Inpatient Admission Overlapping Into Subsequent Episodes

1. If a patient is admitted to an inpatient facility and the inpatient stay overlaps into what would have been the subsequent episode and there is no recertification *assessment* of the patient, then the *new* certification begins with the new start of care date after inpatient discharge.

2. *If a patient is admitted to an inpatient facility and the inpatient stay overlaps into what would have been the subsequent episode and there was a recertification assessment of the patient during days 56-60 and the patient returns home from the inpatient stay on day 61, if the home health resource group (HHRG) remains the same then the second episode of care would be considered continuous and thus be considered a recertification. However, if the HHRG is different, this would result in a new start of care OASIS and thus be considered a new certification and begins with the new start of care date after inpatient discharge.*

3. *If a patient is admitted to an inpatient facility and the inpatient stay overlaps into what would have been the subsequent episode and there was a recertification assessment of the patient during days 56-60 and the patient returns home from the inpatient stay after day 61 (after the first day of the next episode of care), then a new certification begins with the new start of care date after inpatient discharge.*

10.11 - Consolidated Billing
(Rev. 208, Issued: 04-22-15, Effective: 01-01-15, Implementation: 05-11-15)

For individuals under a home health plan of care, payment for all services and supplies, with the exception of osteoporosis drugs and DME, is included in the *HH* PPS *base payment rates*. HHAs must provide the covered home health services (except DME) either directly or under arrangement, and must bill for such covered home health services.

Payment must be made to the HHA.

A. Home Health Services Subject to Consolidated Billing Requirements

The home health services included in the consolidated billing governing *the HH* PPS are:

- Part-time or intermittent skilled nursing services;
- Part-time or intermittent home health aide services;
- Physical therapy;
- Speech-language pathology services;
- Occupational therapy;
- Medical social services;
- Routine and nonroutine medical supplies;
- Covered osteoporosis drug as defined in §1861(kk) of the Act, but excluding other drugs and biologicals;

- Medical services provided by an intern or resident-in-training of the program of the hospital in the case of an HHA that is affiliated or under common control with a hospital with an approved teaching program; and

- Home health services defined in §1861(m) provided under arrangement at hospitals, SNFs, or rehabilitation centers when they involve equipment too cumbersome to bring to the home or are furnished while the patient is at the facility to receive such services.

B. Medical Supplies

The law requires *that* all medical supplies (routine and nonroutine) *be provided by* the *HHA* while the patient is under a home health plan of care. The agency that establishes the episode is the only entity that can bill and receive payment for medical supplies during an episode for a patient under a home health plan of care. Both routine and nonroutine medical supplies are included in the base rates for every Medicare home health patient regardless of whether or not the patient requires medical supplies during the episode.

Due to the consolidated billing requirements, CMS provided additional amounts in the base rates for those nonroutine medical supplies that have a duplicate Part B code that could have been unbundled to Part B prior to *HH* PPS. See §50.4 for detailed discussion of medical supplies.

Medical supplies used by the patient, provider, or other practitioners under arrangement on behalf of the agency (other than physicians) are subject to consolidated billing and bundled *into* the HHA episodic payment rate. Once a patient is discharged from home health and not under a home health plan of care, the HHA is not responsible for medical supplies.

DME, including supplies covered as DME, are paid separately from the *HH* PPS and are excluded from the consolidated billing requirements governing *the HH* PPS. The determining factor is the medical classification of the supply, not the diagnosis of the patient. For example, infusion therapy will continue to be covered under the DME benefit separately and excluded from the consolidated billing requirements governing *the HH* PPS. DME supplies that are currently covered and paid in accordance with the DME fee schedule as category SU are billed under the DME benefit.

The osteoporosis drug *(injectable calcitonin) is* included in consolidated billing under the home health benefit. However, payment is not bundled into the *HH PPS* payment *rates.* HHAs must bill for *the* osteoporosis drug in accordance with billing instructions. Payment is in addition to the *HH PPS* payment.

C. Relationship Between Consolidated Billing Requirements and Part B Supplies and Part B Therapies Included in the Baseline Rates That Could Have Been Unbundled Prior to *HH* PPS That No Longer Can Be Unbundled

The HHA is responsible for the services provided under arrangement on their behalf by other entities. Covered home health services at §1861(m) of the Act (except DME) are included in the baseline *HH* PPS rates and subject to the consolidated billing requirements while the patient is under a plan of care of the HHA. The time the services are bundled is while the patient is under a home health plan of care.

Physician services or nurse practitioner services *paid under* the physician fee schedule are not recognized as home health *services* included in the PPS *rates*. Supplies incident to a physician service or related to a physician service billed to the *Medicare contractor* are not subject to the consolidated billing requirements. The physician would not be acting as a supplier billing the DME *Medicare contractor* in this situation.

Therapies (physical therapy, occupational therapy, and speech-language pathology services) are covered home health services that are included in the baseline rates and subject to the consolidated billing requirements. In addition to therapies that had been paid on a cost basis under home health, CMS has included in the rates additional amounts for Part B therapies that could have been unbundled prior to PPS. These therapies are subject to the consolidated billing requirements. There are revenue center codes that reflect the ranges of outpatient physical therapy, occupational therapy, and speech-language pathology services and *Healthcare Common Procedure Coding System (*HCPCS*)* codes that reflect physician supplier codes that are physical therapy, occupational therapy, and speech-language pathology services by code definition and are subject to the consolidated billing requirements. Therefore, the above-mentioned therapies must be provided directly or under arrangement on behalf of the HHA while a patient is under a home health plan of care *and* cannot be separately billed to Part B during an open 60-day episode.

D. Freedom of Choice Issues

A beneficiary exercises his or her freedom of choice for the services under the home health benefit listed in §1861(m) of the Act, including medical supplies, but excluding DME covered as a home health service by choosing the HHA. Once a home health patient chooses a particular HHA, he or she has clearly exercised freedom of choice with respect to all items and services included within the scope of the Medicare home health benefit (except DME). The HHA's consolidated billing role supersedes all other billing situations the beneficiary may wish to establish for home health services covered under the scope of the Medicare home health benefit during the certified episode.

E. Knowledge of Services Arranged for on Behalf of the HHA

The consolidated billing requirements governing *HH* PPS requires that the HHA provide all covered home health services (except DME) either directly or under arrangement while a patient is under a home health plan of care. Providing services either directly or under arrangement requires knowledge of the services provided during the episode. In addition, in accordance with current Medicare conditions of participation and Medicare coverage guidelines governing home health, the patient's plan of care must reflect the physician ordered services that the HHA provides either directly or under arrangement.

An HHA would not be responsible for payment in the situation in which they have no prior knowledge (unaware of physician orders) of the services provided by an entity during an episode to a patient who is under their home health plan of care. An HHA is responsible for payment in the situation in which services are provided to a patient by another entity, under arrangement with the HHA, during an episode in which the patient is under the HHA's home health plan of care. However, it is in the best interest of future business relationships to discuss the situation with any entity that seeks payment from the HHA during an episode in an effort to resolve any misunderstanding and avoid such situations in the future.

10.12 - Change of Ownership Relationship to Episodes Under PPS
(Rev. 139, Issued: 02-16-11, Effective: 01-01-11, Implementation: 03-10-11)

A. Change of Ownership With Assignment

When there is a change of ownership and the new owner accepts assignment of the existing provider agreement, the new owner is subject to all the terms and conditions under which the existing agreement was issued. The provider number remains the same if the new HHA owner accepts assignment of the existing provider agreement. As long as the new owner complies with the regulations governing home health PPS, billing, and payment for episodes with applicable adjustments for existing patients under an established plan of care will continue on schedule through the change in ownership with assignment. The episode would be uninterrupted spanning the date of sale. The former owner is required to file a terminating cost report. Instructions regarding when a cost report is filed are in the Provider Reimbursement Manual, Part 1, §1500.

B. Change of Ownership Without Assignment

When there is a change of ownership, and the new owner does not take the assignment of the existing provider agreement, the provider agreement and provider number of the former owner is terminated. The former owner will receive partial episode payment adjusted payments in accordance with the methodology set forth in the Medicare Claims Processing Manual, Chapter 10, "Home Health Agency Billing," §40.2, and 42 CFR 484.235, based on the last billable visit date for existing patients under a home health plan of care ending on or before the date of sale. The former owner is required to file a terminating cost report. The new owner cannot bill Medicare for payment until the effective date of the Medicare approval. The new HHA will not be able to participate in the Medicare program without going through the same process as any new provider, which includes an initial survey. Once the new owner is Medicare-approved, the HHA may start a new episode for purposes of payment, OASIS assessment, and certification of the home health plan of care for all new patients in accordance with the regulations governing home health PPS, effective with the date of the new provider certification.

C. Change of Ownership - Mergers

The merger of a provider corporation into another corporation constitutes a change of ownership. For information on specific procedures, refer to Pub. 100-07, State Operations Manual, chapter 2, section 2202.17.

20 - Conditions To Be Met for Coverage of Home Health Services
(Rev. 1, 10-01-03)
A3-3116, HHA-203

Medicare covers HHA services when the following criteria are met:

1. The person to whom the services are provided is an eligible Medicare beneficiary;

2. The HHA that is providing the services to the beneficiary has in effect a valid agreement to participate in the Medicare program;

3. The beneficiary qualifies for coverage of home health services as described in §30;

4. The services for which payment is claimed are covered as described in §§40 and 50;

5. Medicare is the appropriate payer; and

6. The services for which payment is claimed are not otherwise excluded from payment.

20.1 - Reasonable and Necessary Services
(Rev. 1, 10-01-03)
A3-3116.1. HHA-203.1

20.1.1 - Background
(Rev. 1, 10-01-03)
A3-3116.1A, HHA-203.1A

In enacting the Medicare program, Congress recognized that the physician would play an important role in determining utilization of services. The law requires that payment can be made only if a physician certifies the need for services and establishes a plan of care. The Secretary is responsible for ensuring that Medicare covers the claimed services, including determining whether they are "reasonable and necessary."

20.1.2 - Determination of Coverage
(Rev. 208, Issued: 04-22-15, Effective: 01-01-15, Implementation: 05-11-15)

The *Medicare contractor's* decision on whether care is reasonable and necessary is based on information reflected in the home health plan of care, the OASIS as required by 42 CFR 484.55 or a medical record of the individual patient. Medicare does not deny coverage solely on the basis of the reviewer's general inferences about patients with similar diagnoses or on data related to utilization generally, but bases it upon objective clinical evidence regarding the patient's individual need for care. Coverage of skilled nursing care or therapy to perform a maintenance program does not turn on the presence or absence of a patient's potential for improvement from the nursing care or therapy, but rather on the patient's need for skilled care. Skilled care may be necessary to improve a patient's current condition, to maintain the patient's current condition, to prevent or slow further deterioration of the patient's condition.

20.2 - Impact of Other Available Caregivers and Other Available Coverage on Medicare Coverage of Home Health Services
(Rev. 208, Issued: 04-22-15, Effective: 01-01-15, Implementation: 05-11-15)

Where the Medicare criteria for coverage of home health services are met, patients are entitled by law to coverage of reasonable and necessary home health services. Therefore, a patient is entitled to have the costs of reasonable and necessary services reimbursed by Medicare without regard to whether there is someone available to furnish the services. However, where a family member or other person is or will be providing services that adequately meet the patient's needs, it would not be reasonable and necessary for HHA personnel to furnish such services. Ordinarily it can be presumed that there is no able and willing person in the home to provide the services being rendered by the HHA unless the patient or family indicates otherwise and objects to the provision of the services by the HHA, or unless the HHA has first hand knowledge to the contrary.

Similarly, a patient is entitled to reasonable and necessary *Medicare* home health services even if the patient would qualify for institutional care (e.g., hospital care or skilled nursing facility care) *and Medicare payment should be made for reasonable and necessary home health services where the patient is also receiving supplemental services that do not meet Medicare's definition of skilled nursing care or home health aide services.*

EXAMPLE 1:

A patient who lives with an adult daughter and otherwise qualifies for Medicare coverage of home health services, requires the assistance of a home health aide for bathing and assistance with an exercise program to improve endurance. The daughter is unwilling to bathe her elderly father and assist him with the exercise program. Home health aide services would be reasonable and necessary.

EXAMPLE 2:

A patient who is being discharged from a hospital with a diagnosis of osteomyelitis and requires continuation of the I.V. antibiotic therapy that was begun in the hospital was found to meet the criteria for Medicare coverage of skilled nursing facility services. If the patient also meets the qualifying criteria for coverage of home health services, payment may be made for the reasonable and necessary home health services the patient needs, notwithstanding the availability of coverage in a skilled nursing facility.

EXAMPLE 3:

A patient who needs skilled nursing care on an intermittent basis also hires a licensed practical (vocational) nurse to provide nighttime assistance while family members sleep. The care provided by the nurse, as respite to the family members, does not require the skills of a licensed nurse (as defined in §40.1) and therefore has no impact on the beneficiary's eligibility for Medicare payment of home health services even though another third party insurer may pay for that nursing care.

20.3 - Use of Utilization Screens and "Rules of Thumb"
(Rev. 1, 10-01-03)
A3-3116.3, HHA-203.3

Medicare recognizes that determinations of whether home health services are reasonable and necessary must be based on an assessment of each beneficiary's individual care needs. Therefore, denial of services based on numerical utilization screens, diagnostic screens, diagnosis or specific treatment norms is not appropriate.

30 - Conditions Patient Must Meet to Qualify for Coverage of Home Health Services
(Rev. 1, 10-01-03)
A3-3117, HHA-204, A-98-49

To qualify for the Medicare home health benefit, under §§1814(a)(2)(C) and 1835(a)(2)(A) of the Act, a Medicare beneficiary must meet the following requirements:

- Be confined to the home;

- Under the care of a physician;

- Receiving services under a plan of care established and periodically reviewed by a physician;

- Be in need of skilled nursing care on an intermittent basis or physical therapy or speech-language pathology; or

- Have a continuing need for occupational therapy.

For purposes of benefit eligibility, under §§1814(a)(2)(C) and 1835(a)(2)(A) of the Act, "intermittent" means skilled nursing care that is either provided or needed on fewer than 7 days each week or less than 8 hours of each day for periods of 21 days or less (with extensions in exceptional circumstances when the need for additional care is finite and predictable).

A patient must meet each of the criteria specified in this section. Patients who meet each of these criteria are eligible to have payment made on their behalf for services discussed in §§40 and 50.

30.1 - Confined to the Home
(Rev. 1, 10-01-03)
A3-3117.1, HHA-204.1

30.1.1 - Patient Confined to the Home
(Rev. 208, Issued: 04-22-15, Effective: 01-01-15, Implementation: 05-11-15)

For a patient to be eligible to receive covered home health services under both Part A and Part B, the law requires that a physician certify in all cases that the patient is confined to his/her home. For purposes of the statute, an individual shall be considered "confined to the home" (homebound) if the following two criteria are met:

1. Criteria-One:

The patient must either:

- Because of illness or injury, need the aid of supportive devices such as crutches, canes, wheelchairs, and walkers; the use of special transportation; or the assistance of another person in order to leave their place of residence

OR

- Have a condition such that leaving his or her home is medically contraindicated.

If the patient meets one of the Criteria-One conditions, then the patient must ALSO meet two additional requirements defined in Criteria-Two below.

2. Criteria-Two:

- There must exist a normal inability to leave home;

AND

- Leaving home must require a considerable and taxing effort.

If the patient does in fact leave the home, the patient may nevertheless be considered homebound if the absences from the home are infrequent or for periods of relatively short duration, or are attributable to the need to receive health care treatment. Absences attributable to the need to receive health care treatment include, but are not limited to:

- Attendance at adult day centers to receive medical care;

- Ongoing receipt of outpatient kidney dialysis; or

- The receipt of outpatient chemotherapy or radiation therapy.

Any absence of an individual from the home attributable to the need to receive health care treatment, including regular absences for the purpose of participating in therapeutic, psychosocial, or medical treatment in an adult day-care program that is licensed or certified by a State, or accredited to furnish adult day-care services in a State, shall not disqualify an individual from being considered to be confined to his home. Any other absence of an individual from the home shall not so disqualify an individual if the absence is of an infrequent or of relatively short duration. For purposes of the preceding sentence, any absence for the purpose of attending a religious service shall be deemed to be an absence of infrequent or short duration. It is expected that in most instances, absences from the home that occur will be for the purpose of receiving health care treatment. However, occasional absences from the home for nonmedical purposes, e.g., an occasional trip to the barber, a walk around the block or a drive, attendance at a family reunion, funeral, graduation, or other infrequent or unique event would not necessitate a finding that the patient is not homebound if the absences are undertaken on an infrequent basis or are of relatively short duration and do not indicate that the patient has the capacity to obtain the health care provided outside rather than in the home.

Some examples of homebound patients that illustrate the factors used to determine whether a homebound condition exists *are listed below.*

- A patient paralyzed from a stroke who is confined to a wheelchair or requires the aid of crutches in order to walk.

- A patient who is blind or senile and requires the assistance of another person in leaving their place of residence.

- A patient who has lost the use of their upper extremities and, therefore, is unable to open doors, use handrails on stairways, etc., and requires the assistance of another individual to leave their place of residence.

- A patient in the late stages of ALS or neurodegenerative disabilities. In determining whether the patient has the general inability to leave the home and leaves the home only infrequently or for periods of short duration, it is necessary (as is the case in determining whether skilled nursing services are intermittent) to look at the patient's condition over a period of time rather than for short periods within the home health stay. For example, a patient may leave the home *(meeting both criteria listed above)* more frequently during a short period when the *patient has multiple appointments with health care professionals and medical tests in 1 week.* So long as the patient's overall condition and experience is such that he or she meets these qualifications, he or she should be considered confined to the home.

- A patient who has just returned from a hospital stay involving surgery, who may be suffering from resultant weakness and pain *because of the surgery* and; therefore, their actions may be restricted by their physician to certain specified and limited activities *(*such as getting out of bed only for a specified period of time, walking stairs only once a day, etc.*)*.

- A patient with arteriosclerotic heart disease of such severity that they must avoid all stress and physical activity.

- A patient with a psychiatric illness that is manifested in part by a refusal to leave home or is of such a nature that it would not be considered safe for the patient to leave home unattended, even if they have no physical limitations.

The aged person who does not often travel from home because of feebleness and insecurity brought on by advanced age would not be considered confined to the home for purposes of receiving home health services unless they meet one of the above conditions.

Although a patient must be confined to the home to be eligible for covered home health services, some services cannot be provided at the patient's residence because equipment is required that cannot be made available there. If the services required by an individual involve the use of such equipment, the HHA may make arrangements with a hospital, SNF, or a rehabilitation center to provide these services on an outpatient basis. (See §50.6.) However, even in these situations, for the services to be covered as home health services the patient must be considered confined to home *and meet both criteria listed above*.

If a question is raised as to whether a patient is confined to the home, the HHA will be requested to furnish the *Medicare contractor* with the information necessary to establish that the patient is homebound as defined above.

30.1.2 - Patient's Place of Residence
(Rev. 208, Issued: 04-22-15, Effective: 01-01-15, Implementation: 05-11-15)

A patient's residence is wherever he or she makes his or her home. This may be his or her own dwelling, an apartment, a relative's home, a home for the aged, or some other type of institution. However, an institution may not be considered a patient's residence if the institution meets the requirements of §§1861(e)(1) or 1819(a)(1) of the Act. Included in this group are hospitals and skilled nursing facilities, as well as most nursing facilities under Medicaid. (See the Medicare State Operations Manual, §2166.)

Thus, if a patient is in an institution or distinct part of an institution identified above, the patient is not entitled to have payment made for home health services under either Part A or Part B since such an institution may not be considered their residence. When a patient remains in a participating SNF following their discharge from active care, the facility may not be considered their residence for purposes of home health coverage.

A patient may have more than one home and the Medicare rules do not prohibit a patient from having one or more places of residence. A patient, under a Medicare home health plan of care, who resides in more than one place of residence during an episode of Medicare covered home health services will not disqualify the patient's homebound status for purposes of eligibility. For example, a person may reside in a principal home and also a second vacation home, mobile home, or the home of a caretaker relative. The fact that the patient resides in more than one home and, as a result, must transit from one to the other, is not in itself, an indication that the patient is not homebound. The requirements of homebound must be met at each location *(i.e., the patient must meet both criteria listed in section 30.1.1 above).*

A. Assisted Living Facilities, Group Homes, and Personal Care Homes

An individual may be "confined to the home" for purposes of Medicare coverage of home health services if he or she resides in an institution that is not primarily engaged in providing to inpatients:

- Diagnostic and therapeutic services for medical diagnosis;

- Treatment;

- Care of injured, disabled or sick persons;

- Rehabilitation services or other skilled services needed to maintain a patient's current condition or to prevent or slow further deterioration; or

- Skilled nursing care or related services for patients who require medical or nursing care.

If it is determined that the assisted living facility (also called personal care homes, group homes, etc.) in which the individuals reside are not primarily engaged in providing the above services, then Medicare will cover reasonable and necessary home health care furnished to these individuals.

If it is determined that the services furnished by the home health agency are duplicative of services furnished by an assisted living facility when provision of such care is required of the facility under State licensure requirements, claims for such services should be denied under §1862(a)(1)(A) of the Act. Section 1862(a)(1)(A) excludes services that are not necessary for the diagnosis or treatment of illness or injury or to improve the functioning of a malformed body member from Medicare coverage. Services to people who already have access to appropriate care from a willing caregiver would not be considered reasonable and necessary to the treatment of the individual's illness or injury.

Medicare coverage would not be an optional substitute for the services that a facility is required to provide by law to its patients or where the services are included in the base contract of the facility. An individual's choice to reside in such a facility is also a choice to accept the services it holds itself out as offering to its patients.

B. Day Care Centers and Patient's Place of Residence

The current statutory definition of homebound or confined does not imply that Medicare coverage has been expanded to include adult day care services.

The law does not permit an HHA to furnish a Medicare covered billable visit to a patient under a home health plan of care outside his or her home, except in those limited circumstances where the patient needs to use medical equipment that is too cumbersome to bring to the home. Section 1861(m) of the Act stipulates that home health services provided to a patient be provided to the patient on a visiting basis in a place of residence used as the individual's home. A licensed/certified day care center does not meet the definition of a place of residence.

C. State Licensure/Certification of Day Care Facilities

Per Section 1861(m) of the Act, an adult day care center must be either licensed or certified by the State or accredited by a private accrediting body. State licensure or certification as an adult day care facility must be based on State interpretations of its process. For example, several States do not license adult day care facilities as a whole, but do certify some entities as Medicaid certified centers for purposes of providing adult day care under the Medicaid home and community based waiver program. It is the responsibility of the State to determine the necessary criteria for "State certification" in such a situation. A State could determine that Medicaid certification is an acceptable standard and consider its Medicaid certified adult day care facilities to be "State certified." On the other hand, a State could determine Medicaid certification to be insufficient and require other conditions to be met before the adult day care facility is considered "State certified".

D. Determination of the Therapeutic, Medical or Psychosocial Treatment of the Patient at the Day Care Facility

It is not the obligation of the HHA to determine whether the adult day care facility is providing psychosocial treatment, but only to assure that the adult day care center is licensed/certified by the State or accrediting body. The intent of the law, in extending the homebound exception status to attendance at such adult day care facilities, recognizes that they ordinarily furnish psychosocial services.

30.2 - Services Are Provided Under a Plan of Care Established and Approved by a Physician
(Rev. 1, 10-01-03)
A3-3117.2, HHA-204.2

30.2.1 - Content of the Plan of Care
(Rev. 208, Issued: 04-22-15, Effective: 01-01-15, Implementation: 05-11-15)

The HHA must be acting upon a physician plan of care that meets the requirements of this section for HHA services to be covered.

The plan of care must contain all pertinent diagnoses, including:

- The patient's mental status;

- The types of services, supplies, and equipment required;

- The frequency of the visits to be made;

- Prognosis;

- Rehabilitation potential;

- Functional limitations;

- Activities permitted;

- Nutritional requirements;

- All medications and treatments;

- Safety measures to protect against injury;

- Instructions for timely discharge or referral; and

- Any additional items the HHA or physician *chooses* to include.

If the plan of care includes a course of treatment for therapy services:

- The course of therapy treatment must be established by the physician after any needed consultation with the qualified therapist;

- The plan must include measurable therapy treatment goals which pertain directly to the patient's illness or injury, and the patient's resultant impairments;

- The plan must include the expected duration of therapy services; and

- The plan must describe a course of treatment which is consistent with the qualified therapist's assessment of the patient's function.

30.2.2 - Specificity of Orders
(Rev. 1, 10-01-03)
A3-3117.2.B, HHA-204.2.B

The orders on the plan of care must indicate the type of services to be provided to the patient, both with respect to the professional who will provide them and the nature of the individual services, as well as the frequency of the services.

EXAMPLE 1:

SN x 7/wk x 1 wk; 3/wk x 4 wk; 2/wk x 3 wk, (skilled nursing visits 7 times per week for 1 week; 3 times per week for 4 weeks; and 2 times per week for 3 weeks) for skilled observation and evaluation of the surgical site, for teaching sterile dressing changes and to perform sterile dressing changes. The sterile change consists of (detail of procedure).

Orders for care may indicate a specific range in the frequency of visits to ensure that the most appropriate level of services is provided during the 60-day episode to home health patients. When a range of visits is ordered, the upper limit of the range is considered the specific frequency.

EXAMPLE 2:

SN x 2-4/wk x 4 wk; 1-2/wk x 4 wk for skilled observation and evaluation of the surgical site.

Orders for services to be furnished "as needed" or "PRN" must be accompanied by a description of the patient's medical signs and symptoms that would occasion a visit and a specific limit on the number of those visits to be made under the order before an additional physician order would have to be obtained.

30.2.3 - Who Signs the Plan of Care
(Rev. 1, 10-01-03)
A3-3117.2.C, HHA-204-2.C

The physician who signs the plan of care must be qualified to sign the physician certification as described in 42 CFR 424.22.

30.2.4 - Timeliness of Signature
(Rev. 1, 10-01-03)
A3-3117.2.D, HHA-204-2.D

A. Initial Percentage Payment

If a physician signed plan of care is not available at the beginning of the episode, the HHA may submit a RAP for the initial percentage payment based on physician verbal orders OR a referral prescribing detailed orders for the services to be rendered that is signed and dated by the physician. If the RAP submission is based on physician verbal orders, the verbal order must be recorded in the plan of care, include a description of the patient's condition and the services to be provided by the home health agency, include an attestation (relating to the physician's orders and the date received per 42 CFR 409.43), and the plan of care is copied and immediately submitted to the physician. A billable visit must be rendered prior to the submission of a RAP.

B. Final Percentage Payment

The plan of care must be signed and dated by a physician as described who meets the certification and recertification requirements of 42 CFR 424.22 and before the claim for each episode for services is submitted for the final percentage payment. Any changes in the plan of care must be signed and dated by a physician.

30.2.5 - Use of Oral (Verbal) Orders
(Rev. 208, Issued: 04-22-15, Effective: 01-01-15, Implementation: 05-11-15)

When services are furnished based on a physician's oral order, the orders may be accepted and put in writing by personnel authorized to do so by applicable State and Federal laws and regulations as well as by the HHA's internal policies. The orders must be signed and dated with the date of receipt by the registered nurse or qualified therapist (i.e., physical therapist, speech-language pathologist, occupational therapist, or medical social worker) responsible for furnishing or supervising the ordered services. The orders may be signed by the supervising registered nurse or qualified therapist after the services have been rendered, as long as HHA personnel who receive the oral orders notify that nurse or therapist before the service is rendered. Thus, the rendering of a service that is based on an oral order would not be delayed pending signature of the supervising nurse or therapist. Oral orders must be countersigned and dated by the physician before the HHA bills for the care in the same way as the plan of care.

Services which are provided from the beginning of the 60-day episode certification period based on a request for anticipated payment and before the physician signs the plan of care are considered to be provided under a plan of care established and approved by the physician where there is an oral order for the care prior to rendering the services which is documented in the medical record and where the services are included in a signed plan of care.

Services that are provided in the subsequent 60-day episode certification period are considered provided under the plan of care of the subsequent 60-day episode where there is an oral order before the services provided in the subsequent period are furnished and the order is reflected in the medical record. However, services that are provided after the expiration of the plan of care, but before the acquisition of an oral order or a signed plan of care are not considered provided under a plan of care.

EXAMPLE 1:

The HHA acquires an oral order for I.V. medication administration for a patient to be performed on August 1. The HHA provides the I.V. medication administration August 1 and evaluates the patient's need for continued care. The physician signs the plan of care for the I.V. medication administration on August 15. The visit is covered since it is considered provided under a plan of care established and approved by the physician, and the HHA had acquired an oral order prior to the delivery of services.

EXAMPLE 2:

The patient is under a plan of care in which the physician orders I.V. medication administration every 2 weeks. The last day covered by the initial plan of care is July 31. The patient's next I.V. medication administration is scheduled for August 5 and the physician signs the plan of care for the new period on August 1. The I.V. medication administration on August 5 was provided under a plan of care established and approved by the physician. The episode begins on the 61 day regardless of the date of the first covered visit.

EXAMPLE 3:

The patient is under a plan of care in which the physician orders I.V. medication administration every 2 weeks. The last day covered by the plan of care is July 31. The patient's next I.V. medication administration is scheduled for August 5 and the physician does not sign the plan of care until August 6. The HHA acquires an oral order for the I.V. medication administration before the August 5 visit, and therefore the visit is considered to be provided under a plan of care established and approved by the physician. The episode begins on the 61 day regardless of the date of the first covered visit.

Any increase in the frequency of services or addition of new services during a certification period must be authorized by a physician by way of a written or oral order prior to the provision of the increased or additional services

30.2.6 - Frequency of Review of the Plan of Care
(Rev. 1, 10-01-03)
A3-3117.2.F, HHA-204.2.F

The plan of care must be reviewed and signed by the physician who established the plan of care, in consultation with HHA professional personnel, at least every 60 days. Each review of a patient's plan of care must contain the signature of the physician and the date of review.

30.2.7 - Facsimile Signatures
(Rev. 1, 10-01-03)
A3-3117.2.G, HHA-204.2.G

The plan of care or oral order may be transmitted by facsimile machine. The HHA is not required to have the original signature on file. However, the HHA is responsible for obtaining original signatures if an issue surfaces that would require verification of an original signature.

30.2.8 - Alternative Signatures
(Rev. 1, 10-01-03)

A3-3117.2.H, HHA-204.2.H

HHAs that maintain patient records by computer rather than hard copy may use electronic signatures. However, all such entries must be appropriately authenticated and dated. Authentication must include signatures, written initials, or computer secure entry by a unique identifier of a primary author who has reviewed and approved the entry. The HHA must have safeguards to prevent unauthorized access to the records and a process for reconstruction of the records in the event of a system breakdown.

30.2.9 - Termination of the Plan of Care - Qualifying Services
(Rev. 1, 10-01-03)
A3-3117.2.I, HHA-204.2.I

The plan of care is considered to be terminated if the patient does not receive at least one covered skilled nursing, physical therapy, speech-language pathology service, or occupational therapy visit in a 60-day period since these are qualifying services for the home health benefit. An exception is if the physician documents that the interval without such care is appropriate to the treatment of the patient's illness or injury.

30.2.10 - Sequence of Qualifying Services and Other Medicare Covered Home Health Services
(Rev. 1, 10-01-03)
A3-3117.2.J, HHA-204.2.J

Once patient eligibility has been confirmed and the plan of care contains physician orders for the qualifying service as well as other Medicare covered home health services, the qualifying service does not have to be rendered prior to the other Medicare covered home health services ordered in the plan of care. The sequence of visits performed by the disciplines must be dictated by the individual patient's plan of care. For example, for an eligible patient in an initial 60-day episode that has both physical therapy and occupational therapy orders in the plan of care, the sequence of the delivery of the type of therapy is irrelevant as long as the need for the qualifying service is established prior to the delivery of other Medicare covered services and the qualifying discipline provides a billable visit prior to transfer or discharge in accordance with 42 CFR 409.43(f).

NOTE: Dependent services provided after the final qualifying skilled service are not covered under the home health benefit, except when the dependent service was followed by a qualifying skilled service as a result of the unexpected inpatient admission or death of the patient or due to some other unanticipated event.

30.3 - Under the Care of a Physician
(Rev. 208, Issued: 04-22-15, Effective: 01-01-15, Implementation: 05-11-15)

The patient must be under the care of a physician who is qualified to sign the physician certification and plan of care in accordance with 42 CFR 424.22.

A patient is expected to be under the care of the physician who signs the plan of care. It is expected *that in most instances, the physician who certifies the patient's eligibility for Medicare home health services, in accordance with §30.5 below, will be the same physician who establishes and signs the plan of care.*

30.4 - Needs Skilled Nursing Care on an Intermittent Basis (Other than Solely Venipuncture for the Purposes of Obtaining a Blood Sample), Physical Therapy, Speech-Language Pathology Services, or Has Continued Need for Occupational Therapy
(Rev. 1, 10-01-03)
A3-3117.4, HHA-204.4

The patient must need one of the following types of services:

1. Skilled nursing care that is

    -   Reasonable and necessary as defined in §40.1;

    -   Needed on an "intermittent" based as defined in §40.1; and

    -   Not solely needed for venipuncture for the purposes of obtaining blood sample as defined in §40.1.2.13;or

2. Physical therapy as defined in §40.2.2; or

3. Speech-language pathology services as defined in §40.2.3; or

4. Have a continuing need for occupational therapy as defined in §§40.2.4.

The patient has a continued need for occupational therapy when:

1. The services which the patient requires meet the definition of "occupational therapy" services of §40.2, and

2. The patient's eligibility for home health services has been established by virtue of a prior need for skilled nursing care (other than solely venipuncture for the purposes of obtaining a blood sample), speech-language pathology services, or physical therapy in the current or prior certification period.

EXAMPLE: A patient who is recovering from a cerebrovascular accident (CVA) has an initial plan of care that called for physical therapy, speech-language pathology services, and home health aide services. In the next certification period, the physician orders only occupational therapy and home health aide services because the patient no longer needs the skills of a physical therapist or a speech-language pathologist, but needs the services provided by the occupational therapist. The patient's need for occupational therapy qualifies him for home health services, including home health aide services (presuming that all other qualifying criteria are met).

30.5 - Physician Certification *and Recertification of Patient Eligibility for Medicare Home Health Services*
(Rev. 208, Issued: 04-22-15, Effective: 01-01-15, Implementation: 05-11-15)

The HHA must be acting upon a plan of care as described in §30.2, and a physician certification *or recertification that* meets the *requirements* of *the following sections in order* for HHA services to be covered.

30.5.1 - Physician Certification
(Rev. 208, Issued: 04-22-15, Effective: 01-01-15, Implementation: 05-11-15)

A certification (versus recertification) is considered to be anytime that a Start of Care OASIS is completed to initiate care. In such instances, a physician must certify *(attest)* that:

1. The home health services are or were needed because the patient is or was confined to the home as defined in §30.1;

2. The patient needs or needed skilled nursing services on an intermittent basis (other than solely venipuncture for the purposes of obtaining a blood sample), or physical therapy, or speech-language pathology services. Where a patient's sole skilled service need is for skilled oversight of unskilled services (management and evaluation of the care plan as defined in §40.1.2.2), the physician must include a brief narrative describing the clinical justification of this need as part of the certification, or as a signed addendum to the certification;

3. A plan of care has been established and is periodically reviewed by a physician;

4. The services are or were furnished while the patient is or was under the care of a physician;

5. For episodes with starts of care beginning January 1, 2011 and later, *in accordance with §30.5.1.1 below, a face-to-face encounter occurred no more than 90 days prior to or within 30 days after the start of the home health care, was related to the primary reason the patient requires home health services, and was performed by an allowed provider type. The certifying physician must also document the date of the encounter.*

If the patient is starting home health directly after discharge from an acute/post-acute care setting where the physician, with privileges, that cared for the patient in that setting is certifying the patient's eligibility for the home health benefit, but will not be following the patient after discharge, then the certifying physician must identify the community physician who will be following the patient after discharge. One of the criteria that must be met for a patient to be considered eligible for the home health benefit is that the patient must be under the care of a physician (number 4 listed above). Otherwise, the certification is not valid.

The certification must be complete prior to when an HHA bills Medicare for reimbursement; however, physicians should complete the certification when the plan of care is established, or as soon as possible thereafter. This is longstanding CMS policy as referenced in Pub 100-01, Medicare General Information, Eligibility, and Entitlement Manual, chapter 4, section 30.1. It is not acceptable for HHAs to wait until the end of a 60-day episode of care to obtain a completed certification/recertification.

30.5.1.1 – Face-to-Face Encounter
(Rev. 208, Issued: 04-22-15, Effective: 01-01-15, Implementation: 05-11-15)

1. *Allowed Provider Types*

As part of the certification of patient eligibility for the Medicare home health benefit, a face-to-face encounter with the patient must be performed by the certifying physician himself or herself, a physician that cared for the patient in the acute or post-acute care facility (with privileges who cared for the patient in an acute or post-acute care facility from which the patient was directly admitted to home health) or an allowed non-physician practitioner (NPP).

NPPs who are allowed to perform the encounter are:

- A nurse practitioner or a clinical nurse specialist working in accordance with State law and in collaboration with the certifying physician *or in collaboration with an acute or post-acute care physician, with privileges, who cared for the patient in the acute or post-acute care facility from which the patient was directly admitted to home health;*

- A certified nurse midwife, as authorized by State law*, under the supervision of the certifying physician or under the supervision of an acute or post-acute care physician with privileges who cared for the patient in the acute or post-acute care facility from which the patient was directly admitted to home health;*

- A physician assistant under the supervision of the certifying physician *or under the supervision of an acute or post-acute care physician with privileges who cared for the patient in the acute or post-acute care facility from which the patient was directly admitted to home health.*

NPPs performing the encounter are subject to the same financial restrictions with the HHA as the certifying physician, as described in 42 CFR 424.22(d).

2. *Timeframe Requirements*

- The encounter must occur no more than 90 days prior to the home health start of care date or within 30 days after the start of care.

- In situations when a physician orders home health care for the patient based on a new condition that was not evident during a visit within the 90 days prior to start of care, the certifying physician or an allowed NPP must see the patient again within 30 days after admission. Specifically, if a patient saw the certifying physician or NPP within the 90 days prior to start of care, another encounter would be needed if the patient's condition had changed to the extent that standards of practice would indicate that the physician or a non-physician practitioner should examine the patient in order to establish an effective treatment plan.

3. *Exceptional Circumstances*

When a home health patient dies shortly after admission, before the face-to-face encounter occurs, if the contractor determines a good faith effort existed on the part of the HHA to facilitate/coordinate the encounter and if all other certification requirements are met, the certification is deemed to be complete.

4. *Telehealth*

The face-to-face encounter can be performed via a telehealth service, in an approved originating site. An originating site is considered to be the location of an eligible Medicare beneficiary at the time the service being furnished via a telecommunications system occurs. Medicare beneficiaries are eligible for telehealth services only if they are presented from an originating site located in a rural health professional shortage area or in a county outside of a Metropolitan Statistical Area.

Entities that participate in a Federal telemedicine demonstration project approved by (or receiving funding from) the Secretary of the Department of Health and Human Services as of December 31, 2000, qualify as originating sites regardless of geographic location.

The originating sites authorized by law are:

- The office of a physician or practitioner;
- Hospitals;
- Critical Access Hospitals (CAH);
- Rural Health Clinics (RHC);
- Federally Qualified Health Centers (FQHC);
- Hospital-based or CAH-based Renal Dialysis Centers (including satellites);
- Skilled Nursing Facilities (SNF); and
- Community Mental Health Centers (CMHC).

30.5.1.2 – *Supporting Documentation Requirements*
(Rev. 208, Issued: 04-22-15, Effective: 01-01-15, Implementation: 05-11-15)

As of January 1, 2015, documentation in the certifying physician's medical records and/or the acute /post-acute care facility's medical records (if the patient was directly admitted to home health) will be used as the basis upon which patient eligibility for the Medicare home health benefit will be determined. Documentation from the certifying physician's medical records and/or the acute /post-acute care facility's medical records (if the patient was directly admitted to home health) used to support the certification of home health eligibility must be provided, upon request, to the home health agency, review entities, and/or the Centers for Medicare and Medicaid Services (CMS). In turn, an HHA must be able to provide, upon request, the supporting documentation that substantiates the eligibility for the Medicare home health benefit to review entities and/or CMS. If the documentation used as the basis for the certification of eligibility is not sufficient to demonstrate that the patient is or was eligible to receive services under the Medicare home health benefit, payment will not be rendered for home health services provided.

The certifying physician and/or the acute/post-acute care facility medical record (if the patient was directly admitted to home health) for the patient must contain information that justifies the referral for Medicare home health services. This includes documentation that substantiates the patient's:

- *Need for the skilled services; and*
- *Homebound status;*

The certifying physician and/or the acute/post-acute care facility medical record (if the patient was directly admitted to home health) for the patient must contain the actual clinical note for the face-to-face encounter visit that demonstrates that the encounter:

- *Occurred within the required timeframe,*
- *Was related to the primary reason the patient requires home health services; and*
- *Was performed by an allowed provider type.*

This information can be found most often in clinical and progress notes and discharge summaries.

- *Information from the HHA, such as the initial and/or comprehensive assessment of the patient required per 42 CFR 484.55, can be incorporated into the certifying physician's medical record for the patient and used to support the patient's homebound status and need for skilled care. However, this information must be corroborated by other medical record entries in the certifying physician's and/or the acute/post-acute care facility's medical record for the patient.*

30.5.2 - *Physician* Recertification
(Rev. 207, Issued: 04-10-15, Effective: 05-11-15, Implementation: 05-11-15)

At the end of the 60-day episode, a decision must be made whether or not to recertify the patient for a subsequent 60-day episode. An eligible beneficiary who qualifies for a subsequent 60-day episode would start the subsequent 60-day episode on day 61. Under

HH PPS, the plan of care must be reviewed and signed by the physician every 60 days unless one of the following occurs:

- A beneficiary transfers to another HHA; *or*

- A discharge and return to home health during the 60-day episode.

The physician must include an estimate of how much longer the skilled services will be required and must certify (attest) that:

1. The home health services are or were needed because the patient is or was confined to the home as defined in §30.1;

2. The patient needs or needed skilled nursing services on an intermittent basis (other than solely venipuncture for the purposes of obtaining a blood sample), or physical therapy, or speech-language pathology services; or continues to need occupational therapy after the need for skilled nursing care, physical therapy, or speech-language pathology services ceased. Where a patient's sole skilled service need is for skilled oversight of unskilled services (management and evaluation of the care plan as defined in §40.1.2.2), the physician must include a brief narrative describing the clinical justification of this need as part of the recertification, or as a signed addendum to the recertification;

3. A plan of care has been established and is periodically reviewed by a physician; and

4. The services are or were furnished while the patient is or was under the care of a physician.

Medicare does not limit the number of continuous episode recertifications for beneficiaries who continue to be eligible for the home health benefit. The physician certification may cover a period less than but not greater than 60 days.

See §10.4 for counting initial and subsequent 60-day episodes. See §10.5 for recertifications for split percentage payments.

30.5.3 - Who May Sign the Certification *or Recertification*
(Rev. 208, Issued: 04-22-15, Effective: 01-01-15, Implementation: 05-11-15)

The physician who signs the certification *or recertification* must be permitted to do so by 42 CFR 424.22.

30.5.4 – Physician Billing for Certification and Recertification
(Rev. 208, Issued: 04-22-15, Effective: 01-01-15, Implementation: 05-11-15)

Physician certification/recertification claims are Part B physician claims paid for under the Physician Fee Schedule. These claims are billed using HCPCS codes G0180 (certification) or G0179 (re-certification). The descriptions of these two codes indicate that they are used to bill for certification or recertification of patient eligibility "for Medicare-covered home health services under a home health plan of care (patient not present), including contacts with the HHA and review of reports of patient status required by physicians to affirm the initial implementation of the plan of care that meets patient's needs, per certification period". As noted above, these codes are for physician certification or recertification for Medicare-covered home health services. If there are no Medicare-covered home health services, these codes should not be billed or paid. As such, physician claims for certification/recertification of eligibility for home health services (G0180 and G0179, respectively) will not be covered if the HHA claim itself was non-covered because the certification/recertification of eligibility was not complete or because there was insufficient documentation to support that the patient was eligible for the Medicare home health benefit.

40 - Covered Services Under a Qualifying Home Health Plan of Care
(Rev. 1, 10-01-03)
A3-3118, HHA-205

Section 1861(m)of the Act governs the Medicare home health services that may be provided to eligible beneficiaries by or under arrangements made by a participating home health agency (HHA). Section 1861(m) describes home health services as

- Part-time or intermittent skilled nursing care (other than solely venipuncture for the purposes of obtaining a blood sample);

- Part-time or intermittent home health aide services;

- Physical therapy;

- Speech-language pathology;

- Occupational therapy;

- Medical social services;

- Medical supplies (including catheters, catheter supplies, ostomy bags, supplies related to ostomy care, and a covered osteoporosis drug (as defined in §1861(kk) of the Act), but excluding other drugs and biologicals);

- Durable medical equipment while under the plan of care established by physician;

- Medical services provided by an intern or resident-in-training under an approved teaching program of the hospital in the case of an HHA which is affiliated or under common control with a hospital; and

- Services at hospitals, skilled nursing facilities, or rehabilitation centers when they involve equipment too cumbersome to bring to the home.

The term "part-time or intermittent" for purposes of coverage under §1861(m) of the Act means skilled nursing and home health aide services furnished any number of days per week as long as they are furnished (combined) less than 8 hours each day and 28 or fewer hours each week (or, subject to review on a case-by-case basis as to the need for care, less than 8 hours each day and 35 or fewer hours per week). See §50.7.

For any home health services to be covered by Medicare, the patient must meet the qualifying criteria as specified in §30, including having a need for skilled nursing care on an intermittent basis, physical therapy, speech-language pathology services, or a continuing need for occupational therapy as defined in this section.

40.1 - Skilled Nursing Care
(Rev. 179, Issued: 01-14-14, Effective: 01-07-14, Implementation: 01-07-14)
A3-3118.1, HHA-205.1

To be covered as skilled nursing services, the services must require the skills of a registered nurse, or a licensed practical (vocational) nurse under the supervision of a registered nurse, must be reasonable and necessary to the treatment of the patient's illness or injury as discussed in §40.1.1, below, and must be intermittent as discussed in §40.1.3. Coverage of skilled nursing care does not turn on the presence or absence of a patient's potential for improvement from the nursing care, but rather on the patient's need for skilled care.

40.1.1 - General Principles Governing Reasonable and Necessary Skilled Nursing Care
(Rev. 179, Issued: 01-14-14, Effective: 01-07-14, Implementation: 01-07-14)
A3-3118.1, HHA-205.1

If all other eligibility and coverage requirements under the home health benefit are met, skilled nursing services are covered when an individualized assessment of the patient's clinical condition demonstrates that the specialized judgment, knowledge, and skills of a registered nurse or, when provided by regulation, a licensed practical (vocational) nurse ("skilled care") are necessary. Skilled nursing services are covered where such skilled nursing services are necessary to maintain the patient's current condition or prevent or slow further deterioration so long as the beneficiary requires skilled care for the services to be safely and effectively provided. When, however, the individualized assessment does not demonstrate such a necessity for skilled care, including when the services needed do not require skilled nursing care because they could safely and effectively be performed by the patient or unskilled caregivers, such services will not be covered under the home health benefit.

Skilled nursing care is necessary only when (a) the particular patient's special medical complications require the skills of a registered nurse or, when provided by regulation, a licensed practical nurse to perform a type of service that would otherwise be considered non-skilled; or (b) the needed services are of such complexity that the skills of a registered nurse or, when provided by regulation, a licensed practical nurse are required to furnish the services. To be considered a skilled service, the service must be so inherently complex that it can be safely and effectively performed only by, or under the supervision of, professional or technical personnel as provided by regulation, including 42 C.F.R. 409.32.

Some services may be classified as a skilled nursing service on the basis of complexity alone (e.g., intravenous and intramuscular injections or insertion of catheters) and, if reasonable and necessary to the treatment of the patient's illness or injury, would be covered on that basis. If a service can be safely and effectively performed (or self-administered) by an unskilled person, without the direct supervision of a nurse, the service cannot be regarded as a skilled nursing service although a nurse actually provides the service. However, in some cases, the condition of the patient may cause a service that would ordinarily be considered unskilled to be considered a skilled nursing service. This would occur when the patient's condition is such that the service can be safely and effectively provided only by a nurse. A service is not considered a skilled nursing service merely because it is performed by or under the supervision of a nurse. The unavailability of a competent person to provide a non-skilled service, regardless of the importance of the service to the patient, does not make it a skilled service when a nurse provides the service.

A service that, by its nature, requires the skills of a nurse to be provided safely and effectively continues to be a skilled service even if it is taught to the patient, the patient's family, or other caregivers.

The skilled nursing service must be reasonable and necessary to the diagnosis and treatment of the patient's illness or injury within the context of the patient's unique medical condition. To be considered reasonable and necessary for the diagnosis or treatment of the patient's illness or injury, the services must be consistent with the nature and severity of the illness or injury, the patient's particular medical needs, and accepted standards of medical and nursing practice. The determination of whether the services are reasonable and necessary should be made in consideration that a physician has determined that the services ordered are reasonable and necessary. The services must, therefore, be viewed from the perspective of the condition of the patient when the services were ordered and what was, at that time, reasonably expected to be appropriate treatment for the illness or injury throughout the certification period.

A patient's overall medical condition, without regard to whether the illness or injury is acute, chronic, terminal, or expected to extend over a long period of time, should be considered in deciding whether skilled services are needed. A patient's diagnosis should never be the sole factor in deciding that a service the patient needs is either skilled or not skilled. Skilled care may, depending on the unique condition of the patient, continue to be necessary for patients whose condition is stable.

As is outlined in home health regulations, as part of the home health agency (HHA) Conditions of Participation (CoPs), the clinical record of the patient must contain progress and clinical notes. Additionally, in Pub. 100-04, Medicare Claims Processing Manual, Chapter 10; "Home Health Agency Billing", instructions specify that for each claim, HHAs are required to report all services provided to the beneficiary during each episode, which includes reporting each visit in line-item detail. As such, it is expected that the home health records for every visit will reflect the need for the skilled medical care provided. These clinical notes are also expected to provide important communication among all members of the home care team regarding the development, course and outcomes of the skilled observations, assessments, treatment and training performed. Taken as a whole then, the clinical notes are expected to tell the story of the patient's achievement towards his/her goals as outlined in the Plan of Care. In this way, the notes will serve to demonstrate why a skilled service is needed.

Therefore the home health clinical notes must document as appropriate:

- the history and physical exam pertinent to the day's visit, (including the response or changes in behavior to previously administered skilled services) and the skilled services applied on the current visit, and

- the patient/caregiver's response to the skilled services provided, and

- the plan for the next visit based on the rationale of prior results,

- a detailed rationale that explains the need for the skilled service in light of the patient's overall medical condition and experiences,

- the complexity of the service to be performed, and

- any other pertinent characteristics of the beneficiary or home

Clinical notes should be written so that they adequately describe the reaction of a patient to his/her skilled care. Clinical notes should also provide a clear picture of the treatment, as well as "next steps" to be taken. Vague or subjective descriptions of the patient's care should not be used. For example terminology such as the following would not adequately describe the need for skilled care:

- Patient tolerated treatment well
- Caregiver instructed in medication management
- Continue with POC

Objective measurements of physical outcomes of treatment should be provided and/or a clear description of the changed behaviors due to education programs should be recorded in order that all concerned can follow the results of the applied services.

EXAMPLE 1:

The presence of a plaster cast on an extremity generally does not indicate a need for skilled nursing care. However, the patient with a preexisting peripheral vascular or circulatory condition might need skilled nursing care to observe for complications, monitor medication administration for pain control, and teach proper skin care to preserve skin integrity and prevent breakdown. The documentation must support the severity of the circulatory condition that requires skilled care. The clinical notes for each home health visit should document the patient's skin and circulatory examination as well as the patient and/or caregiver application of the educational principles taught since the last visit. The plan for the next visit should describe the skilled services continuing to be required.

EXAMPLE 2:

The condition of a patient, who has irritable bowel syndrome or is recovering from rectal surgery, may be such that he or she can be given an enema safely and effectively only by a nurse. If the enema were necessary to treat the illness or injury, then the visit would be covered as a skilled nursing visit. The documentation must support the skilled need for the enema, and the plan for future visits based on this information.

EXAMPLE 3:

Giving a bath does not ordinarily require the skills of a nurse and, therefore, would not be covered as a skilled nursing service unless the patient's condition is such that the bath could be given safely and effectively only by a nurse (as discussed in §30.1 above).

EXAMPLE 4:

A patient with a well-established colostomy absent complications may require assistance changing the colostomy bag because they cannot do it themselves and there is no one else to change the bag. Notwithstanding the need for the routine colostomy care, changing the colostomy bag does not become a skilled nursing service when the nurse provides it.

EXAMPLE 5:

A patient was discharged from the hospital with an open draining wound that requires irrigation, packing, and dressing twice each day. The HHA has taught the family to perform the dressing changes. The HHA continues to see the patient for the wound care that is needed during the time that the family is not available and willing to provide the dressing changes. The wound care continues to be skilled nursing care, notwithstanding that the family provides it part of the time, and may be covered as long as the patient requires it.

EXAMPLE 6:

A physician has ordered skilled nursing visits for a patient with a hairline fracture of the hip. The home health record must document the reason skilled services are required and why the nursing visits are reasonable and necessary for treatment of the patient's hip injury.

EXAMPLE 7:

A physician has ordered skilled nursing visits for teaching of self-administration and self-management of the medication regimen for a patient, newly diagnosed, with diabetes mellitus in the home health plan of care. Each visit's documentation must describe the patient's progress in this activity.

EXAMPLE 8:

Following a cerebrovascular accident (CVA), a patient has an in-dwelling Foley catheter because of urinary incontinence, and is expected to require the catheter for a long and indefinite period. The medical condition of the patient must be described and documented to support the need for nursing skilled services in the home health plan of care. Periodic visits to change the catheter as needed, treat the symptoms of catheter malfunction, and teach proper catheter care would be covered as long as they are reasonable and necessary, although the patient is stable, even if there is an expectation that the care will be needed for a long and indefinite period. However, at every home health visit, the patient's current medical condition must be described and there must be documentation to support the need for continued skilled nursing services.

EXAMPLE 9:

A patient with advanced multiple sclerosis undergoing an exacerbation of the illness needs skilled teaching of medications, measures to overcome urinary retention, and the establishment of a program designed to minimize the adverse impact of the exacerbation. The clinical notes for each home health visit must describe why skilled nursing services were required. The skilled nursing care received by the patient would be covered despite the chronic nature of the illness.

EXAMPLE 10:

A patient with malignant melanoma is terminally ill, and requires skilled observation, assessment, teaching, and treatment. The patient has not elected coverage under Medicare's hospice benefit. The documentation should describe the goal of the skilled nursing intervention, and at each visit the services provided should support that goal. The skilled nursing care that the patient requires would be covered, notwithstanding that the condition is terminal, because the documentation and description must support that the needed services required the skills of a nurse.

40.1.2 - Application of the Principles to Skilled Nursing Services
(Rev. 1, 10-01-03)
A3-3118.1.B, HHA-205.1.B

The following discussion of skilled nursing services applies the foregoing principles to specific skilled nursing services about which questions are most frequently raised.

40.1.2.1 - Observation and Assessment of the Patient's Condition When Only the Specialized Skills of a Medical Professional Can Determine Patient's Status
(Rev. 179, Issued: 01-14-14, Effective: 01-07-14, Implementation: 01-07-14)

Observation and assessment of the patient's condition by a nurse are reasonable and necessary skilled services where there is a reasonable potential for change in a patient's condition that requires skilled nursing personnel to identify and evaluate the patient's need for possible modification of treatment or initiation of additional medical procedures until the patient's clinical condition and/or treatment regimen has stabilized. Where a patient was admitted to home health care for skilled observation because there was a reasonable potential of a complication or further acute episode, but did not develop a further acute episode or complication, the skilled observation services are still covered for 3 weeks or so long as there remains a reasonable potential for such a complication or further acute episode.

Information from the patient's home health record must document the rationale that demonstrates that there is a reasonable potential for a future complication or acute episode and, therefore, may justify the need for continued skilled observation and assessment beyond the 3-week period. Such signs and symptoms as abnormal/fluctuating vital signs, weight changes, edema, symptoms of drug toxicity, abnormal/fluctuating lab values, and respiratory changes on auscultation may justify skilled observation and assessment. Where these signs and symptoms are such that there is a reasonable potential that skilled observation and assessment by a licensed nurse will result in changes to the treatment of the patient, then the services would be covered. However, observation and assessment by a nurse is not reasonable and necessary for the treatment of the illness or injury where fluctuating signs and symptoms are part of a longstanding pattern of the patient's condition which has not previously required a change in the prescribed treatment.

EXAMPLE 1:

A patient with atherosclerotic heart disease with congestive heart failure requires observation by skilled nursing personnel for signs of decompensation or adverse effects resulting from newly prescribed medication. Skilled observation is needed to determine whether the new drug regimen should be modified or whether other therapeutic measures should be considered until the patient's clinical condition and/or treatment regimen has stabilized. The clinical notes for each home health visit should reflect the deliberations and their outcome.

EXAMPLE 2:

A patient has undergone peripheral vascular disease treatment including a revascularization procedure (bypass). The incision area is showing signs of potential infection, (e.g., heat, redness, swelling, drainage) and the patient has elevated body temperature. For each home health visit, the clinical notes must demonstrate that the skilled observation and monitoring is required.

EXAMPLE 3:

A patient was hospitalized following a heart attack. Following treatment he was discharged home. Because it is not known whether increasing exertion will exacerbate the heart disease, skilled observation is reasonable and necessary as mobilization is initiated in the patient's home. The patient's necessity for skilled observation must be documented at each home health visit until the patient's clinical condition and/or treatment regimen has stabilized.

EXAMPLE 4:

A frail 85-year old man was hospitalized for pneumonia. The infection was resolved, but the patient, who had previously maintained adequate nutrition, will not eat or eats poorly. The patient is discharged to the HHA for monitoring of fluid and nutrient intake and assessment of the need for tube feeding. Observation and monitoring by skilled nurses of the patient's oral intake, output and hydration status is required to determine what further treatment or other intervention is needed. The patient's necessity for skilled observation and treatment must be documented at each home health visit, until the patient's clinical condition and/or treatment regimen has stabilized.

EXAMPLE 5:

A patient with glaucoma and a cardiac condition has a cataract extraction. Because of the interaction between the eye drops for the glaucoma and cataracts and the beta-blocker for the cardiac condition, the patient is at risk for serious cardiac arrhythmia. Skilled observation and monitoring of the drug actions is reasonable and necessary until the patient's condition is stabilized. The patient's necessity for skilled observation must be documented at each home health visit, until the clinical condition and/or patient's treatment regimen has stabilized.

EXAMPLE 6:

A patient with hypertension suffered dizziness and weakness. The physician found that the blood pressure was too low and discontinued the hypertension medication. Skilled observation and monitoring of the patient's blood pressure and medication regimen is required until the blood pressure remains stable and in a safe range. The patient's necessity for skilled observation must be documented at each home health visit, until the patient's clinical condition and/or treatment regimen has stabilized.

EXAMPLE 7:

A patient has chronic non-healing skin ulcers, Diabetes Mellitus Type I, and spinal muscular atrophy. In the past, the patient's wounds have deteriorated, requiring the patient to be hospitalized. Previously, a skilled nurse has trained the patient's wife to perform wound care. The treating physician orders a new episode of skilled care, at a frequency of one visit every 2 weeks to perform observation and assessment of the patient's skin ulcers to make certain that they are not worsening. This order is reasonable and necessary because, although the unskilled family caregiver has learned to care for the wounds, the skilled nurse can use observation and assessment to determine if the condition is worsening.

40.1.2.2 - Management and Evaluation of a Patient Care Plan
(Rev. 179, Issued: 01-14-14, Effective: 01-07-14, Implementation: 01-07-14)
A3-3118.1.B.2, HHA-205.1.B.2

Skilled nursing visits for management and evaluation of the patient's care plan are also reasonable and necessary where underlying conditions or complications require that only a registered nurse can ensure that essential unskilled care is achieving its purpose. For skilled nursing care to be reasonable and necessary for management and evaluation of the patient's plan of care, the complexity of the necessary unskilled services that are a necessary part of the medical treatment must require the involvement of skilled nursing personnel to promote the patient's recovery and medical safety in view of the patient's overall condition.

EXAMPLE 1:

An aged patient with a history of diabetes mellitus and angina pectoris is recovering from an open reduction of the neck of the femur. He requires, among other services, careful skin care, appropriate oral medications, a diabetic diet, a therapeutic exercise program to preserve muscle tone and body condition, and observation to notice signs of deterioration in his condition or complications resulting from his restricted, but increasing mobility. Although a properly instructed person could perform any of the required services, that person would not have the capability to understand the relationship among the services and their effect on each other. Since the combination of the patient's condition, age, and immobility create a high potential for serious complications, such an understanding is essential to ensure the patient's recovery and safety. The management of this plan of care requires skilled nursing personnel until nursing visits are not needed to observe and assess the effects of the non-skilled services being provided to treat the illness or injury until the patient recovers. Where nursing visits are not needed to observe and assess the effects of the non-skilled services being provided to treat the illness or injury, skilled nursing care would not be considered reasonable and necessary, and the management and evaluation of the care plan would not be considered a skilled service.

EXAMPLE 2:

An aged patient with a history of mild dementia is recovering from pneumonia which has been treated at home. The patient has had an increase in disorientation, has residual chest congestion, decreased appetite, and has remained in bed, immobile, throughout the episode with pneumonia. While the residual chest congestion and recovery from pneumonia alone would not represent a high risk factor, the patient's immobility and increase in confusion could create a high probability of a relapse. In this situation, skilled oversight of the unskilled services would be reasonable and necessary pending the elimination of the chest congestion and resolution of the persistent disorientation to ensure the patient's medical safety. For this determination to be made, the home health documentation must describe the complexity of the unskilled services that are a necessary part of the medical treatment and which require the involvement of a registered nurse in order to ensure that essential unskilled care is achieving its purpose. Where visits by a licensed nurse are not needed to observe and assess the effects of the unskilled services being provided to treat the illness or injury, skilled nursing care would not be considered reasonable and necessary to treat the illness or injury.

EXAMPLE 3:

A physician orders one skilled nursing visit every 2 weeks and three home health aide visits each week for bathing and washing hair for a patient whose recovery from a CVA has left him with residual weakness on the left side. The cardiovascular condition is stable and the patient has reached the maximum restoration potential. There are no underlying conditions that would necessitate the skilled supervision of a licensed nurse in assisting with bathing or hair washing. The skilled nursing visits are not necessary to manage and supervise the home health aide services and would not be covered.

40.1.2.3 - Teaching and Training Activities
(Rev. 179, Issued: 01-14-14, Effective: 01-07-14, Implementation: 01-07-14)
A3-3118.1.B.3, HHA-205.1.B.3

Teaching and training activities that require skilled nursing personnel to teach a patient, the patient's family, or caregivers how to manage the treatment regimen would constitute skilled nursing services. Where the teaching or training is reasonable and necessary to the treatment of the illness or injury, skilled nursing visits for teaching would be covered. The test of whether a nursing service is skilled relates to the skill required to teach and not to the nature of what is being taught. Therefore, where skilled nursing services are necessary to teach an unskilled service, the teaching may be covered. Skilled nursing visits for teaching and training activities are reasonable and necessary where the teaching or training is appropriate to the patient's functional loss, illness, or injury.

Where it becomes apparent after a reasonable period of time that the patient, family, or caregiver will not or is not able to be trained, then further teaching and training would cease to be reasonable and necessary. **The reason why the training was unsuccessful should be documented in the record.** Notwithstanding that the teaching or training was unsuccessful, the services for teaching and training would be considered to be reasonable and necessary prior to the point that it became apparent that the teaching or training was unsuccessful, as long as such services were appropriate to the patient's illness, functional loss, or injury.

In determining the reasonable and necessary number of teaching and training visits, consideration must be given to whether the teaching and training provided constitutes reinforcement of teaching provided previously in an institutional setting or in the home or whether it represents initial instruction. Where the teaching represents initial instruction, the complexity of the activity to be taught and the unique abilities of the patient are to be considered. Where the teaching constitutes reinforcement, an analysis of the patient's retained knowledge and anticipated learning progress is necessary to determine the appropriate number of visits. Skills taught in a controlled institutional setting often need to be reinforced when the patient returns home. Where the patient needs reinforcement of the institutional teaching, additional teaching visits in the home are covered.

Re-teaching or retraining for an appropriate period may be considered reasonable and necessary where there is a change in the procedure or the patient's condition that requires re-teaching, or where the patient, family, or caregiver is not properly carrying out the task. The medical record should document the reason that the re-teaching or retraining is required and the patient/caregiver response to the education.

EXAMPLE 1:

A physician has ordered skilled nursing care for teaching a diabetic who has recently become insulin dependent. The physician has ordered teaching of self-injection and management of insulin, signs, and symptoms of insulin shock, and actions to take in emergencies. The education is reasonable and necessary to the treatment of the illness or injury, and the teaching services and the patient/caregiver responses must be documented.

EXAMPLE 2:

A physician has ordered skilled nursing care to teach a patient to follow a new medication regimen in which there is a significant probability of adverse drug reactions due to the nature of the drug and the patient's condition, to recognize signs and symptoms of adverse reactions to new medications, and to follow the necessary dietary restrictions. After it becomes apparent that the patient remains unable to take the medications properly, cannot demonstrate awareness of potential adverse reactions, and is not following the necessary dietary restrictions, skilled nursing care for further teaching would not be reasonable and necessary, since the patient has demonstrated an inability to be taught. The documentation must thoroughly describe all efforts that have been made to educate the patient/caregiver, and their responses. The health record should also describe the reason for the failure of the educational attempts.

EXAMPLE 3:

A physician has ordered skilled nursing visits to teach self-administration of insulin to a patient who has been self-injecting insulin for 10 years and there is no change in the patient's physical or mental status that would require re-teaching. The skilled nursing visits would not be considered reasonable and necessary since the patient has a longstanding history of being able to perform the service.

EXAMPLE 4:

A physician has ordered skilled nursing visits to teach self-administration of insulin to a patient who has been self-injecting insulin for 10 years because the patient has recently lost the use of the dominant hand and must be retrained to use the other hand. Skilled nursing visits to re-teach self-administration of the insulin would be reasonable and necessary. The patient's response to teaching must be documented at each home health visit, until the patient has learned how to self-administer.

EXAMPLE 5:

A patient recovering from pneumonia is being sent home requiring I.V. infusion of antibiotics four times per day. The patient's spouse has been shown how to administer the drug during the hospitalization and has been told the signs and symptoms of infection. The physician has ordered home health services for a nurse to teach the administration of the drug and the signs and symptoms requiring immediate medical attention.

EXAMPLE 6:

A spouse who has been taught to perform a dressing change for a post-surgical patient may need to be re-taught wound care if the spouse demonstrates improper performance of wound care. The medical record should document the reason that the re-teaching or retraining is required and the patient/caregiver response to the education.

NOTE: There is no requirement that the patient, family or other caregiver be taught to provide a service if they cannot or choose not to provide the care.

Teaching and training activities that require the skills of a licensed nurse include, but **are not limited to**, the following:

1. Teaching the self-administration of injectable medications, or a complex range of medications;

2. Teaching a newly diagnosed diabetic or caregiver all aspects of diabetes management, including how to prepare and to administer insulin injections, to prepare and follow a diabetic diet, to observe foot-care precautions, and to observe for and understand signs of hyperglycemia and hypoglycemia;

3. Teaching self-administration of medical gases;

4. Teaching wound care where the complexity of the wound, the overall condition of the patient or the ability of the caregiver makes teaching necessary;

5. Teaching care for a recent ostomy or where reinforcement of ostomy care is needed;

6. Teaching self-catheterization;

7. Teaching self-administration of gastrostomy or enteral feedings;

8. Teaching care for and maintenance of peripheral and central venous lines and administration of intravenous medications through such lines;

9. Teaching bowel or bladder training when bowel or bladder dysfunction exists;

10. Teaching how to perform the activities of daily living when the patient or caregiver must use special techniques and adaptive devices due to a loss of function;

11. Teaching transfer techniques, e.g., from bed to chair, that are needed for safe transfer;

12. Teaching proper body alignment and positioning, and timing techniques of a bed-bound patient;

13. Teaching ambulation with prescribed assistive devices (such as crutches, walker, cane, etc.) that are needed due to a recent functional loss;

14. Teaching prosthesis care and gait training;

15. Teaching the use and care of braces, splints and orthotics and associated skin care;

16. Teaching the preparation and maintenance of a therapeutic diet; and

17. Teaching proper administration of oral medication, including signs of side-effects and avoidance of interaction with other medications and food.

18. Teaching the proper care and application of any special dressings or skin treatments, (for example, dressings or treatments needed by patients with severe or widespread fungal infections, active and severe psoriasis or eczema, or due to skin deterioration due to radiation treatments)

40.1.2.4 - Administration of Medications
(Rev. 1, 10-01-03)
A3-3118.1.B.4, HHA-205.1.B.4

Although drugs and biologicals are specifically excluded from coverage by the statute (§1861(m)(5) of the Act, the services of a nurse that are required to administer the medications safely and effectively may be covered if they are reasonable and necessary to the treatment of the illness or injury.

A. Injections

Intravenous, intramuscular, or subcutaneous injections and infusions, and hypodermoclysis or intravenous feedings require the skills of a licensed nurse to be performed (or taught) safely and effectively. Where these services are reasonable and necessary to treat the illness or injury, they may be covered. For these services to be reasonable and necessary, the medication being administered must be accepted as safe and effective treatment of the patient's illness or injury, and there must be a medical

351

reason that the medication cannot be taken orally. Moreover, the frequency and duration of the administration of the medication must be within accepted standards of medical practice, or there must be a valid explanation regarding the extenuating circumstances to justify the need for the additional injections.

1. Vitamin B-12 injections are considered specific therapy only for the following conditions:

- Specified anemias: pernicious anemia, megaloblastic anemias, macrocytic anemias, fish tapeworm anemia;

- Specified gastrointestinal disorders: gastrectomy, malabsorption syndromes such as sprue and idiopathic steatorrhea, surgical and mechanical disorders such as resection of the small intestine, strictures, anastomosis and blind loop syndrome, and

- Certain neuropathies: posterolateral sclerosis, other neuropathies associated with pernicious anemia, during the acute phase or acute exacerbation of a neuropathy due to malnutrition and alcoholism.

For a patient with pernicious anemia caused by a B-12 deficiency, intramuscular or subcutaneous injection of vitamin B-12 at a dose of from 100 to 1000 micrograms no more frequently than once monthly is the accepted reasonable and necessary dosage schedule for maintenance treatment. More frequent injections would be appropriate in the initial or acute phase of the disease until it has been determined through laboratory tests that the patient can be sustained on a maintenance dose.

2. Insulin Injections

Insulin is customarily self-injected by patients or is injected by their families. However, where a patient is either physically or mentally unable to self-inject insulin and there is no other person who is able and willing to inject the patient, the injections would be considered a reasonable and necessary skilled nursing service.

EXAMPLE: A patient who requires an injection of insulin once per day for treatment of diabetes mellitus, also has multiple sclerosis with loss of muscle control in the arms and hands, occasional tremors, and vision loss that causes inability to fill syringes or self-inject insulin. If there weren't an able and willing caregiver to inject her insulin, skilled nursing care would be reasonable and necessary for the injection of the insulin.

The prefilling of syringes with insulin (or other medication that is self-injected) does not require the skills of a licensed nurse and, therefore, is not considered to be a skilled nursing service. If the patient needs someone only to prefill syringes (and therefore needs no skilled nursing care on an intermittent basis, physical therapy, or speech-language pathology services), the patient, therefore, does not qualify for any Medicare coverage of home health care. Prefilling of syringes for self-administration of insulin or other medications is considered to be assistance with medications that are ordinarily self-administered and is an appropriate home health aide service. (See §50.2.) However, where State law requires that a licensed nurse prefill syringes, a skilled nursing visit to prefill syringes is paid as a skilled nursing visit (if the patient otherwise needs skilled nursing care, physical therapy, or speech-language pathology services), but is not considered to be a skilled nursing service.

B. Oral Medications

The administration of oral medications by a nurse is not reasonable and necessary skilled nursing care except in the specific situation in which the complexity of the patient's condition, the nature of the drugs prescribed, and the number of drugs prescribed require the skills of a licensed nurse to detect and evaluate side effects or reactions. The medical record must document the specific circumstances that cause administration of an oral medication to require skilled observation and assessment.

C. Eye Drops and Topical Ointments

The administration of eye drops and topical ointments does not require the skills of a nurse. Therefore, even if the administration of eye drops or ointments is necessary to the treatment of an illness or injury and the patient cannot self-administer the drops, and there is no one available to administer them, the visits cannot be covered as a skilled nursing service. This section does not eliminate coverage for skilled nursing visits for observation and assessment of the patient's condition. (See §40.2.1.)

EXAMPLE 1:

A physician has ordered skilled nursing visits to administer eye drops and ointments for a patient with glaucoma. The administration of eye drops and ointments does not require the skills of a nurse. Therefore, the skilled nursing visits cannot be covered as skilled nursing care, notwithstanding the importance of the administration of the drops as ordered.

EXAMPLE 2:

A physician has ordered skilled nursing visits for a patient with a reddened area under the breast. The physician instructs the patient to wash, rinse, and dry the area daily and apply vitamin A and D ointment. Skilled nursing care is not needed to provide this treatment and related services safely and effectively.

40.1.2.5 - Tube Feedings
(Rev. 1, 10-01-03)
A3-3118.1.B.5, HHA-205.1.B.5

Nasogastric tube, and percutaneous tube feedings (including gastrostomy and jejunostomy tubes), and replacement, adjustment, stabilization. and suctioning of the tubes are skilled nursing services, and if the feedings are required to treat the patient's illness or injury, the feedings and replacement or adjustment of the tubes would be covered as skilled nursing services.

40.1.2.6 - Nasopharyngeal and Tracheostomy Aspiration
(Rev. 1, 10-01-03)
A3-4118.1.B.6, HHA-205.1.B.6

Nasopharyngeal and tracheostomy aspiration are skilled nursing services and, if required to treat the patient's illness or injury, would be covered as skilled nursing services.

40.1.2.7 - Catheters
(Rev. 179, Issued: 01-14-14, Effective: 01-07-14, Implementation: 01-07-14)
A3-3118.1.B.7, HHA-205.1.B.7

Insertion and sterile irrigation and replacement of catheters, care of a suprapubic catheter, and in selected patients, urethral catheters, are considered to be skilled nursing services. Where the catheter is necessitated by a permanent or temporary loss of bladder control, skilled nursing services that are provided at a frequency appropriate to the type of catheter in use would be considered reasonable and necessary. Absent complications, Foley catheters generally require skilled care once approximately every 30 days and silicone catheters generally require skilled care once every 60-90 days and this frequency of service would be considered reasonable and necessary. However, where there are complications that require more frequent skilled care related to the catheter, such care would, with adequate documentation, be covered.

EXAMPLE: A patient who has a Foley catheter due to loss of bladder control because of multiple sclerosis has a history of frequent plugging of the catheter and urinary tract infections. The physician has ordered skilled nursing visits once per month to change the catheter, and has left a "PRN" order for up to three additional visits per month for skilled observation and evaluation and/or catheter changes if the patient or caregiver reports signs and symptoms of a urinary tract infection or a plugged catheter. During the certification period, the patient's family contacts the HHA because the patient has an elevated temperature, abdominal pain, and scant urine output. The nurse visits the patient and determines that the catheter is plugged and there are symptoms of a urinary tract infection. The nurse changes the catheter and contacts the physician to report findings and discuss treatment. The skilled nursing visit to change the catheter and to evaluate the patient would be reasonable and necessary to the treatment of the illness or injury. The need for the skilled services must be documented.

40.1.2.8 - Wound Care
(Rev. 179, Issued: 01-14-14, Effective: 01-07-14, Implementation: 01-07-14)
A3-3118.1.B.8, HHA-205.1.B.8

Care of wounds, (including, but not limited to, ulcers, burns, pressure sores, open surgical sites, fistulas, tube sites, and tumor erosion sites) when the skills of a licensed nurse are needed to provide safely and effectively the services necessary to treat the illness or injury, is considered to be a skilled nursing service. For skilled nursing care to be reasonable and necessary to treat a wound, the size, depth, nature of drainage (color, odor, consistency, and quantity), and condition and appearance of the skin surrounding the wound must be documented in the clinical findings so that an assessment of the need for skilled nursing care can be made. Coverage or denial of skilled nursing visits for wound care may not be based solely on the stage classification of the wound, but rather must be based on all of the documented clinical findings. Moreover, the plan of care must contain the specific instructions for the treatment of the wound. Where the physician has ordered appropriate active treatment (e.g., sterile or complex dressings, administration of prescription medications, etc.) of wounds with the following characteristics, the skills of a licensed nurse are usually reasonable and necessary:

- Open wounds which are draining purulent or colored exudate or have a foul odor present or for which the patient is receiving antibiotic therapy;

- Wounds with a drain or T-tube with requires shortening or movement of such drains;

- Wounds which require irrigation or instillation of a sterile cleansing or medicated solution into several layers of tissue and skin and/or packing with sterile gauze;

- Recently debrided ulcers;

- Pressure sores (decubitus ulcers) with the following characteristics:

  o There is partial tissue loss with signs of infection such as foul odor or purulent drainage; or

  o There is full thickness tissue loss that involves exposure of fat or invasion of other tissue such as muscle or bone.

  NOTE: Wounds or ulcers that show redness, edema, and induration, at times with epidermal blistering or desquamation do not ordinarily require skilled nursing care.

- Wounds with exposed internal vessels or a mass that may have a proclivity for hemorrhage when a dressing is changed (e.g., post radical neck surgery, cancer of the vulva);

- Open wounds or widespread skin complications following radiation therapy, or which result from immune deficiencies or vascular insufficiencies;

- Post-operative wounds where there are complications such as infection or allergic reaction or where there is an underlying disease that has a reasonable potential to adversely affect healing (e.g., diabetes);

- Third degree burns, and second degree burns where the size of the burn or presence of complications causes skilled nursing care to be needed;

- Skin conditions that require application of nitrogen mustard or other chemotherapeutic medication that present a significant risk to the patient;

- Other open or complex wounds that require treatment that can only be provided safely and effectively by a licensed nurse.

EXAMPLE 1:

A patient has a second-degree burn with full thickness skin damage on the back. The wound is cleansed, followed by an application of Sulfamylon. While the wound requires skilled monitoring for signs and symptoms of infection or complications, the dressing change requires skilled nursing services. The home health record at each visit must document the need for the skilled nursing services.

EXAMPLE 2:

A patient experiences a decubitus ulcer where the full thickness tissue loss extends through the dermis to involve subcutaneous tissue. The wound involves necrotic tissue with a physician's order to apply a covering of a debriding ointment following vigorous irrigation. The wound is then packed loosely with wet to dry dressings or continuous moist dressing and covered with dry sterile gauze. Skilled nursing care is necessary for proper treatment. The home health record at each visit must document the need for the skilled nursing services.

NOTE: This section relates to the direct, hands on skilled nursing care provided to patients with wounds, including any necessary dressing changes on those wounds. While a wound might not require this skilled nursing care, the wound may still require skilled monitoring for signs and symptoms of infection or complication (See §40.1.2.1) or skilled teaching of wound care to the patient or the patient's family. (See §40.1.2.3.)

40.1.2.9 - Ostomy Care
(Rev. 179, Issued: 01-14-14, Effective: 01-07-14, Implementation: 01-07-14)
A3-3118.1.B.9, HHA-205.1.B.9

Ostomy care during the post-operative period and in the presence of associated complications where the need for skilled nursing care is clearly documented is a skilled nursing service. Teaching ostomy care remains skilled nursing care regardless of the presence of complications. The teaching services and the patient/caregiver responses must be documented.

40.1.2.10 - Heat Treatments
(Rev. 1, 10-01-03)
A3-3118.1.B.10, HHA-205.1.B.10

Heat treatments that have been specifically ordered by a physician as part of active treatment of an illness or injury and require observation by a licensed nurse to adequately evaluate the patient's progress would be considered a skilled nursing service.

40.1.2.11 - Medical Gases
(Rev. 1, 10-01-03)
A3-3118.1.B.11, HHA-205.1.B.11

Initial phases of a regimen involving the administration of medical gases that are necessary to the treatment of the patient's illness or injury, would require skilled nursing care for skilled observation and evaluation of the patient's reaction to the gases, and to teach the patient and family when and how to properly manage the administration of the gases.

40.1.2.12 - Rehabilitation Nursing
(Rev. 1, 10-01-03)
A3-3118.1.B.12, HHA-205.1.B.12

Rehabilitation nursing procedures, including the related teaching and adaptive aspects of nursing that are part of active treatment (e.g., the institution and supervision of bowel and bladder training programs) would constitute skilled nursing services.

40.1.2.13 - Venipuncture
(Rev. 179, Issued: 01-14-14, Effective: 01-07-14, Implementation: 01-07-14)
A3-3118.1.B.13, HHA-205.1.B.13

Effective February 5, 1998, venipuncture for the purposes of obtaining a blood sample can no longer be the sole reason for Medicare home health eligibility. However, if a beneficiary qualifies for home health eligibility based on a skilled need other than solely venipuncture (e.g., eligibility based on the skilled nursing service of wound care and meets all other Medicare home health eligibility criteria), medically reasonable and necessary venipuncture coverage may continue during the 60-day episode under a home health plan of care.

Sections 1814(a)(2)(C) and 1835(a)(2)(A) of the Act specifically exclude venipuncture, as a basis for qualifying for Medicare home health services if this is the sole skilled service the beneficiary requires. However, the Medicare home health benefit will continue to pay for a blood draw if the beneficiary has a need for another qualified skilled service and meets all home health eligibility criteria. This specific requirement applies to home health services furnished on or after February 5, 1998.

For venipuncture to be reasonable and necessary:

1. The physician order for the venipuncture for a laboratory test should be associated with a specific symptom or diagnosis, or the documentation should clarify the need for the test when it is not diagnosis/illness specific. In addition, the treatment must be recognized (in the Physician's Desk Reference, or other

authoritative source) as being reasonable and necessary to the treatment of the illness or injury for venipuncture and monitoring the treatment must also be reasonable and necessary.

2. The frequency of testing should be consistent with accepted standards of medical practice for continued monitoring of a diagnosis, medical problem, or treatment regimen. Even where the laboratory results are consistently stable, periodic venipuncture may be reasonable and necessary because of the nature of the treatment.

3. The home health record must document the rationale for the blood draw as well as the results.

Examples of reasonable and necessary venipuncture for stabilized patients include, but are not limited to those described below.

a. Captopril may cause side effects such as leukopenia and agranulocytosis and it is standard medical practice to monitor the white blood cell count and differential count on a routine basis (every 3 months) when the results are stable and the patient is asymptomatic.

b. In monitoring phenytoin (e.g., Dilantin) administration, the difference between a therapeutic and a toxic level of phenytoin in the blood is very slight and it is therefore appropriate to monitor the level on a routine basis (every 3 months) when the results are stable and the patient is asymptomatic.

c. Venipuncture for fasting blood sugar (FBS)

   • An unstable insulin dependent or noninsulin dependent diabetic would require FBS more frequently than once per month if ordered by the physician.

   • Where there is a new diagnosis or where there has been a recent exacerbation, but the patient is not unstable, monitoring once per month would be reasonable and necessary.

   • A stable insulin or noninsulin dependent diabetic would require monitoring every 2-3 months.

d. Venipuncture for prothrombin

   • Where the documentation shows that the dosage is being adjusted, monitoring would be reasonable and necessary as ordered by the physician.

- Where the results are stable within the therapeutic ranges, monthly monitoring would be reasonable and necessary.

- Where the results remain within nontherapeutic ranges, there must be specific documentation of the factors that indicate why continued monitoring is reasonable and necessary.

EXAMPLE: A patient with coronary artery disease was hospitalized with atrial fibrillation and subsequently discharged to the HHA with orders for anticoagulation therapy as well as other skilled nursing care. If indicated, monthly venipuncture to report prothrombin (protime) levels to the physician would be reasonable and necessary even though the patient's prothrombin time tests indicate essential stability. The home health record must document the rationale for the blood draw as well as the results.

40.1.2.14 - Student Nurse Visits
(Rev. 179, Issued: 01-14-14, Effective: 01-07-14, Implementation: 01-07-14)
A3-3118.1.B.14, HHA-205.1.B.14

Visits made by a student nurse may be covered as skilled nursing care when the HHA participates in training programs that utilize student nurses enrolled in a school of nursing to perform skilled nursing services in a home setting. To be covered, the services must be reasonable and necessary skilled nursing care and must be performed under the general supervision of a registered or licensed nurse. The supervising nurse need not accompany the student nurse on each visit. All documentation requirements must be fulfilled by student nurses.

40.1.2.15 - Psychiatric Evaluation, Therapy, and Teaching
(Rev. 208, Issued: 04-22-15, Effective: 01-01-15, Implementation: 05-11-15)

The evaluation, psychotherapy, and teaching needed by a patient suffering from a diagnosed psychiatric disorder that requires active treatment by a psychiatrically trained nurse and the costs of the psychiatric nurse's services may be covered as a skilled nursing service. Psychiatrically trained nurses are nurses who have special training and/or experience beyond the standard curriculum required for a registered nurse. The services of the psychiatric nurse are to be provided under a plan of care established and reviewed by a physician.

Because the law precludes agencies that primarily provide care and treatment of mental diseases from participating as HHAs, psychiatric nursing must be furnished by an agency that does not primarily provide care and treatment of mental diseases. If a substantial number of an HHA's patients attend partial hospitalization programs or receive outpatient mental health services, the *Medicare contractor* will verify whether the patients meet the eligibility requirements specified in §30 and whether the HHA is primarily engaged in care and treatment of mental disease.

Services of a psychiatric nurse would not be considered reasonable and necessary to assess or monitor use of psychoactive drugs that are being used for nonpsychiatric diagnoses or to monitor the condition of a patient with a known psychiatric illness who is on treatment but is considered stable. A person on treatment would be considered stable if their symptoms were absent or minimal or if symptoms were present but were relatively stable and did not create a significant disruption in the patient's normal living situation.

EXAMPLE 1:

A patient is homebound for medical conditions, but has a psychiatric condition for which he has been receiving medication. The patient's psychiatric condition has not required a change in medication or hospitalization for over 2 years. During a visit by the nurse, the patient's spouse indicates that the patient is awake and pacing most of the night and has begun ruminating about perceived failures in life. The nurse observes that the patient does not exhibit an appropriate level of hygiene and is dressed inappropriately for the season. The nurse comments to the patient about her observations and tries to solicit information about the patient's general medical condition and mental status. The nurse advises the physician about the patient's general medical condition and the new symptoms and changes in the patient's behavior. The physician orders the nurse to check blood levels of medication used to treat the patient's medical and psychiatric conditions. The physician then orders the psychiatric nursing service to evaluate the patient's mental health and communicate with the physician about whether additional intervention to deal with the patient's symptoms and behaviors is warranted. The home health record at each visit should document the need for the psychiatric skilled nursing services and treatment. The home health record must also reflect the patient/caregiver response to any interventions provided.

EXAMPLE 2:

A patient is homebound after discharge following hip replacement surgery and is receiving skilled therapy services for range of motion exercise and gait training. In the past, the patient had been diagnosed with clinical depression and was successfully stabilized on medication. There has been no change in her symptoms. The fact that the patient is taking an antidepressant does not indicate a need for psychiatric nursing services.

EXAMPLE 3:

A patient was discharged after 2 weeks in a psychiatric hospital with a new diagnosis of major depression. The patient remains withdrawn; in bed most of the day, and refusing to leave home. The patient has a depressed affect and continues to have thoughts of suicide, but is not considered to be suicidal. Psychiatric skilled nursing services are necessary for supportive interventions until antidepressant blood levels are reached and the suicidal thoughts are diminished further, to monitor suicide ideation, ensure medication compliance and patient safety, perform suicidal assessment, and teach crisis management and symptom management to family members. The home health record at each visit should document the need for the psychiatric skilled nursing services and treatment. The home health record must also reflect the patient/caregiver response to any interventions provided.

40.1.3 - Intermittent Skilled Nursing Care
(Rev. 208, Issued: 04-22-15, Effective: 01-01-15, Implementation: 05-11-15)

The law, at §1861(m) of the Act defines intermittent, for the purposes of §§1814(a)(2) and 1835(a)(2)(A), as skilled nursing care that is either provided or needed on fewer than 7 days each week, or less than 8 hours each day for periods of 21 days or less (with extensions in exceptional circumstances when the need for additional care is finite and predictable.)

To meet the requirement for "intermittent" skilled nursing care, a patient must have a medically predictable recurring need for skilled nursing services. In most instances, this definition will be met if a patient requires a skilled nursing service at least once every 60 days. The exception to the intermittent requirement is daily skilled nursing services for diabetics unable to administer their insulin (when there is no able and willing caregiver).

Since the need for "intermittent" skilled nursing care makes the patient eligible for other covered home health services, the *Medicare contractor* should evaluate each claim involving skilled nursing services furnished less frequently than once every 60 days. In such cases, payment should be made only if documentation justifies a recurring need for reasonable, necessary, and medically predictable skilled nursing services. The following are examples of the need for infrequent, yet intermittent, skilled nursing services:

1. The patient with an indwelling **silicone** catheter who generally needs a catheter change only at 90-day intervals;

2. The patient who experiences a fecal impaction (i.e., loss of bowel tone, restrictive mobility, and a breakdown in good health habits) and must receive care to manually relieve the impaction. Although these impactions are likely to recur, it is not possible to pinpoint a specific timeframe; or

3. The blind diabetic who self-injects insulin may have a medically predictable recurring need for a skilled nursing visit at least every 90 days. These visits, for example, would be to observe and determine the need for changes in the level and type of care which have been prescribed thus supplementing the physician's contacts with the patient.

There is a possibility that a physician may order a skilled visit less frequently than once every 60 days for an eligible beneficiary if there exists an extraordinary circumstance of anticipated patient need that is documented in the patient's plan of care in accordance with 42 CFR 409.43(b). A skilled visit frequency of less than once every 60 days would only be covered if it is specifically ordered by a physician in the patient's plan of care and is considered to be a reasonable, necessary, and medically predictable skilled need for the patient in the individual circumstance.

Where the need for "intermittent" skilled nursing visits is medically predictable but a situation arises after the first visit making additional visits unnecessary, e.g., the patient is institutionalized or dies, the one visit would be paid at the wage-adjusted LUPA amount for that discipline type. However, a one-time order; e.g., to give gamma globulin following exposure to hepatitis, would not be considered a need for "intermittent" skilled nursing care since a recurrence of the problem that would require this service is not medically predictable.

Although most patients require services no more frequently than several times a week, Medicare will pay for part-time (as defined in §50.7) medically reasonable and necessary skilled nursing care 7 days a week for a short period of time (2 to 3 weeks). There may also be a few cases involving unusual circumstances where the patient's prognosis indicates the medical need for daily skilled services will extend beyond 3 weeks. As soon as the patient's physician makes this judgment, which usually should be made before the end of the 3-week period, the HHA must forward medical documentation justifying the need for such additional services and include an estimate of how much longer daily skilled services will be required.

A person expected to need more or less full-time skilled nursing care over an extended period of time, i.e., a patient who requires institutionalization, would usually not qualify for home health benefits.

40.2 - Skilled Therapy Services
(Rev. 179, Issued: 01-14-14, Effective: 01-07-14, Implementation: 01-07-14)
A3-3118.2, HHA-205.2

To be covered as skilled therapy, the services must require the skills of a qualified therapist and must be reasonable and necessary for the treatment of the patient's illness or injury as discussed below. Coverage does not turn on the presence or absence of an individual's potential for improvement, but rather on the beneficiary's need for skilled care.

40.2.1 - General Principles Governing Reasonable and Necessary Physical Therapy, Speech-Language Pathology Services, and Occupational Therapy
(Rev. 208, Issued: 04-22-15, Effective: 01-01-15, Implementation: 05-11-15)

The service of a physical therapist, speech-language pathologist, or occupational therapist is a skilled therapy service if the inherent complexity of the service is such that it can be performed safely and/or effectively only by or under the general supervision of a skilled therapist. To be covered, assuming all other eligibility and coverage criteria have been met, the skilled services must also be reasonable and necessary to the treatment of the patient's illness or injury or to the restoration or maintenance of function affected by the patient's illness or injury. It is necessary to determine whether individual therapy services are skilled and whether, in view of the patient's overall condition, skilled management of the services provided is needed.

The development, implementation, management, and evaluation of a patient care plan based on the physician's orders constitute skilled therapy services when, because of the patient's clinical condition, those activities require the specialized skills, knowledge, and judgment of a qualified therapist to ensure the effectiveness of the treatment goals and ensure medical safety. Where the specialized skills, knowledge, and judgment of a therapist are needed to manage and periodically reevaluate the appropriateness of a maintenance program, such services would be covered, even if the skills of a therapist were not needed to carry out the activities performed as part of the maintenance program.

While a patient's particular medical condition is a valid factor in deciding if skilled therapy services are needed, a patient's diagnosis or prognosis should never be the sole factor in deciding that a service is or is not skilled. The key issue is whether the skills of a therapist are needed to treat the illness or injury, or whether the services can be carried out by unskilled personnel.

A service that is ordinarily considered unskilled could be considered a skilled therapy service in cases where there is clear documentation that, because of special medical complications, skilled rehabilitation personnel are required to perform the service. However, the importance of a particular service to a patient or the frequency with which it must be performed does not, by itself, make an unskilled service into a skilled service.

Assuming all other eligibility and coverage criteria have been met, the skilled therapy services must be reasonable and necessary to the treatment of the patient's illness or injury within the context of the patient's unique medical condition. To be considered reasonable and necessary for the treatment of the illness or injury:

a. The services must be consistent with the nature and severity of the illness or injury, the patient's particular medical needs, including the requirement that the amount, frequency, and duration of the services must be reasonable; and

b. The services must be considered, under accepted standards of medical practice, to be specific, safe, and effective treatment for the patient's condition, meeting the standards noted below. The home health record must specify the purpose of the skilled service provided.

To ensure therapy services are effective, at defined points during a course of treatment, for each therapy discipline for which services are provided, a qualified therapist (instead of an assistant) must perform the ordered therapy service. During this visit, the therapist must assess the patient using a method which allows for objective measurement of function and successive comparison of measurements. The therapist must document the measurement results in the clinical record. Specifically:

i.   **Initial Therapy Assessment**

- For each therapy discipline for which services are provided, a qualified therapist (instead of an assistant) must assess the patient's function using a method which objectively measures activities of daily living such as, but not limited to, eating, swallowing, bathing, dressing, toileting, walking, climbing stairs, using assistive devices, and mental and cognitive factors. The measurement results must be documented in the clinical record.

- Where more than one discipline of therapy is being provided, a qualified therapist from each of the disciplines must functionally assess the patient. The therapist must document the measurement results which correspond to the therapist's discipline and care plan goals in the clinical record.

ii. **Reassessment at least every 30 days (performed in conjunction with an ordered therapy service)**

- At least once every 30 days, for each therapy discipline for which services are provided, a qualified therapist (instead of an assistant) must provide the ordered therapy service, functionally reassess the patient, and compare the resultant measurement to prior assessment measurements. The therapist must document in the clinical record the measurement results along with the therapist's determination of the effectiveness of therapy, or lack thereof.

- *For multi-discipline therapy cases, a qualified therapist from each of the disciplines must functionally reassess the patient. The therapist must document the measurement results which correspond to the therapist's discipline and care plan goals in the clinical record.*

- The 30-day clock begins with the first therapy service (of that discipline) and the clock resets with each therapist's visit/assessment/measurement/documentation (of that discipline).

c. Services involving activities for the general welfare of any patient, e.g., general exercises to promote overall fitness or flexibility and activities to provide diversion or general motivation do not constitute skilled therapy. Unskilled individuals without the supervision of a therapist can perform those services.

d. Assuming all other eligibility and coverage requirements have been met, in order for therapy services to be covered, one of the following three conditions must be met:

1. The skills of a qualified therapist are needed to restore patient function:

- To meet this coverage condition, therapy services must be provided with the expectation, based on the assessment made by the physician of the patient's restorative potential that the condition of the patient will improve materially in a reasonable and generally predictable period of time. Improvement is evidenced by objective successive measurements.

- Therapy is not considered reasonable and necessary under this condition if the patient's expected restorative potential would be insignificant in relation to the extent and duration of therapy services required to reach such potential.

- Therapy is not required to effect improvement or restoration of function where a patient suffers a transient or easily reversible loss of function (such as temporary weakness following surgery) which could reasonably be expected to improve spontaneously as the patient gradually resumes normal activities. Therapy in such cases is not considered reasonable and necessary to treat the patient's illness or injury, under this condition. However, if the criteria for maintenance therapy described in (3) below is met, therapy could be covered under that condition.

2. The patient's clinical condition requires the specialized skills, knowledge, and judgment of a qualified therapist to establish or design a maintenance program, related to the patient's illness or injury, in order to ensure the safety of the patient and the effectiveness of the program, to the extent provided by regulation,

    - For patients receiving rehabilitative/restorative therapy services, if the specialized skills, knowledge, and judgment of a qualified therapist are required to develop a maintenance program, the expectation is that the development of that maintenance program would occur during the last visit(s) for rehabilitative/restorative treatment. The goals of a maintenance program would be to maintain the patient's current functional status or to prevent or slow further deterioration.

    - Necessary periodic reevaluations by a qualified therapist of the beneficiary and maintenance program are covered if the specialized skills, knowledge, and judgment of a qualified therapist are required.

    - Where a maintenance program is not established until after the rehabilitative/restorative therapy program has been completed, or where there was no rehabilitative/restorative therapy program, and the specialized skills, knowledge, and judgment of a qualified therapist are required to develop a maintenance program, such services would be considered reasonable and necessary for the treatment of the patient's condition in order to ensure the effectiveness of the treatment goals and ensure medical safety. When the development of a maintenance program could not be accomplished during the last visits(s) of rehabilitative/restorative treatment, the therapist must document why the maintenance program could not be developed during those last rehabilitative/restorative treatment visit(s).

    - When designing or establishing a maintenance program, the qualified therapist must teach the patient or the patient's family or caregiver's necessary techniques, exercises or precautions as necessary to treat the illness or injury. The instruction of the beneficiary or appropriate caregiver by a qualified therapist regarding a maintenance program is covered if the specialized skills, knowledge, and judgment of a qualified therapist are required. However, visits made by skilled therapists to a patient's home solely to train other HHA staff (e.g., home health aides) are not billable as visits since the HHA is responsible for ensuring that its staff is properly trained to perform any service it furnishes. The cost of a skilled therapist's visit for the purpose of training HHA staff is an administrative cost to the agency.

3. The skills of a qualified therapist (not an assistant) are needed to perform maintenance therapy:

- Coverage of therapy services to perform a maintenance program is not determined solely on the presence or absence of a beneficiary's potential for improvement from the therapy, but rather on the beneficiary's need for skilled care. Assuming all other eligibility and coverage requirements are met, skilled therapy services are covered when an individualized assessment of the patient's clinical condition demonstrates that the specialized judgment, knowledge, and skills of a qualified therapist ("skilled care") are necessary for the performance of a safe and effective maintenance program. Such a maintenance program to maintain the patient's current condition or to prevent or slow further deterioration is covered so long as the beneficiary requires skilled care for the safe and effective performance of the program. When, however, the individualized assessment does not demonstrate such a necessity for skilled care, including when the performance of a maintenance program does not require the skills of a therapist because it could safely and effectively be accomplished by the patient or with the assistance of non-therapists, including unskilled caregivers, such maintenance services will not be covered.

- Further, under the standard set forth in the previous paragraph, skilled care is necessary for the performance of a safe and effective maintenance program only when (a) the particular patient's special medical complications require the skills of a qualified therapist to perform a therapy service that would otherwise be considered non-skilled; or (b) the needed therapy procedures are of such complexity that the skills of a qualified therapist are required to perform the procedure.

e. The amount, frequency, and duration of the services must be reasonable.

As is outlined in home health regulations, as part of the home health agency (HHA) Conditions of Participation (CoPs), the clinical record of the patient must contain progress and clinical notes. Additionally, in Pub. 100-04, Medicare Claims Processing Manual, Chapter 10; "Home Health Agency Billing", instructions specify that for each claim, HHAs are required to report all services provided to the beneficiary during each episode, this includes reporting each visit in line-item detail. As such, it is expected that the home health records for every visit will reflect the need for the skilled medical care provided. These clinical notes are also expected to provide important communication among all members of the home care team regarding the development, course and outcomes of the skilled observations, assessments, treatment and training performed. Taken as a whole then, the clinical notes are expected to tell the story of the patient's achievement towards his/her goals as outlined in the Plan of Care. In this way, the notes will serve to demonstrate why a skilled service is needed.

Therefore the home health clinical notes must document as appropriate:

- the history and physical exam pertinent to the day's visit , (including the response or changes in behavior to previously administered skilled services) and

- the skilled services applied on the current visit, and

- the patient/caregiver's immediate response to the skilled services provided, and

- the plan for the next visit based on the rationale of prior results.

Clinical notes should be written such that they adequately describe the reaction of a patient to his/her skilled care. Clinical notes should also provide a clear picture of the treatment, as well as "next steps" to be taken. Vague or subjective descriptions of the patient's care should not be used. For example terminology such as the following would not adequately describe the need for skilled care:

- Patient tolerated treatment well
- Caregiver instructed in medication management
- Continue with POC

Objective measurements of physical outcomes of treatment should be provided and/or a clear description of the changed behaviors due to education programs should be recorded in order that all concerned can follow the results of the applied services.

When the skilled service is being provided to either maintain the patient's condition or prevent or slow further deterioration, the clinical notes must also describe:

- A detailed rationale that explains the need for the skilled service in light of the patient's overall medical condition and experiences,

- the complexity of the service to be performed, and

- any other pertinent characteristics of the beneficiary or home.

40.2.2 - Application of the Principles to Physical Therapy Services
(Rev. 179, Issued: 01-14-14, Effective: 01-07-14, Implementation: 01-07-14)

The following discussion of skilled physical therapy services applies the principles in §40.2.1 to specific physical therapy services about which questions are most frequently raised.

A. Assessment

Assuming all other eligibility and coverage requirements have been met, the skills of a physical therapist to assess and periodically reassess a patient's rehabilitation needs and potential or to develop and/or implement a physical therapy program are covered when they are reasonable and necessary because of the patient's condition. Skilled rehabilitation services concurrent with the management of a patient's care plan include objective tests and measurements such as, but not limited to, range of motion, strength, balance, coordination, endurance, or functional ability.

As described in section 40.2.1(b), at defined points during a course of therapy, the qualified physical therapist (instead of an assistant) must perform the ordered therapy service visit, assess the patient's function using a method which allows for objective measurement of function and comparison of successive measurements, and document the results of the assessments, corresponding measurements, and effectiveness of the therapy in the patient's clinical record. Refer to §40.2.1(b) for specific timing and documentation requirements associated with these requirements.

B. Therapeutic Exercises

Therapeutic exercises, which require the skills of a qualified physical therapist to ensure the safety of the beneficiary and the effectiveness of the treatment constitute skilled physical therapy, when the criteria in §40.2.1(d) above are met.

C. Gait Training

Gait evaluation and training furnished to a patient whose ability to walk has been impaired by neurological, muscular or skeletal abnormality require the skills of a qualified physical therapist and constitute skilled physical therapy and are considered reasonable and necessary if they can be expected to materially improve or maintain the patient's ability to walk or prevent or slow further deterioration of the patient's ability to walk. Gait evaluation and training which is furnished to a patient whose ability to walk has been impaired by a condition other than a neurological, muscular, or skeletal abnormality would nevertheless be covered where physical therapy is reasonable and necessary to restore or maintain function or to prevent or slow further deterioration. Refer to §40.2.1(d)(1) for the reasonable and necessary coverage criteria associated with restoring patient function.

EXAMPLE 1:

A physician has ordered gait evaluation and training for a patient whose gait has been materially impaired by scar tissue resulting from burns. Physical therapy services to evaluate the beneficiary's gait, establish a gait training program, and provide the skilled services necessary to implement the program would be covered. The patient's response to therapy must be documented. At appropriate intervals (see above), the qualified therapist must assess the patient with objective measurements of function.

EXAMPLE 2:

A patient who has had a total hip replacement is ambulatory but demonstrates weakness and is unable to climb stairs safely. Physical therapy would be reasonable and necessary to teach the patient to climb and descend stairs safely. Once the patient has reached the goal of climbing and descending stairs safely, additional therapy services are no longer required, and thus would not be covered.

EXAMPLE 3:

A patient who has received gait training has reached their maximum restoration potential, and the physical therapist is teaching the patient and family how to safely perform the activities that are a part of the maintenance program. The visits by the physical therapist to demonstrate and teach the activities (which by themselves do not require the skills of a therapist) would be covered since they are needed to establish the program (refer to §40.2.1(d)(2)). The patient's and caregiver's understanding and implementation of the maintenance program must be documented. After the establishment of the maintenance program, any further visits would need to document why the skilled services of a physical therapist are still required.

D. Range of Motion

Only a qualified physical therapist may perform range of motion tests and, therefore, such tests are skilled physical therapy.

Range of motion exercises constitute skilled physical therapy only if they are part of an active treatment for a specific disease state, illness, or injury that has resulted in a loss or restriction of mobility (as evidenced by physical therapy notes showing the degree of motion lost and the degree to be restored). Unskilled individuals may provide range of motion exercises unrelated to the restoration of a specific loss of function often safely and effectively. Passive exercises to maintain range of motion in paralyzed extremities that can be carried out by unskilled persons do not constitute skilled physical therapy.

However, if the criteria in §40.2.1(d)(3) are met, where there is clear documentation that, because of special medical complications (e.g., susceptible to pathological bone fractures), the skills of a therapist are needed to provide services which ordinarily do not need the skills of a therapist, and then the services would be covered.

E. Maintenance Therapy

Where services that are required to maintain the patient's current function or to prevent or slow further deterioration are of such complexity and sophistication that the skills of a qualified therapist are required to perform the procedure safely and effectively, the services would be covered physical therapy services. Further, where the particular patient's special medical complications require the skills of a qualified therapist to perform a therapy service safely and effectively that would otherwise be considered unskilled, such services would be covered physical therapy services. Refer to §40.2.1(d)(3).

EXAMPLE 4:

Where there is an unhealed, unstable fracture that requires regular exercise to maintain function until the fracture heals, the skills of a physical therapist would be needed to ensure that the fractured extremity is maintained in proper position and alignment during maintenance range of motion exercises.

EXAMPLE 5:

A Parkinson's patient or a patient with rheumatoid arthritis who has not been under a restorative physical therapy program may require the services of a physical therapist to determine what type of exercises are required to maintain the patient's present level of function or to prevent or slow further deterioration. The initial evaluation of the patient's needs, the designing of a maintenance program appropriate to the patient's capacity and tolerance and to the treatment objectives of the physician, the instruction of the patient, family or caregivers to carry out the program safely and effectively, and such reevaluations as may be required by the patient's condition, would constitute skilled physical therapy. Each component of this process must be documented in the home health record.

While a patient is under a restorative physical therapy program, the physical therapist should regularly reevaluate the patient's condition and adjust any exercise program the patient is expected to carry out alone or with the aid of supportive personnel to maintain the function being restored. Consequently, by the time it is determined that no further restoration is possible (i.e., by the end of the last restorative session) the physical therapist will already have designed the maintenance program required and instructed the patient or caregivers in carrying out the program.

F. Ultrasound, Shortwave, and Microwave Diathermy Treatments

These treatments must always be performed by or under the supervision of a qualified physical therapist and are skilled therapy.

G. Hot Packs, Infra-Red Treatments, Paraffin Baths and Whirlpool Baths

Heat treatments and baths of this type ordinarily do not require the skills of a qualified physical therapist. However, the skills, knowledge, and judgment of a qualified physical therapist might be required in the giving of such treatments or baths in a particular case, e.g., where the patient's condition is complicated by circulatory deficiency, areas of desensitization, open wounds, fractures, or other complications. There must be clear documentation in the home health record, of the special medical complications that describe the need for the skilled services provided by the therapist.

H. Wound Care Provided Within Scope of State Practice Acts

If wound care falls within the auspice of a physical therapist's State Practice Act, then the physical therapist may provide the specific type of wound care services defined in the State Practice Act. However, such visits in this specific situation would be a covered therapy service when there is documentation in the home health record that the skills of a therapist are required to perform the service. The patient's response to therapy must be documented.

40.2.3 - Application of the General Principles to Speech-Language Pathology Services
(Rev. 179, Issued: 01-14-14, Effective: 01-07-14, Implementation: 01-07-14)

The following discussion of skilled speech-language pathology services applies the principles to specific speech-language pathology services about which questions are most frequently raised. Coverage of speech-language pathology services is not determined solely on the presence or absence of a beneficiary's potential for improvement from the therapy, but rather on the beneficiary's need for skilled care. Assuming all other eligibility and coverage requirements have been met, skilled speech-language pathology services are covered when the individualized assessment of the patient's clinical condition demonstrates that the specialized judgment, knowledge, and skills of a qualified speech-language pathologist are necessary.

As described in §40.2.1(b), at defined points during a course of therapy, the qualified speech-language pathologist must perform the ordered therapy service visit, assess the patient's function using a method which allows for objective measurement of function and comparison of successive measurements, and document the results of the assessments, corresponding measurements, and effectiveness of therapy in the patient's clinical record. Refer to §40.2.1(b) for specific timing and documentation requirements associated with these requirements.

1. The skills of a speech-language pathologist are required for the assessment of a patient's rehabilitation needs (including the causal factors and the severity of the speech and language disorders), and rehabilitation potential. Reevaluation would be considered reasonable and necessary only if the patient exhibited:

   - A change in functional speech or motivation;

   - Clearing of confusion; or

- The remission of some other medical condition that previously contraindicated speech-language pathology services.

Where a patient is undergoing restorative speech-language pathology services, routine reevaluations are considered to be a part of the therapy and cannot be billed as a separate visit.

2. The services of a speech-language pathologist would be covered if they are needed as a result of an illness or injury and are directed towards specific speech/voice production.

3. Speech-language pathology would be covered where a skilled service can only be provided by a speech-language pathologist and where it is reasonably expected that the skilled service will improve, maintain, or prevent or slow further deterioration in the patient's ability to carry out communication or feeding activities.

4. The services of a speech-language pathologist to establish a hierarchy of speech-voice-language communication tasks and cueing that directs a patient toward speech-language communication goals in the plan of care would be covered speech-language pathology.

5. The services of a speech-language pathologist to train the patient, family, or other caregivers to augment the speech-language communication, treatment, to establish an effective maintenance program, or carry out a safe and effective maintenance program when the particular patient's special medical complications require the skills of a qualified therapist (not an assistant) to perform a therapy service that would otherwise be considered unskilled or the needed therapy procedures are of such complexity that the skills of a qualified therapist are required to perform the procedures, would be covered speech-language pathology services.

6. The services of a speech-language pathologist to assist patients with aphasia in rehabilitation of speech and language skills are covered when needed by a patient.

7. The services of a speech-language pathologist to assist patients with voice disorders to develop proper control of the vocal and respiratory systems for correct voice production are covered when needed by a patient.

40.2.4 - Application of the General Principles to Occupational Therapy
(Rev. 179, Issued: 01-14-14, Effective: 01-07-14, Implementation: 01-07-14)
A3-3118.2.D, HHA-205.2.D

The following discussion of skilled occupational therapy services applies the principles to specific occupational therapy services about which questions are most frequently raised. Coverage of occupational therapy services is not determined solely on the presence or absence of a beneficiary's potential for improvement from the therapy, but rather on the beneficiary's need for skilled care. Assuming all other eligibility and coverage requirements have been met, skilled occupational therapy services are covered when the individualized assessment of the patient's clinical condition demonstrates that the specialized judgment, knowledge, and skills of a qualified occupational therapist are necessary.

40.2.4.1 - Assessment
(Rev. 179, Issued: 01-14-14, Effective: 01-07-14, Implementation: 01-07-14)

Assuming all other eligibility and coverage requirements are met, the skills of an occupational therapist to assess and reassess a patient's rehabilitation needs and potential or to develop and/or implement an occupational therapy program are covered when they are reasonable and necessary because of the patient's condition.

As described in §40.2.1(b), at defined points during a course of therapy, the qualified occupational therapist (instead of an assistant) must perform the ordered therapy service visit, assess the patient's function using a method which allows for objective measurement of function and comparison of successive measurements, and document the results of the assessments, corresponding measurements, and effectiveness of therapy in the patient's clinical record. Refer to §40.2.1(b) for specific timing and documentation requirements associated with these requirements.

40.2.4.2 - Planning, Implementing, and Supervision of Therapeutic Programs
(Rev. 1, 10-01-03)
A3-3118.2.D.2, HHA-205.2.D.2

The planning, implementing, and supervision of therapeutic programs including, but not limited to those listed below are skilled occupational therapy services, and if reasonable and necessary to the treatment of the patient's illness or injury would be covered.

A. Selecting and Teaching Task Oriented Therapeutic Activities Designed to Restore Physical Function.

EXAMPLE: Use of woodworking activities on an inclined table to restore shoulder, elbow, and wrist range of motion lost as a result of burns.

B. Planning, Implementing, and Supervising Therapeutic Tasks and Activities Designed to Restore Sensory-Integrative Function.

EXAMPLE: Providing motor and tactile activities to increase sensory output and improve response for a stroke patient with functional loss resulting in a distorted body image.

C. Planning, Implementing, and Supervising of Individualized Therapeutic Activity Programs as Part of an Overall "Active Treatment" Program for a Patient With a Diagnosed Psychiatric Illness.

EXAMPLE: Use of sewing activities that require following a pattern to reduce confusion and restore reality orientation in a schizophrenic patient.

D. Teaching Compensatory Techniques to Improve the Level of Independence in the Activities of Daily Living.

EXAMPLE: Teaching a patient who has lost use of an arm how to pare potatoes and chop vegetables with one hand.

EXAMPLE: Teaching a stroke patient new techniques to enable them to perform feeding, dressing, and other activities of daily living as independently as possible.

E. The Designing, Fabricating, and Fitting of Orthotic and Self-Help Devices.

EXAMPLE: Construction of a device which would enable a patient to hold a utensil and feed themselves independently.

EXAMPLE: Construction of a hand splint for a patient with rheumatoid arthritis to maintain the hand in a functional position.

F. Vocational and Prevocational Assessment and Training

Vocational and prevocational assessment and training that is directed toward the restoration of function in the activities of daily living lost due to illness or injury would be covered. Where vocational or prevocational assessment and training is related solely to specific employment opportunities, work skills, or work settings, such services would not be covered because they would not be directed toward the treatment of an illness or injury.

40.2.4.3 - Illustration of Covered Services
(Rev. 179, Issued: 01-14-14, Effective: 01-07-14, Implementation: 01-07-14)
A3-3118.2.D.3, HHA-205.2.D.3

EXAMPLE 1:

A physician orders occupational therapy for a patient who is recovering from a fractured hip and who needs to be taught compensatory and safety techniques with regard to lower extremity dressing, hygiene, toileting, and bathing. The occupational therapist will establish goals for the patient's rehabilitation (to be approved by the physician), and will undertake teaching techniques necessary for the patient to reach the goals. Occupational therapy services would be covered at a duration and intensity appropriate to the severity of the impairment and the patient's response to treatment. Such visits would be considered covered when the skills of a therapist are required to perform the services. The patient's needs in response to therapy must be documented.

EXAMPLE 2:

A physician has ordered occupational therapy for a patient who is recovering from a CVA. The patient has decreased range of motion, strength, and sensation in both the upper and lower extremities on the right side. In addition, the patient has perceptual and cognitive deficits resulting from the CVA. The patient's condition has resulted in decreased function in activities of daily living (specifically bathing, dressing, grooming, hygiene, and toileting). The loss of function requires assistive devices to enable the patient to compensate for the loss of function and maximize safety and independence. The patient also needs equipment such as himi-slings to prevent shoulder subluxation and a hand splint to prevent joint contracture and deformity in the right hand. The services of an occupational therapist would be necessary to:

- Assess the patient's needs;

- Develop goals (to be approved by the physician);

- Manufacture or adapt the needed equipment to the patient's use;

- Teach compensatory techniques;

- Strengthen the patient as necessary to permit use of compensatory techniques; and

- Provide activities that are directed towards meeting the goals governing increased perceptual and cognitive function.

Occupational therapy services would be covered at a duration and intensity appropriate to the severity of the impairment and the patient's response to treatment. Such visits would be considered covered therapy services when the skills of a therapist are required to perform the services. The patient's needs, course of therapy and response to therapy must be documented.

50 - Coverage of Other Home Health Services
(Rev. 1, 10-01-03)
A3-3119, HHA-206

50.1 - Skilled Nursing, Physical Therapy, Speech-Language Pathology Services, and Occupational Therapy
(Rev. 1, 10-01-03)
A3-3119.1, HHA-206.1

Where the patient meets the qualifying criteria in §30, Medicare covers skilled nursing services that meet the requirements of §§40.1 and 50.7, physical therapy that meets the requirements of §40.2, speech-language pathology services that meets the requirements of §40.2, and occupational therapy that meets the requirements of §40.2.

Home health coverage is not available for services furnished to a qualified patient who is no longer in need of one of the qualifying skilled services specified in §30. Therefore, dependent services furnished after the final qualifying skilled service are not covered under the home health benefit, except when the dependent service was followed by a qualifying skilled service as a result of the unexpected inpatient admission or death of the patient or due to some other unanticipated event.

50.2 - Home Health Aide Services
(Rev. 1, 10-01-03)
A3-3119.2, HHA-206.2

For home health aide services to be covered:

- The patient must meet the qualifying criteria as specified in §30;

- The services provided by the home health aide must be part-time or intermittent as discussed in §50.7;

- The services must meet the definition of home health aide services of this section; and

- The services must be reasonable and necessary to the treatment of the patient's illness or injury.

NOTE: A home health aide must be certified consistent the competency evaluation requirements.

The reason for the visits by the home health aide must be to provide hands-on personal care of the patient or services needed to maintain the patient's health or to facilitate treatment of the patient's illness or injury.

The physician's order should indicate the frequency of the home health aide services required by the patient. These services may include but are not limited to:

A. Personal Care

Personal care means:

1. Bathing, dressing, grooming, caring for hair, nail, and oral hygiene which are needed to facilitate treatment or to prevent deterioration of the patient's health, changing the bed linens of an incontinent patient, shaving, deodorant application, skin care with lotions and/or powder, foot care, and ear care; and

2. Feeding, assistance with elimination (including enemas unless the skills of a licensed nurse are required due to the patient's condition, routine catheter care and routine colostomy care), assistance with ambulation, changing position in bed, assistance with transfers.

EXAMPLE 1:

A physician has ordered home health aide visits to assist the patient in personal care because the patient is recovering from a stroke and continues to have significant right side weakness that causes the patient to be unable to bathe, dress or perform hair and oral care. The plan of care established by the HHA nurse sets forth the specific tasks with which the patient needs assistance. Home health aide visits at an appropriate frequency would be reasonable and necessary to assist in these tasks.

EXAMPLE 2:

A physician ordered four home health aide visits per week for personal care for a multiple sclerosis patient who is unable to perform these functions because of increasing debilitation. The home health aide gave the patient a bath twice per week and washed hair on the other two visits each week. Only two visits are reasonable and necessary since the services could have been provided in the course of two visits.

EXAMPLE 3:

A physician ordered seven home health aide visits per week for personal care for a bed-bound, incontinent patient. All visits are reasonable and necessary because the patient has extensive personal care needs.

EXAMPLE 4:

A patient with a well established colostomy forgets to change the bag regularly and has difficulty changing the bag. Home health aide services at an appropriate frequency to change the bag would be considered reasonable and necessary to the treatment of the illness or injury.

B. Simple Dressing Changes That Do Not Require the Skills of a Licensed Nurse
EXAMPLE 5:

A patient who is confined to the bed has developed a small reddened area on the buttocks. The physician has ordered home health aide visits for more frequent repositioning, bathing and the application of a topical ointment and a gauze 4x4. Home health aide visits at an appropriate frequency would be reasonable and necessary.

C. Assistance With Medications Which Are Ordinarily Self-Administered and Do Not Require the Skills of a Licensed Nurse to Be Provided Safely and Effectively

NOTE: Prefilling of insulin syringes is ordinarily performed by the diabetic as part of the self-administration of the insulin and, unlike the injection of the insulin, does not require the skill of a licensed nurse to be performed properly. Therefore, if HHA staff performs the prefilling of insulin syringes, it is considered to be a home health aide service. However, where State law precludes the provision of this service by other than a licensed nurse or physician, Medicare will make payment for this service, when covered, as though it were a skilled nursing service. Where the patient needs only prefilling of insulin syringes and does not need skilled nursing care on an intermittent basis, physical therapy, speech-language pathology services, or have a continuing need for occupational therapy, then Medicare cannot cover any home health services to the patient (even if State law requires that the insulin syringes be filled by a licensed nurse).

Home health aide services are those services ordered in the plan of care that the aide is permitted to perform under State law. Medicare coverage of the administration of insulin by a home health aide will depend on whether or not the agency is in compliance with all Federal and State laws and regulations related to this task. However, when the task of insulin administration has been delegated to the home health aide, the task must be considered and billed as a Medicare home health aide service. By a State allowing the delegation of insulin administration to home health aides, the State has extended the role of aides, not equated aide services with the services of a registered nurse.

D. Assistance With Activities which Are Directly Supportive of Skilled Therapy Services but Do Not Require the Skills of a Therapist to Be Safely and Effectively Performed Such as Routine Maintenance Exercises and Repetitive Practice of Functional Communication Skills to Support Speech-Language Pathology Services

E. Provision of Services Incidental to Personal Care Services not Care of Prosthetic and Orthotic Devices

When a home health aide visits a patient to provide a health related service as discussed above, the home health aide may also perform some incidental services which do not meet the definition of a home health aide service (e.g., light cleaning, preparation of a meal, taking out the trash, shopping, etc.) However, the purpose of a home health aide visit may not be to provide these incidental services since they are not health related services, but rather are necessary household tasks that must be performed by anyone to maintain a home.

EXAMPLE 1:

A home health aide visits a recovering stroke patient whose right side weakness and poor endurance cause her to be able to leave the bed and chair only with extreme difficulty. The physician has ordered physical therapy and speech-language pathology services for the patient and home health aide services three or four times per week for personal care, assistance with ambulation as mobility increases, and assistance with repetitive speech exercises as her impaired speech improves. The home health aide also provides incidental household services such as preparation of meals, light cleaning and taking out the trash. The patient lives with an elderly frail sister who is disabled and who cannot perform either the personal care or the incidental tasks. The home health aide visits at a frequency appropriate to the performance of the health related services would be covered, notwithstanding the incidental provision of noncovered services (i.e., the household services) in the course of the visits.

EXAMPLE 2:

A physician orders home health aide visits three times per week. The only services provided are light housecleaning, meal preparation and trash removal. The home health aide visits cannot be covered, notwithstanding their importance to the patient, because the services provided do not meet Medicare's definition of "home health aide services."

50.3 - Medical Social Services
(Rev. 1, 10-01-03)
A3-3119.3, HHA-206.3

Medical social services that are provided by a qualified medical social worker or a social work assistant under the supervision of a qualified medical social worker may be covered as home health services where the beneficiary meets the qualifying criteria specified in §30, and:

1. The services of these professionals are necessary to resolve social or emotional problems that are or are expected to be an impediment to the effective treatment of the patient's medical condition or rate of recovery; and

2. The plan of care indicates how the services which are required necessitate the skills of a qualified social worker or a social work assistant under the supervision of a qualified medical social worker to be performed safely and effectively.

Where both of these requirements for coverage are met, services of these professionals which may be covered include, but are not limited to:

1. Assessment of the social and emotional factors related to the patient's illness, need for care, response to treatment and adjustment to care;

2. Assessment of the relationship of the patient's medical and nursing requirements to the patient's home situation, financial resources and availability of community resources;

3. Appropriate action to obtain available community resources to assist in resolving the patient's problem (**NOTE:** Medicare does not cover the services of a medical social worker to complete or assist in the completion of an application for Medicaid because Federal regulations require the State to provide assistance in completing the application to anyone who chooses to apply for Medicaid.);

4. Counseling services that are required by the patient; and

5. Medical social services furnished to the patient's family member or caregiver on a short-term basis when the HHA can demonstrate that a brief intervention (that is, two or three visits) by a medical social worker is necessary to remove a clear and direct impediment to the effective treatment of the patient's medical condition or to the patient's rate of recovery. To be considered "clear and direct," the behavior or actions of the family member or caregiver must plainly obstruct, contravene, or prevent the patient's medical treatment or rate of recovery. Medical social

services to address general problems that do not clearly and directly impede treatment or recovery as well as long-term social services furnished to family members, such as ongoing alcohol counseling, are not covered.

NOTE: Participating in the development of the plan of care, preparing clinical and progress notes, participating in discharge planning and in-service programs, and acting as a consultant to other agency personnel are appropriate administrative costs to the HHA.

EXAMPLE 1:

The physician has ordered a medical social worker assessment of a diabetic patient who has recently become insulin dependent and is not yet stabilized. The nurse, who is providing skilled observation and evaluation to try to restabilize the patient notices during her visits that the supplies left in the home for the patient's use appear to be frequently missing, and the patient is not compliant with the regimen although she refuses to discuss the matter. The assessment by a medical social worker would be reasonable and necessary to determine if there are underlying social or emotional problems impeding the patient's treatment.

EXAMPLE 2:

A physician ordered an assessment by a medical social worker for a multiple sclerosis patient who was unable to move anything but her head and who had an indwelling catheter. The patient had experienced recurring urinary tract infections and multiple infected ulcers. The physician ordered medical social services after the HHA indicated to him that the home was not well cared for, the patient appeared to be neglected much of the time, and the relationship between the patient and family was very poor. The physician and HHA were concerned that social problems created by family caregivers were impeding the treatment of the recurring infections and ulcers. The assessment and follow-up for counseling both the patient and the family by a medical social worker were reasonable and necessary.

EXAMPLE 3:

A physician is aware that a patient with atherosclerosis and hypertension is not taking medications as ordered and adhering to dietary restrictions because he is unable to afford the medication and is unable to cook. The physician orders several visits by a medical social worker to assist in resolving these problems. The visits by the medical social worker to review the patient's financial status, discuss options, and make appropriate contacts with social services agencies or other community resources to arrange for medications and meals would be a reasonable and necessary medical social service.

EXAMPLE 4:

A physician has ordered counseling by a medical social worker for a patient with cirrhosis of the liver who has recently been discharged from a 28-day inpatient alcohol treatment program to her home which she shares with an alcoholic and neglectful adult child. The physician has ordered counseling several times per week to assist the patient in remaining free of alcohol and in dealing with the adult child. The services of the medical social worker would be covered until the patient's social situation ceased to impact on her recovery and/or treatment.

EXAMPLE 5:

A physician has ordered medical social services for a patient who is worried about his financial arrangements and payment for medical care. The services ordered are to arrange Medicaid if possible and resolve unpaid medical bills. There is no evidence that the patient's concerns are adversely impacting recovery or treatment of his illness or injury. Medical social services cannot be covered.

EXAMPLE 6:

A physician has ordered medical social services for a patient of extremely limited income who has incurred large unpaid hospital and other medical bills following a significant illness. The patient's recovery is adversely affected because the patient is not maintaining a proper therapeutic diet, and cannot leave the home to acquire the medication necessary to treat their illness. The medical social worker reviews the patient's financial status, arranges meal service to resolve the dietary problem, arranges for home delivered medications, gathers the information necessary for application to Medicaid to acquire coverage for the medications the patient needs, files the application on behalf of the patient, and follows up repeatedly with the Medicaid State agency.

The medical social services that are necessary to review the financial status of the patient, arrange for meal service and delivery of medications to the home, and arrange for the Medicaid State agency to assist the patient with the application for Medicaid are covered. The services related to the assistance in filing the application for Medicaid and the follow-up on the application are not covered since they must be provided by the State agency free of charge, and hence the patient has no obligation to pay for such assistance.

EXAMPLE 7:

A physician has ordered medical social services for an insulin dependent diabetic whose blood sugar is elevated because she has run out of syringes and missed her insulin dose for two days. Upon making the assessment visit, the medical social worker learns that the patient's daughter, who is also an insulin dependent diabetic, has come to live with the patient because she is out of work. The daughter is now financially dependent on the patient for all of her financial needs and has been using the patient's insulin syringes. The social worker assesses the patient's financial resources and determines that they are adequate to support the patient and meet her own medical needs, but are not sufficient to support the daughter. She also counsels the daughter and helps her access community resources. These visits would be covered, but only to the extent that the services are necessary to prevent interference with the patient's treatment plan.

EXAMPLE 8:

A wife is caring for her husband who is an Alzheimer's patient. The nurse learns that the wife has not been giving the patient his medication correctly and seems distracted and forgetful about various aspects of the patient's care. In a conversation with the nurse, the wife relates that she is feeling depressed and overwhelmed by the patient's illness. The nurse contacts the patient's physician who orders a social work evaluation. In her assessment visit, the social worker learns that the patient's wife is so distraught over her situation that she cannot provide adequate care to the patient. While there, the social worker counsels the wife and assists her with referrals to a support group and her private physician for evaluation of her depression. The services would be covered.

EXAMPLE 9:

The parent of a dependent disabled child has been discharged from the hospital following a hip replacement. Although arrangements for care of the disabled child during the hospitalization were made, the child has returned to the home. During a visit to the patient, the nurse observes that the patient is transferring the child from bed to a wheelchair. In an effort to avoid impeding the patient's recovery, the nurse contacts the patient's physician to order a visit by a social worker to mobilize family members or otherwise arrange for temporary care of the disabled child. The services would be covered.

50.4 - Medical Supplies (Except for Drugs and Biologicals Other Than Covered Osteoporosis Drugs) and the Use of Durable Medical Equipment
(Rev.26, Issued 11-05-04, Effective: 01-01-05, Implementation: 04-04-05)

50.4.1 - Medical Supplies
(Rev. 1, 10-01-03)
A3-3119.4.A, HHA-206.4.A

Medical supplies are items that, due to their therapeutic or diagnostic characteristics, are essential in enabling HHA personnel to conduct home visits or to carry out effectively the care the physician has ordered for the treatment or diagnosis of the patient's illness or injury. All supplies which would have been covered under the cost-based reimbursement system are bundled under home health PPS. Payment for the cost of supplies has been incorporated into the per visit and episode payment rates. Supplies fit into two categories. They are classified as:

- **Routine** - because they are used in small quantities for patients during the usual course of most home visits; or

- **Nonroutine** - because they are needed to treat a patient's specific illness or injury in accordance with the physician's plan of care and meet further conditions discussed in more detail below.

All HHAs are expected to separately identify in their records the cost of medical and surgical supplies that are not routinely furnished in conjunction with patient care visits and the use of which are directly identifiable to an individual patient.

50.4.1.1 - The Law, Routine and Nonroutine Medical Supplies, and the Patient's Plan of Care
(Rev. 1, 10-01-03)
A3-3119.4A.2, HHA-206.4A3, 4, 5

A. The Law

The Medicare law governing the home health PPS is specific to the type of items and services bundled to the HHA and the time the services are bundled. Medical supplies are bundled while the patient is under a home health plan of care. If a patient is admitted for a condition which is related to a chronic condition that requires a medical supply (e.g., ostomy patient) the HHA is required to provide the medical supply while the patient is under a home health plan of care during an open episode. The physician orders in the plan of care must reflect all nonroutine medical supplies provided and used while the patient is under a home health plan of care during an open 60-day episode. The consolidated billing requirement is not superseded by the exclusion of certain medical supplies from the plan of care and then distinguishing between medical supplies that are related and unrelated to the plan of care. Failure to include medical supplies on the plan of care does not relieve HHAs from the obligation to comply with the consolidated billing requirements. The comprehensive nature of the current patient assessment and plan of care requirements looks at the totality of patient needs. However, there could be a circumstance where a physician could be uncomfortable with writing orders for a preexisting condition unrelated to the reason for home health care. In those circumstances, PRN orders for such supplies may be used in the plan of care by a physician.

Thus, all medical supplies are bundled while the patient is under a home health plan of care during an open 60-day episode. This includes, but is not limited to, the above listed medical supplies as well as the Part B items provided in the final PPS rule. The latter item lists are subsequently updated in accordance with the current process governing the deletion, replacement and revision of Medicare Part B codes. Parenteral and enteral nutrition, prosthetics, orthotics, DME and DME supplies are not considered medical supplies and therefore not subject to bundling while the patient is under a home health plan of care during an open episode. However, §1834(h)(4)(c) of the Act specifically excludes from the term "orthotics and prosthetics" medical supplies including catheters, catheter supplies, ostomy bags and supplies related to ostomy care furnished by an HHA under §1861(m) of the Act. Therefore, these items are bundled while a patient is under a home health plan of care.

B. Relationship Between Patient Choice and Veterans Benefits

For veterans, both Medicare and Veteran's Administration (VA) benefits are primary. Therefore, the beneficiary who is a veteran has some choices in cases where the benefits overlap. The beneficiary, however, must select one or the other program as primary when obtaining active care. If the VA is selected as primary for home health care, then Medicare becomes a secondary payer. An HHA must provide the medical supplies a Medicare beneficiary needs no matter the payer; it is not obligated to provide medical supplies that are not needed. If a patient has medical supplies provided by the VA because of the patient's preference, then the HHA must not duplicate the supplies under Medicare. The beneficiary's choice is controlling. The HHA may not require the beneficiary to obtain or use medical supplies covered by the primary payer from any other source, including the VA.

C. Medical Supplies Purchased by the Patient Prior to the Start of Care

A patient may have acquired medical supplies prior to his/her Medicare home health start of care date. If a patient prefers to use his or her own medical supplies after having been offered appropriate supplies by the HHA and it is determined by the HHA that the patient's medical supplies are clinically appropriate, then the patient's choice is controlling. The HHA is not required to duplicate the medical supplies if the patient elects to use his or her own medical supplies. However, if the patient prefers to have the HHA provide medical supplies while the patient is under a Medicare home health plan of care during an open episode, then the HHA must provide the medical supplies. The HHA may not require that the patient obtain or use medical supplies from any other source. Given the possibility of subsequent misunderstandings arising between the HHA and the patient on this issue, the HHA should document the beneficiary's decision to decline HHA furnished medical supplies and use their own resources.

50.4.1.2 - Routine Supplies (Nonreportable)
(Rev. 1, 10-01-03)
A3-3119.4.A.1, HHA-206.4.A.1

Routine supplies are supplies that are customarily used in small quantities during the course of most home care visits. They are usually included in the staff's supplies and not designated for a specific patient. These supplies are included in the cost per visit of home health care services. Routine supplies would not include those supplies that are specifically ordered by the physician or are essential to HHA personnel in order to effectuate the plan of care.

Examples of supplies which are usually considered routine include, but are not limited to:

A. Dressings and Skin Care

- Swabs, alcohol preps, and skin prep pads;
- Tape removal pads;
- Cotton balls;
- Adhesive and paper tape;
- Nonsterile applicators; and

- 4 x 4's.

B. Infection Control Protection

- Nonsterile gloves;
- Aprons;
- Masks; and
- Gowns.

C. Blood Drawing Supplies

- Specimen containers.

D. Incontinence Supplies

- Incontinence briefs and Chux Covered in the normal course of a visit. For example, if a home health aide in the course of a bathing visit to a patient determines the patient requires an incontinence brief change, the incontinence brief in this example would be covered as a routine medical supply.

E. Other

- Thermometers; and
- Tongue depressors.

There are occasions when the supplies listed in the above examples would be considered nonroutine and thus would be considered a billable supply, i.e., if they are required in quantity, for recurring need, and are included in the plan of care. Examples include, but are not limited to, tape, and 4x4s for major dressings.

50.4.1.3 - Nonroutine Supplies (Reportable)
(Rev. 1, 10-01-03)
A3-3119.4.A.2, HHA-206.4.A.2

Nonroutine supplies are identified by the following conditions:

1. The HHA follows a consistent charging practice for Medicare and other patients receiving the item;

2. The item is directly identifiable to an individual patient;

3. The cost of the item can be identified and accumulated in a separate cost center; and

4. The item is furnished at the direction of the patient's physician and is specifically identified in the plan of care.

All nonroutine supplies must be specifically ordered by the physician or the physician's order for services must require the use of the specific supplies to be effectively furnished.

The charge for nonroutine supplies is excluded from the per visit costs.

Examples of supplies that can be considered nonroutine include, but are not limited to:

1. Dressings/Wound Care

- Sterile dressings;
- Sterile gauze and toppers;
- Kling and Kerlix rolls;
- Telfa pads;
- Eye pads;
- Sterile solutions, ointments;
- Sterile applicators; and
- Sterile gloves.

2. I.V. Supplies

3. Ostomy Supplies

4. Catheters and Catheter Supplies

- Foley catheters; and
- Drainage bags, irrigation trays.

5. Enemas and Douches

6. Syringes and Needles

7. Home Testing

- Blood glucose monitoring strips; and
- Urine monitoring strips.

Consider other items that are often used by persons who are not ill or injured to be medical supplies only where:

- The item is recognized as having the capacity to serve a therapeutic or diagnostic purpose in a specific situation; and

- The item is required as a part of the actual physician-prescribed treatment of a patient's existing illness or injury.

For example, items that generally serve a routine hygienic purpose, e.g., soaps and shampoos and items that generally serve as skin conditioners, e.g., baby lotion, baby oil, skin softeners, powders, lotions, are not considered medical supplies unless the particular item is recognized as serving a specific therapeutic purpose in the physician's prescribed treatment of the patient's existing skin (scalp) disease or injury.

Limited amounts of medical supplies may be left in the home between visits where repeated applications are required and rendered by the patient or other caregivers. These items must be part of the plan of care in which the home health staff is actively involved. For example, the patient is independent in insulin injections but the nurse visits once a day to change wound dressings. The wound dressings/irrigation solution may be left in the home between visits. Supplies such as needles, syringes, and catheters that require administration by a nurse should not be left in the home between visits.

50.4.2 - Durable Medical Equipment
(Rev. 1, 10-01-03)
A3-3119.4.B, HHA-206.4.B

Durable medical equipment which meets the requirements of the Medicare Benefit Policy Manuals, Chapter 6, "Hospital Services Covered Under Part B," §80, and Chapter 15, "Covered Medical and Other Health Services" §110, is covered under the home health benefit with the beneficiary responsible for payment of a 20 percent coinsurance.

50.4.3 – Covered Osteoporosis Drugs
(Rev. 26, Issued 11-05-04, Effective: 01-01-05, Implementation: 04-04-05)

Sections 1861(m) and 1861(kk) of the Act provide for coverage of FDA approved injectable drugs for the treatment of osteoporosis. These drugs are expected to be provided by an HHA to female beneficiaries who are currently receiving services under an open home health plan of care, who meet existing coverage criteria for the home health benefit and who meet the criteria listed below. These drugs are covered on a cost basis when provided by an HHA under the circumstances listed below.

The home health visit (i.e., the skilled nurse's visit) to administer the drug is covered under all fee-for-service Medicare (Part A or Part B) home health coverage rules (see section 30 above). Coverage of the drug is limited to female beneficiaries who meet each of the following criteria:

- The individual is eligible for Medicare Part B coverage of home health services (the nursing visit to perform the injection may be the individual's qualifying service);

o The individual sustained a bone fracture that a physician certifies was related to post-menopausal osteoporosis; and

o The individual's physician certifies that she is unable to learn the skills needed to self-administer the drug or is otherwise physically or mentally incapable of administering the drug, and that her family or caregivers are unable or unwilling to administer the drug.

This drug is considered part of the home health benefit under Part B. Therefore, Part B deductible and coinsurance apply regardless of whether home health visits for the administration of the drug are covered under Part A or Part B.

For instructions on billing for covered osteoporosis drugs, see Pub. 100-04, Medicare Claims Processing Manual, chapter 10, section 90.1.

50.5 - Services of Interns and Residents
(Rev. 1, 10-01-03)
A3-3119.5, HHA-206.5

Home health services include the medical services of interns and residents-in-training under an approved hospital teaching program if the services are ordered by the physician who is responsible for the plan of care and the HHA is affiliated with or is under common control of a hospital furnishing the medical services. Approved means:

- Approved by the Accreditation Council for Graduate Medical Education;

- In the case of an osteopathic hospital, approved by the Committee on Hospitals of the Bureau of Professional Education of the American Osteopathic Association;

- In the case of an intern or resident-in-training in the field of dentistry, approved by the Council on Dental Education of the American Dental Association; or

- In the case of an intern or resident-in-training in the field of podiatry, approved by the Council on Podiatric Education of the American Podiatric Association.

50.6 - Outpatient Services
(Rev. 1, 10-01-03)
A3-3119.6, HHA-206.6

Outpatient services include any of the items or services described above which are provided under arrangements on an outpatient basis at a hospital, skilled nursing facility, rehabilitation center, or outpatient department affiliated with a medical school, and (1) which require equipment which cannot readily be made available at the patient's place of residence, or (2) which are furnished while the patient is at the facility to receive the services described in (1). The hospital, skilled nursing facility, or outpatient department affiliated with a medical school must all be qualified providers of services. However, there are special provisions for the use of the facilities of rehabilitation centers. The cost of transporting an individual to a facility cannot be reimbursed as home health services.

50.7 - Part-Time or Intermittent Home Health Aide and Skilled Nursing Services
(Rev. 1, 10-01-03)
A3-3119.7, HHA-206.7, A3-3119.7A, HHA-206.7A, A3-3119.7.B, HHA-206.7.B

Where a patient is eligible for coverage of home health services, Medicare covers either part-time or intermittent home health aide services or skilled nursing services subject to the limits below. The law at §1861(m) of the Act clarified: "the term "part-time or intermittent services" means skilled nursing and home health aide services furnished any number of days per week as long as they are furnished (combined) less than 8 hours each day and 28 or fewer hours each week (or, subject to review on a case-by-case basis as to the need for care, less than 8 hours each day and 35 or fewer hours each week).

50.7.1 - Impact on Care Provided in Excess of "Intermittent" or "Part-Time" Care
(Rev. 208, Issued: 04-22-15, Effective: 01-01-15, Implementation: 05-11-15)

Home health aide and/or skilled nursing care, in excess of the amounts of care that meet the definition of part-time or intermittent, may be provided to a home care patient or purchased by other payers without bearing on whether the home health aide and skilled nursing care meets the Medicare definitions of part-time or intermittent.

EXAMPLE: A patient needs skilled nursing care monthly for a catheter change and the home health agency also renders needed daily home health aide services 24 hours per day that will be needed for a long and indefinite period of time. The HHA bills Medicare for the skilled nursing and home health aide services, which were provided before the 35th hour of service each week, and bills the beneficiary (or another payer) for the remainder of the care. If the *Medicare contractor* determines that the 35 hours of care are reasonable and necessary, Medicare would cover the 35 hours of skilled nursing and home health aide visits.

50.7.2 - Application of this Policy Revision
(Rev. 1, 10-01-03)
A3-3119.7.D, HHA-206.7.D

Additional care covered by other payers discussed in §50.7.1 does not affect Medicare coverage when the conditions listed below apply. A patient must meet the criteria for Medicare coverage of home health services, before this policy revision becomes applicable to skilled nursing services and/or home health aide services. The definition of "intermittent" with respect to the need for skilled nursing care where the patient qualifies for coverage based on the need for "skilled nursing care on an intermittent basis" remains unchanged. Specifically:

1. This policy revision always applies to home health aide services when the patient qualifies for coverage;

2. This policy revision applies to skilled nursing care only when the patient needs physical therapy or speech-language pathology services or continued occupational therapy, and also needs skilled nursing care; and

3. If the patient needs skilled nursing care but does not need physical therapy or speech-language pathology services or occupational therapy, the patient must still meet the longstanding and unchanged definition of "intermittent" skilled nursing care in order to qualify for coverage of any home health services.

60 - Special Conditions for Coverage of Home Health Services Under Hospital Insurance (Part A) and Supplementary Medical Insurance (Part B)
(Rev. 1, 10-01-03)
A3-3122, HHA-212

60.1 - Post-Institutional Home Health Services Furnished During A Home Health Benefit Period - Beneficiaries Enrolled in Part A and Part B
(Rev. 1, 10-01-03)
A3-3122.1, HHA-212.1, A3-3122.1, HHA-212.2, PMs A-97-12, A-97-16, A-98-49

Section 1812(a)(3) of the Act provides post-institutional home health services for individuals enrolled in Part A and Part B and home health services for individuals who are eligible for Part A only. For beneficiaries who are enrolled in Part A and Part B, Part A finances post-institutional home health services furnished during a home health spell of illness for up to 100 visits during a spell of illness.

Part A finances up to 100 visits furnished during a home health spell of illness if the following criteria are met:

- Beneficiaries are enrolled in Part A **and** Part B and qualify to receive the Medicare home health benefit;

- Beneficiaries must have at least a three consecutive day stay in a hospital or rural primary care hospital; and

- Home health services must be initiated and the first covered home health visit must be rendered within 14 days of discharge from a 3 consecutive day stay in a hospital or rural primary care hospital or within 14 days of discharge from a skilled nursing facility in which the individual was provided post-hospital extended care services. If the first home health visit is not initiated within 14 days of discharge, then home health services are financed under Part B.

After an individual exhausts 100 visits of Part A post-institutional home health services, Part B finances the balance of the home health spell of illness. A home health spell of illness is a period of consecutive days beginning with the first day not included in a previous home health spell of illness on which the individual is furnished post-institutional home health services which occurs in a month the individual is entitled to Part A. The home health spell of illness ends with the close of the first period of 60 consecutive days in which the individual is neither an inpatient of a hospital or rural primary care hospital nor an inpatient of a skilled nursing facility (in which the individual was furnished post-hospital extended care services) nor provided home health services.

EXAMPLE 1:

An individual is enrolled in Part A and Part B, qualifies for the Medicare home health benefit, has a three consecutive day stay in a hospital, and is discharged on May 1. On May 5, the individual receives the first skilled nursing visit under the plan of care. Therefore, post-institutional home health services have been initiated within 14 days of discharge. The individual is later hospitalized on June 2. Prior to the June 2 hospitalization, the individual received 12 home health visits. The individual stays in the hospital for four consecutive days, is discharged and receives home health services. That individual continues the May 5 home health spell of illness and would have 88 visits left under that home health spell of illness under Part A. That individual could not start another home health spell of illness (100 visits under Part A) until a 60-day consecutive period in which the individual was not an inpatient of a hospital, rural primary care hospital, an inpatient of a skilled nursing facility (in which the individual was furnished post-hospital extended care services), or provided home health services had passed.

EXAMPLE 2:

An individual is enrolled in Part A and Part B, qualifies for the Medicare home health benefit, has a three consecutive day stay in a hospital, and home health is initiated within 14 days of discharge. The individual exhausts the 100 visits under Part A post-institutional home health services, continues to need home health services, and receives home health services under Part B. The individual is then hospitalized for 4 consecutive days. The individual is again discharged and receives home health services. The individual cannot begin a new home health spell of illness because 60 days did not pass in which the individual was not an inpatient of a hospital or rural primary care hospital or an inpatient of a skilled nursing facility in which the individual was furnished post-hospital extended care services. The individual would be discharged and Part B would continue to finance the home health services.

60.2 - Beneficiaries Who Are Enrolled in Part A and Part B, but Do Not Meet Threshold for Post-Institutional Home Health Services
(Rev. 1, 10-01-03)
A3-3122.1, HHA-212.3

If beneficiaries are enrolled in Part A and Part B and are eligible for the Medicare home health benefit, but do not meet the three consecutive day stay requirement or the 14 day initiation of care requirement, then all of their home health services would be financed under Part B. For example, this situation would include, but is not limited to, beneficiaries enrolled in Part A and Part B who are coming from the community to a home health agency in need of home health services or who stay less than three consecutive days in a hospital and are discharged. Any home health services received after discharge would be financed under Part B.

60.3 - Beneficiaries Who Are Part A Only or Part B Only
(Rev. 1, 10-01-03)
A3-3122.1, HHA-212.4

If a beneficiary is enrolled **only** in Part A and qualifies for the Medicare home health benefit, then all of the home health services are financed under Part A. The 100-visit limit does **not** apply to beneficiaries who are only enrolled in Part A. If a beneficiary is enrolled **only** in Part B and qualifies for the Medicare home health benefit, then all of the home health services are financed under Part B. There is no 100-visit limit under Part B. The new definition of post-institutional home health services provided during a home health spell of illness **only** applies to those beneficiaries who are enrolled in **both** Part A and Part B and qualify for the Medicare home health benefit.

60.4 - Coinsurance, Copayments, and Deductibles
(Rev. 1, 10-01-03)
A3-3122.1, HHA-212.5

There is no coinsurance, copayment, or deductible for home health services and supplies other than the following:

- coinsurance required for durable medical equipment (DME) covered as a home health service and

- deductible and coinsurance for the osteoporosis drug, which is part of the home health benefit only paid under Part B.

The coinsurance liability of the beneficiary for DME and osteoporosis drug furnished as a home health service is 20 percent of the fee schedule amount for the services.

70 - Duration of Home Health Services
(Rev. 1, 10-01-03)
A3-3123, HHA-215, A3-3123.1, HHA-215.1

70.1 - Number of Home Health Visits Under Supplementary Medical Insurance (Part B)
(Rev. 1, 10-01-03)
A3-3123.2, HHA-215.2

To the extent that all coverage requirements are met, payment may be made on behalf of eligible beneficiaries under Part B for an unlimited number of covered home health visits. The determination of Part A or Part B Trust Fund financing and coverage is made in accordance with the financing shift required by the BBA described above in §60.

70.2 - Counting Visits Under the Hospital and Medical Plans
(Rev. 208, Issued: 04-22-15, Effective: 01-01-15, Implementation: 05-11-15)

The number of visits are counted in the same way whether paid under the hospital (Part A) or supplemental medical (Part B) Medicare trust funds

A. Visit Defined

A visit is an episode of personal contact with the patient by staff of the HHA, or others under arrangements with the HHA, for the purpose of providing a covered home health service. Though visits are provided under the HH benefit as part of episodes, and episodes are unlimited, each visit must be uniquely billed as a separate line item on a Medicare HH claim, and data on visit charges is still used in formulating payment rates.

B. Counting Visits

Generally, one visit may be covered each time an HHA employee, or someone providing home health services under arrangements with the HHA, enters the patient's home and provides a covered service to a patient who meets the criteria in §30.

If the HHA furnishes services in an outpatient facility under arrangements with the facility, one visit may be covered for each type of service provided.

If two individuals are needed to provide a service, two visits may be covered. If two individuals are present, but only one is needed to provide the care, only one visit may be covered.

A visit is initiated with the delivery of covered home health services and ends at the conclusion of delivery of covered home health services. In those circumstances in which all reasonable and necessary home health services cannot be provided in the course of a single visit, HHA staff or others providing services under arrangements with the HHA may remain at the patient's home between visits (e.g., to provide noncovered services). However, if all covered services could be provided in the course of one visit, only one visit may be covered.

EXAMPLES:

1. If an occupational therapist and an occupational therapy assistant visit the patient together to provide therapy and the therapist is there to supervise the assistant, **one** visit is counted.

2. If a nurse visits the patient in the morning to dress a wound and later must return to replace a catheter, **two** visits are counted.

3. If the therapist visits the patient for treatment in the morning and the patient is later visited by the assistant for additional treatment, **two** visits are counted.

4. If an individual is taken to a hospital to receive outpatient therapy that could not be furnished in their own home (e.g., hydrotherapy) and, while at the hospital receives speech-language pathology services and other services, **two or more** visits would be charged.

5. Many home health agencies provide home health aide services on an hourly basis (ranging from 1 to 8 hours a day). However, in order to allocate visits properly against a patient's maximum allowable visits, home health aide services are to be counted in terms of visits. Thus, regardless of the number of continuous hours a home health aide spends in a patient's home on any given day, one "visit" is counted for each such day. If, in a rare situation, a home health aide visits a patient for an hour or two in the morning, and again for an hour or two in the afternoon, two visits are counted.

C. Evaluation Visits

The HHAs are required by regulations to have written policies concerning the acceptance of patients by the agency. These include consideration of the physical facilities available in the patient's place of residence, the homebound status, and the attitudes of family members for the purpose of evaluating the feasibility of meeting the patient's medical needs in the home health setting. When personnel of the agency make such an initial evaluation visit, the cost of the visit is considered an administrative cost of the agency and is not chargeable as a visit since at this point the patient has not been accepted for care. If, however, during the course of this initial evaluation visit, the patient is determined suitable for home health care by the agency, and is also furnished the first skilled service as ordered under the physician's plan of care, the visit would become the first billable visit in the 60-day episode.

The *Medicare contractor* will cover an observation and evaluation (or reevaluation) visit made by a nurse (see §40.1.2.1 for a further discussion of skilled nursing observation and evaluation visits) or other appropriate personnel, ordered by the physician for the purpose of evaluating the patient's condition and continuing need for skilled services, as a skilled visit.

A supervisory visit made by a nurse or other appropriate personnel (as required by the conditions of participation) to evaluate the specific personal care needs of the patient or to review the manner in which the personal care needs of the patient are being met by the aide is an administrative function, not a skilled visit.

80 - Specific Exclusions From Coverage as Home Health Services
(Rev. 1, 10-01-03)

A3-3125, HHA-230.A

In addition to the general exclusions from coverage under health insurance listed in the Medicare Benefit Policy Manual, Chapter 16, "General Exclusions from Coverage," the following are also excluded from coverage as home health services:

80.1 - Drugs and Biologicals
(Rev. 1, 10-01-03)
A3-3125.A, HHA-230.A

Drugs and biologicals are excluded from payment under the Medicare home health benefit.

A drug is any chemical compound that may be used on or administered to humans or animals as an aid in the diagnosis, treatment, prevention of disease or other condition, for the relief of pain or suffering, or to control or improve any physiological pathologic condition.

A biological is any medicinal preparation made from living organisms and their products including, but not limited to, serums, vaccines, antigens, and antitoxins. The one drug exception is the osteoporosis drug, which is part of the home health benefit, and home health agencies may provide services such as vaccines outside the home health benefit.

80.2 - Transportation
(Rev. 1, 10-01-03)
A3-3125.B, HHA-230.B

The transportation of a patient, whether to receive covered care or for other purposes, is excluded from home health coverage. Costs of transportation of equipment, materials, supplies, or staff may be allowable as administrative costs, but no separate payment is made.

80.3 - Services That Would Not Be Covered as Inpatient Services
(Rev. 1, 10-01-03)
A3-3125C, HHA-230.C

Services that would not be covered if furnished as inpatient hospital services are excluded from home health coverage.

80.4 - Housekeeping Services
(Rev. 1, 10-01-03)
A3-3125D, HHA-230D

Services for which the sole purpose is to enable the patient to continue residing in their home (e.g., cooking, shopping, Meals on Wheels, cleaning, laundry) are excluded from home health coverage.

80.5 - Services Covered Under *the* End Stage Renal Disease (ESRD) Program
(Rev. 208, Issued: 04-22-15, Effective: 01-01-15, Implementation: 05-11-15)

Renal dialysis services that are covered *and paid for* under the ESRD *PPS, which include* any *item or* service furnished to an ESRD beneficiary that is directly related to that individual's dialysis, are excluded from coverage under the Medicare home health benefit. However, to the extent *that other requirements for coverage are met, an item or* service *that* is not directly related to a patient's dialysis would be covered *(*e.g., *a skilled* nursing visit to furnish wound care for an abandoned shunt site*)*. Within these restrictions, beneficiaries may simultaneously receive items and services under the ESRD *PPS through their ESRD facility* at home at the same time as receiving *items and* services under the home health benefit *that are* not related to ESRD.

80.6 - Prosthetic Devices
(Rev. 1, 10-01-03)
A3-3125F, HHA-230F

Prosthetic items are excluded from home health coverage. However, catheters, catheter supplies, ostomy bags, and supplies related to ostomy care are not considered prosthetic devices if furnished under a home health plan of care and are not subject to this exclusion from coverage but are bundled while a patient is under a HH plan of care.

80.7 - Medical Social Services Furnished to Family Members
(Rev. 1, 10-01-03)
A3-3125G, HHA-230G

Except as provided in §50.3, medical social services furnished solely to members of the patient's family and that are not incidental to covered medical social services being furnished to the patient are not covered.

80.8 - Respiratory Care Services
(Rev. 1, 10-01-03)
A3-3125.H, HHA-230.H

If a respiratory therapist is used to furnish overall training or consultative advice to HHA staff and incidentally furnishes respiratory therapy services to patients in their homes, the costs of the respiratory therapist's services are allowable only as administrative costs to the HHA. Visits by a respiratory therapist to a patient's home are not separately billable during a HH episode when a HH plan of care is in effect. However, respiratory therapy services furnished as part of a plan of care other than a home health plan of care by a licensed nurse or physical therapist and that constitute skilled care may be covered and separately billed as skilled visits when the beneficiary is not in a home health episode. Note that Medicare billing does not recognize respiratory therapy as a separate discipline, but rather sees the services in accordance with the revenue code used on the claims (i.e. 042x).

80.9 - Dietary and Nutrition Personnel
(Rev. 1, 10-01-03)
A3-3125.I, HHA-230.I

If dieticians or nutritionists are used to furnish overall training or consultative advice to HHA staff and incidentally furnish dietetic or nutritional services to patients in their homes, the costs of these professional services are allowable only as administrative costs. Visits by a dietician or nutritionist to a patient's home are not separately billable.

90 - Medical and Other Health Services Furnished by Home Health Agencies
(Rev. 208, Issued: 04-22-15, Effective: 01-01-15, Implementation: 05-11-15)

Payment may be made by *Medicare contractors* to a home health agency which furnishes either directly or under arrangements with others the following "medical and other health services" to beneficiaries with Part B coverage in accordance with Part B billing and payment rules other than when a home health plan of care is in effect.

1. Surgical dressings (for a patient who is not under a home health plan of care), and splints, casts, and other devices used for reduction of fractures and dislocations;

2. Prosthetic (Except for items excluded from the term "orthotics and prosthetics" in accordance with §1834(h)(4)(C) of the Act for patients who are under a home health plan of care);

3. Leg, arm, back, and neck braces, trusses, and artificial legs, arms, and eyes and adjustments to these items when ordered by a physician. (See *Pub 100-02,* Medicare Benefit Policy Manual, Chapter 15);

4. Outpatient physical therapy, outpatient occupational therapy, and outpatient speech-language pathology services (for a patient not under a home health plan of care). (See *Pub 100-02,* Medicare Benefit Policy Manual, Chapter 15); and

5. Rental and purchase of durable medical equipment. (See *Pub 100-02,* Medicare Benefit Policy Manual, Chapter 15.) If a beneficiary meets all of the criteria for coverage of home health services and the HHA is providing home health care under the Hospital Insurance Program (Part A), any DME provided and billed to the *Medicare contractor* by the HHA to that patient must also be provided under Part A. Where the patient meets the criteria for coverage of home health services and the HHA is providing the home health care under the Supplementary Medical Insurance Program (Part B) because the patient is not eligible for Part A, the DME provided by the HHA may, at the beneficiary's option, be furnished under the Part B home health benefit or as a medical and other health service.

Irrespective of how the DME is furnished, the beneficiary is responsible for a 20 percent coinsurance.

6. Ambulance service. (See *Pub 100-02,* Medicare Benefit Policy Manual, Chapter 10, Ambulance Services)

7. Hepatitis B Vaccine. Hepatitis B vaccine and its administration are covered under Part B for patients who are at high or intermediate risk of contracting hepatitis B. High risk groups currently identified include: end-stage renal disease (ESRD) patients, hemophiliacs who receive factor VIII or IX concentrates, clients of institutions for the mentally retarded, persons who live in the same household as a hepatitis B virus carrier, homosexual men, illicit injectable drug users. Intermediate risk groups currently identified include staff in institutions for the mentally retarded, workers in health care professions who have frequent contact with blood or blood-derived body fluids during routine work. Persons in the above listed groups would not be considered at high or intermediate risk of contracting hepatitis B, however, if there is laboratory evidence positive for antibodies to hepatitis B. ESRD patients are routinely tested for hepatitis B antibodies as part of their continuing monitoring and therapy. The vaccine may be administered, upon the order of a doctor of medicine or osteopathy, by home health agencies.

8. Hemophilia clotting factors. Blood clotting factors for hemophilia patients competent to use such factors to control bleeding without medical or other supervision and items related to the administration of such factors are covered under Part B.

9. Pneumococcal and influenza vaccines. See *Pub 100-02,* Medicare Benefit Policy Manual, Chapter 15, "Covered Medical and Other Health Services," §50.4.2 "Immunizations."

10. Splints, casts. See *Pub 100-02,* Medicare Benefit Policy Manual, Chapter 15, "Covered Medical and Other Health Services."

11. Antigens. See *Pub 100-02,* Medicare Benefit Policy Manual, Chapter 15, "Covered Medical and Other Health Services."

100 - Physician Certification for Medical and Other Health Services Furnished by Home Health Agency (HHA)
(Rev. 208, Issued: 04-22-15, Effective: 01-01-15, Implementation: 05-11-15)

A physician must certify that the medical and other health services covered by medical insurance, which were provided by (or under arrangements made by) the HHA, were medically required. This certification needs to be made only once where the patient may require over a period of time the furnishing of the same item or service related to one diagnosis. There is no requirement that the certification be entered on any specific form or handled in any specific way as long as the approach adopted by the HHA permits the

Medicare contractor to determine that the certification requirement is, in fact, met. A written physician's order designating the services required would also be an acceptable certification.

110 - Use of Telehealth in Delivery of Home Health Services
(Rev. 1, 10-01-03)
PM A-01-02, HHA-201.13

Section 1895(e) of the Act governs the home health prospective payment system (PPS) and provides that telehealth services are outside the scope of the Medicare home health benefit and home health PPS.

This provision does not provide coverage or payment for Medicare home health services provided via a telecommunications system. The law does not permit the substitution or use of a telecommunications system to provide any covered home health services paid under the home health PPS, or any covered home health service paid outside of the home health PPS. As stated in 42 CFR 409.48(c), a visit is an episode of personal contact with the beneficiary by staff of the home health agency (HHA), or others under arrangements with the HHA for the purposes of providing a covered service. The provision clarifies that there is nothing to preclude an HHA from adopting telemedicine or other technologies that they believe promote efficiencies, but that those technologies will not be specifically recognized or reimbursed by Medicare under the home health benefit. This provision does not waive the current statutory requirement for a physician certification of a home health plan of care under current §§1814(a)(2)(C) or 1835(a)(2)(A) of the Act.

Transmittals Issued for this Chapter

Rev #	Issue Date	Subject	Impl Date	CR#
R208BP	04/22/2015	Manual Updates to Clarify Requirements for Physician Certification and Recertification of Patient Eligibility for Home Health Services	05/11/2015	9119
R207BP	04/10/2015	Manual Updates to Clarify Requirements for Physician Certification and Recertification of Patient Eligibility for Home Health Services – Rescinded and replaced by Transmittal 208	05/11/2015	9119
R179BP	01/14/2014	Manual Updates to Clarify Skilled Nursing Facility (SNF), Inpatient Rehabilitation Facility (IRF), Home Health (HH), and Outpatient (OPT) Coverage Pursuant to Jimmo vs. Sebelius	01/07/2014	8458
R176BP	12/13/2013	Manual Updates to Clarify Skilled Nursing Facility (SNF), Inpatient Rehabilitation Facility (IRF), Home Health (HH), and Outpatient (OPT) Coverage Pursuant to Jimmo vs. Sebelius – Rescinded and replaced by Transmittal 179	01/07/2014	8458
R172BP	10/18/2013	Home Health - Clarification to Benefit Policy Manual Language on Confined to the Home Definition	11/19/2013	8444
R144BP	05/06/2011	Home Health Therapy Services	05/05/2011	7374
R142BP	04/15/2011	Home Health Therapy Services – Rescinded and replaced by Transmittal 144	05/05/2011	7374
R139BP	02/16/2011	Clarifications for Home Health Face-to Face Encounter Provisions	03/10/2011	7329
R37BP	08/12/2005	Conforming Changes for Change Request 3648 to Pub. 100-02	09/12/2005	3912
R26BP	11/05/2004	Inclusion of Forteo as a Covered Osteoporosis Drug and Clarification of Manual Instructions Regarding Osteoporosis Drugs	04/04/2004	3524

Index

A

B

C

I

J–K–L

M

N

O

P

Q

INDEX

T

U

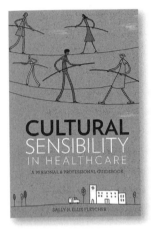
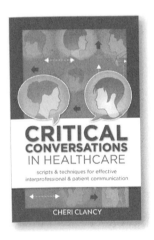
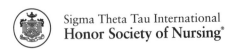
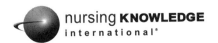

End-of-Life Comfort and Care

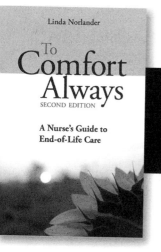
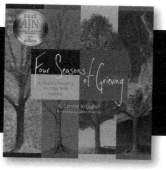
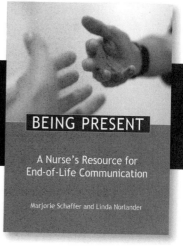

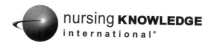

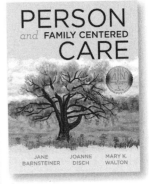
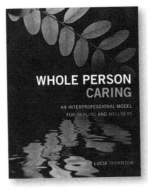
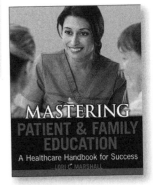
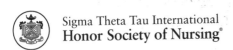
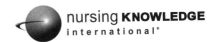